1st Signed 25.—

To Howard
with friendship and
appreciation,

Shifra Shvarts
Oct. 2003

The Workers' Health Fund in Eretz Israel

Rochester Studies in Medical History

Senior Editor: Theodore M. Brown
Professor of History and Preventive Medicine
University of Rochester

Mechanization of the Heart:
Harvey and Descartes
Thomas Fuchs
Translated from the German by Majorie Grene

The Workers' Health Fund in Eretz Israel
Kupat Holim, 1911-1937
Shifra Shvarts

The Workers' Health Fund in Eretz Israel

Kupat Holim, 1911-1937

Shifra Shvarts

The University of Rochester Press

First published 2002
by the University of Rochester Press

The University of Rochester Press is an imprint of Boydell & Brewer, Inc.
668 Mount Hope Avenue
Rochester, NY 14620, USA
and of Boydell & Brewer, Ltd.
P.O. Box 9
Woodbridge, Suffolk 1P12 3DF, UK

Library of Congress Cataloging-in-Publication Data

Shvarts, Shifra.
The workers' health fund in Eretz Israel Kupat Holim, 1911-1937 / Shifra Shvarts.
p.cm.
ISBN 1-58046-122-0
1. Medicine—Israel—History. 2. Medical care—Israel—History. 3. Public health—Israel—History. 4. Federal aid to health facilities—Israel—History. 5. Public health—Israel—Finance. I. Title.

R644.P3 S54 2002
610'.95694—dc21

2002074262

British Library Cataloging-in-Publication Data
A catalogue record for this item is available from the British Library.

Designed and typeset by Christine Menendez
Printed in the United States of America
This publication is printed is on acid-free paper.

To my husband Dov and my daughters, Michal, Tal, and Naama, whose patience, emotional support, and encouragement sustained me in this endeavor.

"ERETZ ISRAEL" (PALESTINE) 1914

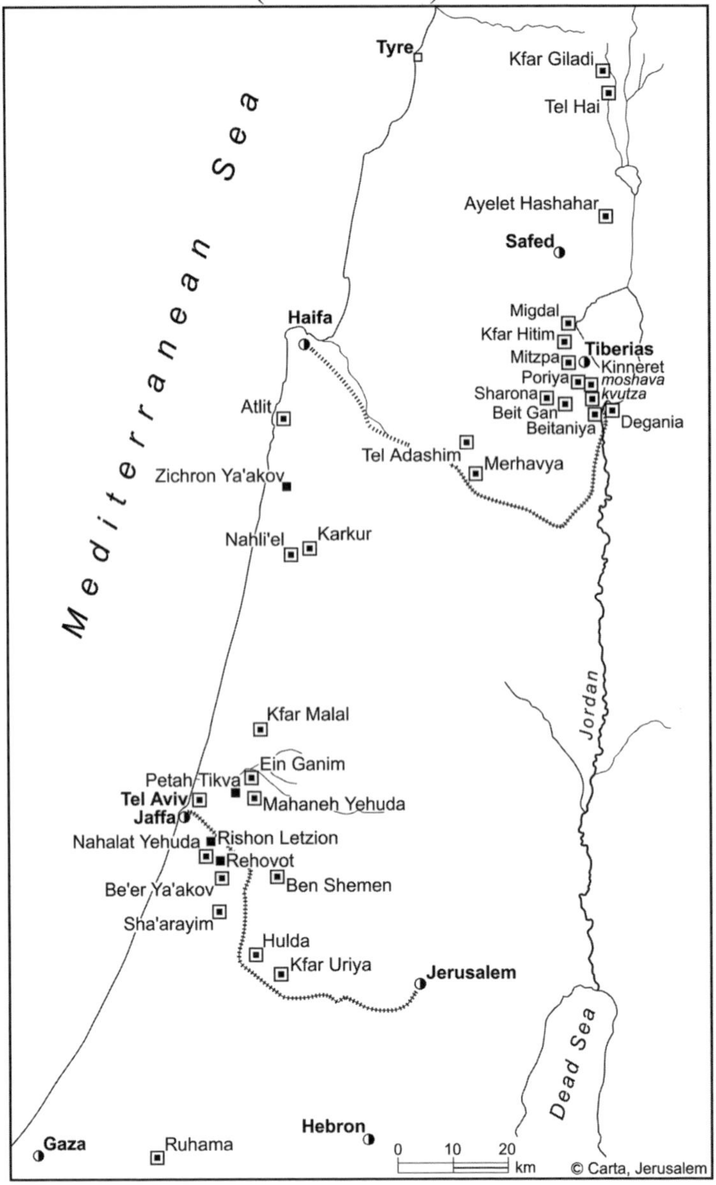

- Settlement founded during Second Aliyah
- Mixed (Jewish-Arab) town existing before Second Aliyah
- Jewish Settlement existing before Second Aliyah
- Railway

Contents

Map of Eretz Israel (Palestine) 1914 *vi*

Illustrations *ix*

Foreword *xi*

Acknowledgments *xiii*

Note on Sources *xv*

Introduction: Kupat Holim Then and Now *1*

1. Health Services in Eretz Israel (Palestine) in the Nineteenth Century *7*
2. The Workers' Health Fund: Ideology and Beginnings, 1903-1914 *20*
3. The Workers' Health Funds in the First World War *55*
4. The Health System Under British Military Government *70*
5. The General Health Fund of Workers in Israel: Kupat Holim *93*
6. According to Needs or According to Ability: Kupat Holim, 1924-1930 *113*
7. Confrontation and Cooperation Between Kupat Holim and Hadassah, 1920-1930 *177*
8. The Emek (Jezreel Valley) Hospital *202*
9. Kupat Holim and the British Mandate Government *225*
10. Kupat Holim and the Federation of Labor: Reciprocal Membership and the Joint Dues *249*

Epilogue: Summary and Conclusions *291*

Notes *301*

Glossary *319*

Works Cited *327*

Index *331*

Illustrations

Map of Eretz Israel (1914) *vi*

1. Workers from the Second Aliyah (1905) *169*
2. Kinnereth, the Women Workers' Farm (1907) *169*
3. Kupat Holim's First Clinic in Petach Tikva (1912) *170*
4. Living Conditions at Kinnereth (1907) *170*
5. Berl Katznelson, Kupat Holim Founder *170*
6. The American Zionist Unit to Palestine (1919) *171*
7. Dr. Isaac Max Rubinow *171*
8. Women Workers at the Kinneret Farm (1913) *171*
9. A Jewish Watchman-worker (early 1920s) *172*
10. Kibbutz Ein Harod in the Jezreel Valley (1921) *172*
11. The Workers' Hospital in Ein Harod (1924) *173*
12. Workers' Sick Room in the Kibbutz Ein Harod (1924) *173*
13. Nurses at The Workers' Hospital Give Children a Sunbath (1926) *174*
14. The Opening Ceremony of "Haemek" Hospital (1930) *174*
15. Tipat Halav Maternal and Child Care Center (early 1930s) *175*
16. Kupat Holim Membership Card *175*
17. Vintage Advertisement for Kupat Holim (1936) *175*
18. Bedside Teaching at Beilinson Hospital Near Tel Aviv (1936) *176*
19. Kupat Holim Primary Care Clinic, Jezreel Valley (late 1930s) *176*

Foreward

On the eve of the one-hundredth anniversary of its founding, the Kupat Holim Clalit—the General Health Fund of the past and General Health Services today—is in the midst of a revolutionary process that involves fundamental and significant changes in the way it will function and the direction it will take in the future.

From solely a "workers' sick fund," the *Clalit* has been transformed into a "general multi-scope organization" that encourages a healthy lifestyle among its members, and views them as full partners in their own health maintenance. The fact that the name of the organization was changed of late from "Kupat Holim Clalit" to "Clalit Health Services" is not coincidental. The change reflects a fundamental change in the essence of the organization.

The *Clalit* is the largest health organization in Israel and one of the largest in the world. The overwhelming majority of Israel's population are insured under its auspices, and receive health services through the *Clalit's* thirteen-hundred clinics, fourteen hospitals, and hundreds of pharmacies, institutes, and labs throughout the country—in the center and on the periphery, in the city and village.

This book describes the stages of the birth and development of the *Clalit* during its formative years. It covers its modest beginnings, with approximately 150 members, and follows its growth to more than 3.5 million members. It traces its evolution from a handful of makeshift "sick rooms" into a comprehensive network of hospitals, clinics, institutes, and labs that apply the latest state-of-the-art technological innovations in the field of medicine, including revolutionary applications in online medical services through the Internet, video conferencing, and so forth.

In the process of describing key junctures and processes in the *Clalit's* development, this volume sheds light on a host of interesting facets of the crystallization of Jewish society in Eretz Israel under the

Ottoman Turks and the British Mandate. At the same time, the history of the *Clalit* reflects differences of political opinion, contrasting views among leaders, and personal and ideological rivalries at different junctures in the organization's development.

In its focus on the development of the General Health Fund in the period in which the social system of the young Jewish community in Eretz Israel was in the formative stages—a time when the social contract of the "General Health Fund" set forth the principle of "health for all, in all locations"—this book reveals a host of factors that impacted on the crystallization of the health system in Israel and the decisive part played by the Health Fund in this process. Moreover, the work is instructive regarding various quandaries faced and plans ultimately formulated for dealing with numerous medical, political, and bureaucratic issues: organizing emergency medical services, establishing a basic governmental health system, coping with immigration, struggling over salaries, mapping a hospital network, shaping the roles of the physician and medical staff, and many other issues, some of which continue to occupy leaders of the health system to this day.

The history of the establishment, crystallization, and development of the *Clalit* is closely bound to the fascinating and unique story of the State of Israel. As one of the biggest economic organizations in Israel—perhaps even the biggest—the *Clalit*, along with the State of Israel as a whole, continues to grapple with budgetary challenges. Even after ninety years of existence, *Clalit* continues to cope with the challenge of reconciling the need to provide advanced and universally accessible medical services in the face of economic restraints and budgetary deficits.

Nevertheless, despite the quandaries and the difficulties, the *Clalit* has the right to be proud of the level of advanced medical services it is able to provide to its members and the leading role it plays in the health system.

The sense of mission that motivated its founders and that continues to guide those who follow in their footsteps is what has preserved the place of honor the *Clalit* continues to hold as a broad-based, modern, and sophisticated health service-provider.

Dr. Y. Petersberg
General Manager, *Clalit*
General Health Services

Acknowledgments

This book is based on a Ph.D. thesis in health sciences done at Ben-Gurion University of the Negev, work supported in part by the research fund of the Ben-Zvi Institute and the higher education department of the Federation of Labor. It was previously published (in 1997) in Hebrew as *Kupat-Holim Ha-Clalit, 1911-1937* and is here translated into English by Daniella Ashkenazy.

I wish to thank Professor Zeev Tzachor and Professor Shmuel Kottek, who served as my advisors in this work, for their devoted guidance; Professor Shimon Glick, who opened the door for me in the pursuit of this topic, for his attentive ear, assistance, encouragement, and unbridled empathy and support; Professor Theodore Brown and Professor Chaim Doron, for the countless hours they devoted to me, discussing the development of health services in Israel, broadening my understanding of the subject; the employees of Kupat Holim throughout the country who assisted me in locating and gathering material at the source; the staff at the Lavon Institute-Labor Archive for their unstinting assistance guiding me through a bulk of documentation; and the staff at the Ben-Gurion Heritage Center and Institute for their expert guidance in charting the way to relevant passages in the voluminous diaries and papers of David Ben-Gurion.

I thank my devoted assistant Ilanit Sarder and my friends the Schneiders for their personal warmth and assistance throughout preparation of the manuscript for publication. I wish to thank Tim Madigan, Editorial Director and Molly Cort, Production Manager for their support at the University of Rochester Press. Special thanks to John Blanpied for his copyediting expertise and to Christine Menendez for her design skills.

Last but not least, to my parents, Batya and Yehezkeel Leider, for their assistance in gathering materials and completing this work; and to my late grandmother Bruria and my late grandfather Dov, Zionist pioneers from the Third Aliyah who dedicated their lives to the realization of a Jewish state and were privileged to be among the founding members of Kupat Holim.

Shifra Shvarts
Beer-Sheva-Omer
September, 2002

Note on Sources

Structure of the Research and Source Material

The primary source of material for this study was archival documentation. I reviewed most of Kupat Holim's papers and documents stored in the Lavon Institute-Labor Archive (ALM) in Tel Aviv, including daily correspondence, decisions of Kupat Holim's directorate ("merkaz"), protocols of deliberations of Kupat Holim's supervisory committee, and various internal reports, budgets, and working papers. I found other archival material—specifically throwing light on the ties between Kupat Holim and the Yishuv's health committee and the Zionist movement's executive committee—in the Central Zionist Archive (CZA) in Jerusalem. This material included decisions of the Yishuv's health committee, deliberations over health matters in the Zionist Federation, and documents tied to working relationships between Kupat Holim and Mandate authorities, mediated by Zionist institutions.

In order to examine relations between Kupat Holim and Hadassah, I examined various papers in the Hadassah Archives in New York City, as well as papers found in the Central Zionist Archive in Jerusalem—primarily the letters of Henrietta Szold from the 1920s.

Besides archival material, I also examined David Ben-Gurion's diary, preserved at the Ben-Gurion Heritage Institute at Sede Boker. Passages in Ben-Gurion's diary illuminated a host of political issues that impacted on the development of Kupat Holim and served as undercurrents in Kupat Holim's relationship with the Federation of Labor during the years covered by this volume. Books written by other contemporaries of the period under study (memoirs, diaries, and so forth) and scholarly works focusing on personalities and the period, all cited in the bibliography, were of great assistance in writing this work.

Finally, a great deal of material concerning Kupat Holim was published in Hebrew newspapers and periodicals of the time (*Hapoel Hatzair, Contras, He'achdut, Me'chiyenu, Davar, Ha'aretz, Davar Hayom, Hayarden, Briut Haoved and others*). Review of the print media provided me with a picture of the ongoing work of Kupat Holim as it was reflected in the public eye, from the viewpoint of all political persuasions, within the context of life as a whole within the Yishuv, including public discourse of controversies and quandaries facing the health fund, thus serving as both a record of events as they unfolded and a prism to the social climate surrounding Kupat Holim in its formative years.

INTRODUCTION

Kupat Holim Then and Now

Kupat Holim—whose full name in Hebrew is Kupat Holim Ha-Clalit or the General Health Fund but is referred to in this volume simply as "Kupat Holim"—originally defined itself, in 1911, as "the emissary of the organized working public in the Federation of Labor in matters of health in Israel." Its role was to extend medical assistance to its members, their families and parents; extend financial assistance to its members in times of illness; organize the workers' health matters; and serve as social-medical insurance for the working public in Israel.

Although the majority of the citizenry of the state of Israel are insured by the health fund, even today questions tied to Kupat Holim's place, function, and effectiveness remain solidly on the public agenda. These issues are not solely the domain of Left or Right, but rather occupy all those involved in health: the ministry of health, the Federation of Labor and its institutions, and Kupat Holim itself. At the heart of deliberations are challenges to the health system stemming from implementation of the National Health Insurance Law and recommendations of the national inquiry commission on the functioning and efficiency of the health system in Israel—the Natanyahu Commission (1990) and the Tzadkah Commission (1993).

In January 1995, the National Health Insurance Law was implemented. The law's main clauses stipulate that financing health services would be carried out through the auspices of National Insurance and that health services would be provided by currently existing health funds. Thus, the direct linkage between Kupat Holim and the Federation of Labor—a tie between the two bodies that had prevailed since 1937 based on a direct levy of what was termed *Mas Achid*, or joint dues to the two organizations—was severed. With enactment of a national compulsory health system, the government of Israel approved a fiscal and organizational rehabilitation plan for Kupat Holim that entailed reduction in wages, cutbacks in job posts, sale of assets, efficiency moves, and reorganization of Kupat Holim.

Ironically, this rehabilitation plan and the initiative for passage of national health insurance legislation was very similar to recommendations made in 1926 by the first legislative committee to scrutinize Kupat Holim. That body, established by the Zionist movement's executive committee (i.e., the administrative arm of the World Zionist Movement) was formed to examine why Kupat Holim was incurring such large deficits and how such deficits could be contained.

It is still unclear whether passage of a national health insurance law and rehabilitation of Kupat Holim are signals of a truly new path or are merely a hiatus in Kupat Holim's history. Should the latter be the case—should legislation and rehabilitation fail to solve the fundamental problems that have plagued the fund—under certain political and economic circumstances, the question of the performance and the very existence of Kupat Holim as we know it could again command a high place on the agenda of Israeli society.

Kupat Holim had its beginnings in the second convention of the Federation of Workers in Judea in December 1911. The absence of health services at a cost within the means of laborers from the Second Aliyah brought the Judea workers to the conclusion that establishment of a workers' health fund was an imperative. The exigency for such a move was underscored by a tragic work accident in which a laborer's hand was severed by a pump engine.

In the founding resolution of the Judea Worker's Health Fund it was stated that "the Convention confirms the vital need for a joint health fund for the workers of Eretz Israel and workers abroad regarding matters common to all." The resolution ultimately led to the establishment of Kupat Holim in 1920, a core social institution that today insures at least 60 percent of all inhabitants of the state of Israel.

The Judea Workers faced two main approaches toward organization of medical services when they began to establish their health funds for workers in Eretz Israel at the outset of the twentieth century: The first approach was the traditional Jewish attitude toward health care with which the Zionist pioneers were familiar from the

Jewish *shtetl* or township in Eastern Europe where most had grown up. This model held the community as a whole responsible for its sick, and care was provided through institutions such as "linat tzedek" (tending to the sick at night) and "bikur holim" (visiting the sick and fulfilling their needs). The second approach was compulsory health insurance on a class basis under governmental supervision, as manifested in the health funds that operated under Bismarck, and then spread to the rest of Europe.

The agricultural workers, proponents of European socialism, were familiar with health organizations for workers in Europe and viewed them as a worthy model. The workers' press in Eretz Israel carried in-depth reports on a regular basis about the activities in labor movements around the world, including their health organizations.

Despite their familiarity with health insurance in Europe, the first institution that members of the Judea Workers established in Eretz Israel was a "linat tzedek" format—a solution that sprung from the traditional Jewish way of caring for the sick and the needy in the community and that was well suited to the small-group frameworks in which the laborers lived. Only later, when they came to the conclusion that this method was insufficient, did the founders seek other ways and new ideas for solving their problems in health matters. At this point, the workers turned to the idea of health funds as they had crystallized at the close of the nineteenth century in Europe, but they still did not abandon the institution of "linat zedek," which was a core element and not merely an appendage in the charters of the health funds for laborers that they had established, largely due to the absence of other normative "support systems," such as family, among the groups that were mostly made up of "singles."

Even if the European method manifested itself in the principles behind the health fund in Eretz Israel, from an *organizational* standpoint they were very different:

First, the ties to other social institutions, particularly the government, were different. The European governments played a core role in organization of the health insurance, while in Eretz Israel the health funds were the fruit of independent enterprise. In Europe, in many cases, the organization enjoyed government support and was accompanied by legislation, following the growth of an urban proletariat of factory workers. The initiative for organization in Europe was based either on political considerations or affiliation, or on a common occupation. In Eretz Israel, organization took place against the backdrop of the growth of the New Yishuv—an "independent" emerging Zionist-oriented society—without any governmental intervention by Ottoman authorities.

Second, size and initial target population was different. In Europe, the funds were large-scope urban frameworks with thousands of members. In Eretz Israel the initiative sprang forth from among agricultural workers in a rural setting who operated in small groups to solve "local" problems that were not shared by the urban Jewish community. Only after the 1920 amalgamation of workers' health funds into one united health fund, Kupat Holim, did it become an arm and organizing tool of the General Federation of Labor.

Third, parallel to this, the fundamental structure and organizational role of Kupat Holim underwent a fundamental change early in its evolution that set it apart from the European approach. Unlike the European pattern, which was based solely on providing medical coverage, Kupat Holim became a health-service provider in its own right, with its own salaried teams of doctors and nurses, and then hospitals. Furthermore, the diffused geographical pattern of small clinics and health centers in Israel was unique, based on community ambulatory services that literally "brought health services to the workers" wherever they lived. In terms of role, the European health insurance plans were part of a larger scheme—a social security insurance policy—while the health fund in Eretz Israel originally dealt solely with curative medicine and care for members in cases of illness. Elements of social security and preventive medicine such as education and inoculation became a part of the health fund's agenda only after the establishment of the state of Israel.

Thus, in many respects,[1] organization of the health fund among agricultural workers was essentially different from the patterns of health insurance as they took shape in Europe.

Today, Kupat Holim's services are comprehensive and multifaceted, encompassing hospitals, clinics, pharmacies, laboratories, x-ray labs, mother-and-child clinics, maternity facilities, and convalescent homes. Even from its beginnings, Kupat Holim viewed itself as the central national agency for health services within the Yishuv. This "national outlook" expressed itself primarily in times of crisis: during the First World War when workers' health funds extended medical assistance to all in need within the Yishuv; under the British Mandate, when Kupat Holim took upon itself to provide health services to encampments of laborers such as the Labor Battalion (*Gdud ha*

Avodah), to collectives and other rural settlements, to new immigrants and to unemployed workers from all socioeconomic classes within the Yishuv; during the Second World War; and throughout the struggle for establishment of a Jewish state and the first years following statehood when Kupat Holim ensured medical assistance to members of the Yishuv in the armed forces and their families and to masses of new immigrants arriving in the country.

With the establishment of the state of Israel, one of the issues on the public agenda was, quite naturally, the health system and the roles of its institutions. One of the most controversial aspects was the place of Kupat Holim within the constellation of health care in the new state. National leaders such as David Ben-Gurion, public figures, and many physicians held that, with the establishment of the state, the health system should be retooled into a unified governmental framework, as was the case with the education and welfare systems. The opposition of the Federation of Labor to unification of all health services led to the formation of two parallel health systems: health services under the auspices of Kupat Holim side by side with health services under the auspices of the Ministry of Health—a legacy that remains to this day.

Kupat Holim from its conception perceived itself as a body with a mission and responsibilities of a national scope, struggling to fulfill humanitarian and national missions, bearing the brunt of assuring the health and well-being of the Yishuv in Eretz Israel. Following the establishment of the state, Kupat Holim came under the jurisdiction of the Ministry of Health, a body thrust into competition with Kupat Holim for economic resources and hegemony in setting health policy. As a consequence, perceptions of the role of Kupat Holim in ensuring medical services underwent a metamorphosis—first and foremost in the eyes of the public and the country's leadership as to the role of the health fund within the health system, but also among Kupat Holim's senior management's and the leadership of the Federation of Labor. There was also a significant change in the manner in which Kupat Holim operated—raising a quandary that had accompanied Kupat Holim from its birth. As the health fund's first director, Eliezer Perlson put it: "Would Kupat Holim provide services 'according to needs' or 'according to [the health fund's] abilities'?" Prior to the establishment of the state, Kupat Holim policy was set according to needs, while after 1948, and particularly in recent years, criteria have shifted toward "ability."

This volume is devoted to examining key junctures in the history and development of Kupat Holim, under the assumption that these issues can serve to illuminate and understand the essence, the power, and the role of Kupat Holim and the difficulties it encountered as the core body in health services in the country. A study of Kupat Holim's history can assist in uncovering the roots of the difficulties it faces today, and perhaps in finding a few answers to the questions and the problems with which it struggles and is likely to continue to struggle within the foreseeable future.

1

Health Services in Eretz Israel in the Nineteenth Century

Up to the year 1837, there was not one hospital, clinic, or even one certified physician in the Jewish community[1] in Eretz Israel[2] under Ottoman Turk rule. Seventy-six years later—in 1913 on the eve of the First World War—there were already sixteen hospitals operating in the country, ten of them in Jerusalem. Among the sixteen facilities, ten were Jewish hospitals, five situated in Jerusalem. The Jewish medical community was organized within the Hebrew Medical Federation with headquarters in Jaffa. Three health funds operated in the Galilee, Judea, and Samaria and tens of certified Jewish doctors practiced medicine throughout the country.

First Medical Institutions in Eretz Israel in the Nineteenth Century

The first health and medical institutions in Eretz Israel were the offspring of political upheavals and social change that the Yishuv underwent in the nineteenth century. At the turn of the century, after three hundred years of Turkish rule, there were approximately six thousand Jewish inhabitants in the entire country—two thousand in Jerusalem and the remainder in the holy cities of Hebron, Safed, and Tiberias.[3] Most were Sfardi Jews of North African and Middle Eastern origin and a minority were Ashkenazi Jews from diverse ethnic backgrounds in Europe. Their livelihoods were dependent for the most part on a biannual living stipend based on donations from Jewish communities in the Diaspora called the Haluka (allocation) that was allocated to family units on the basis of ethnic association. This dispensation was barely sufficient for sustenance, but its regularity served as a buffer against starvation for the Jewish community. The state of sanitation was horrendous: Sewage ran in the streets, garbage was not collected regularly, water came primarily from cisterns, and the community was plagued by outbreaks of numerous epidemics, particularly during the summer. The health and economic circumstances of Jerusalemites was particularly bad. They lived in the Jewish Quarter of the Old City under severely crowded conditions, in homes lacking any sanitary provisions whatsoever. Average mortality in Jerusalem approached 40%, and among children, 70%.[4]

The harsh health circumstances of the Jews of Eretz Israel were not exceptional for their place and times, and were similar to those of Moslem and Christians in the country. The only medical services were provided by witch doctors, amateur pharmacists, and traditional healers armed with herbs, amulets, and incantations, augmented by community assistance and charity societies—Bikur Holim (visiting the sick) and Linat Tzedek (night watch of the sick)—that engaged volunteers among members of the community to succor and care for the indigent sick.

According to the descriptions of researcher Amally Kass, Eretz Israel under the Ottomans was a backwash of civilization, of little note except for its religious significance. The country's inhabitants had been totally passed over by advances in science and technology made during the eighteenth and nineteenth centuries, and still lived in a manner reminiscent of the Middle Ages.

Nissim Levi quotes K. Bazili, the General Consul for Russia in Beirut in the 1830s and 1840s: "Every European looked to the inhabitants like a doctor, and a European headdress was held as if it was a medical diploma."[5]

Ben-Zion Gat noted that during his sojourn in Israel, Ibrahim Pacha (i.e., the son of Muhammad Ali who conquered Eretz Israel from the Turks in 1831) sought the medical services of Rabbi Israel Bek, a printer by profession and amateur healer from Safed, for not even one certified doctor could be found in the country at the time.

The Mission Clinics and the Montefiore Clinic

The first attempt to improve the health of the Jews in Eretz Israel and establish a Jewish medical institution came as the initiative of Moshe Montefiore in 1828, during the renowned philanthropist's first visit to Eretz Israel. Montefiore, who had journeyed to Eretz Israel as president of the Committee of Community Emissaries in England, proposed to the heads of the Jewish community in Jerusalem that a hospital be established in Jerusalem that would be managed by a certified Jewish doctor who would provide organized medical assistance gratis to all in need. His proposal was not realized due to the opposition of Jewish religious elements in Eretz Israel and abroad who claimed that introduction of modern medicine would bring about general modernization of Jewish community life in the country and undermine religious values and the traditional lifestyle of the community. Moreover, the opponents fought the idea with claims that there was "no need for a hospital because what exists is sufficient for every indigent ill person and collection of funding [for such] would be a waste of money."[6]

Reservations among Jerusalemites regarding establishment of regular medical services for members of city's Jews also influenced the small Jewish communities in Tiberias, Safed, and Hebron, who also abstained from establishing medical institutions. The researcher Yehoshua Leibowitz wrote that compared to Christian and Moslem society, the Jews were late in establishing hospitals.[7] Leibowitz believed the roots of such behavior are linked to the mitzva or Jewish religious commandment to visit the sick—an obligation that encompassed all, not just relatives and friends of the patient. Thus, to a great extent fulfillment of this mitzva served as an alternative public institution to hospitals.

In 1837, however, the plight of the Jewish community worsened. Safed was decimated by a major earthquake and many of the survivors fled to Jerusalem; war broke out between Turkey and Egypt over control of Eretz Israel, and revolts by Arab peasants and Druze eroded conditions in the country even more. Epidemics of cholera, yellow fever, and typhus took a heavy toll among members of the Jewish community. In 1840, Egypt lost control of Eretz Israel and Turkey reestablished its hegemony over the region with the assistance and support of the European powers.

The European powers subsequently exploited the weakness of the "sick man of Europe," as the Ottoman Empire was labeled, demanding and receiving capitulations—privileges granted to foreign governments, giving them rights to engage in extensive religious and cultural activities and to establish autonomous institutions that entrenched and enhanced their status in the Holy Land. The European power whose grip and influence was the greatest ultimately would inherit control of Eretz Israel when the Ottoman Empire finally fell. The policy of capitulations led to the establishment of six consulates in Jerusalem within a decade (1842–1852). Jerusalem was the center of activity among the foreign consuls, each actively seeking areas where they could exert influence that would serve their country's interests and enhance its diplomatic status in the city.

The first to inaugurate such activities were the British. In order to heighten sympathy for the English among the Jews of Jerusalem, the British decided to provide assistance in an area in which the Jewish community was most in need—medical assistance. With the assistance of the London Society for the Jews, a Christian missionary fellowship whose mission was to spread Christianity among the Jews, two missionaries were sent to Jerusalem in 1838—Dr. Albert Gerstmann, a physician, and Melville Bergheim, a pharmacist. The pair opened a clinic and began providing medical services gratis to all in need. By 1844, the clinic had become a small twenty-four-bed hospital. High morbidity and economic distress forced many Jews to seek medical assistance at the mission. Historian Mordechi Eliav writes that a thousand Jewish patients were hospitalized in the mission hospital annually.[8]

The opening of the British clinic had a far-reaching impact on the heads of the Jewish community in Jerusalem. Local Jewish leadership feared expansion of missionary activity among the Jews of Jerusalem under the guise of medical assistance; consequently, they decided, despite their previous objections, to establish a clinic headed by a Jewish doctor that would free the Jewish community in the city from their exclusive dependence on the British mission. For this purpose, they turned to Moshe Montefiore, who sent Dr. Shimon Frankel, a Jewish doctor from Germany who was close to ultra-orthodox Jewish circles, to Jerusalem. Dr. Frankel arrived in Eretz Israel in 1843, and established the first Jewish medical clinic in the country, a facility which he operated for fifteen years. The success of the British clinic and the Montefiore clinic prompted other European powers to follow suit. Between the years 1838 and 1914, six hospitals and many clinics were established in Jerusalem. The thriving competition that developed between "Christian missionary medicine" and "Jewish medicine" in Eretz Israel was at times accompanied by clashes between the two camps, but the rivalry also fueled the establishment, expansion, and ultimate hegemony of Jewish-Zionist foundations of medical practice in the country in the nineteenth century.

The First Jewish Hospitals

The outbreak of the Crimean War in 1853 had a profound impact on the economic welfare of the Jewish community. Heads of the community turn to the Rothschild family in Paris to request medical and material assistance. Baron Jacob Rothschild of France[9] responded favorably to their request. After consulting with the European consuls in Jerusalem, the Baron established in 1884 the first Jewish hospital in Eretz Israel under the auspices of the Austrian government. Following the Rothschild hospital, between 1854 and 1914 another four Jewish hospitals were established in Jerusalem: Bikur Holim (Visiting the sick, 1857); Misgav Ladach (1879); Ezrat Nashim (women help, 1895); and Shaarei Tzedek (the gates of justice, 1902). All the hospitals were established along religious and ethnic lines, under the auspices of the consulates. In a similar manner, clinics and hospitals were subsequently founded elsewhere in the Jewish community—in Jaffa (1891), Tiberias (1897), and Safed (1912).

The Shaar Zion Community Hospital

The Shaar Zion Hospital in Jaffa, established in 1891, was an exception in the network of hospitals founded at the close of the nineteenth century by the Old Yishuv. The hospital was established on the initiative of the local Jaffa Community Governing Committee—an exceptional body in terms of local norms, for it was comprised jointly of Sfardi and Ashkenazi Jews rather than along ethnic lines. The funding to establish the facility was procured from donors abroad, but unlike the hospitals among Jewish communities in the holy cities, treatment was not free. Fees were progressive, based on means, and the budget was complemented through community taxes. The hospital was unique not only due to its non-sectarian policies, but also in its decidedly pro-

Zionist character that attracted Zionist-motivated physicians such as Dr. Alexandra Belkind, Dr. Haim Hissin, and others. Adjacent to the hospital the Hebrew Medical Federation was founded in 1912 (today the Israel Medical Federation, the professional organization of Israeli physicians). The organization initiated the first doctors' conferences in the country. The Shaar Zion Hospital was also the first to employ women doctors (Dr. Alexandra Belkind and Dr. Bat-sheva Yunis-Gutmann).

The Shaar Zion Hospital treated Jewish laborers at reduced fees, particularly those who were not eligible for medical assistance in the Jewish agricultural settlements established by the Baron de Rothschild, thus serving as a regional hospital in the full sense of the word.[10] The reports of the Community Governing Committee demonstrate that less than half the patients treated at the hospital were residents of Jaffa. The majority were Jewish laborers from throughout the country who were aware that at Shaar Zion they would receive good care without discrimination or religious coercion; they were willing to wait in rented rooms in Jaffa for an available bed in Shaar Zion rather than be hospitalized in other Jewish hospitals where a religious lifestyle was mandatory and the secular Socialist labors felt unwelcome. Moreover, Shaar Zion did not turn away laborers unable to pay so long as a free bed was available. The hospital physicians even conducted regular biweekly visits to the Jewish agricultural settlements in the vicinity to treat sick Jewish agricultural workers who were unable to travel to Jaffa. Among those who received hospitalization services at Shaar Zion were not only Jews, but also Arab residents in the vicinity.

The Shaar Zion hospital operated in collaboration with Zionist institutions that funneled funding to support the hospital through the "Eretz Israel Office" of the World Zionist Organization,[11] located in Jaffa. During the years 1905 to 1914 Jaffa in general was a center of Zionist activity in the country, and the hospital served as one of the focal points for Zionist endeavor. When the first workers' health funds were founded, the hospital became the provider of hospitalization services, serving in this capacity until the year 1917. The hospital not only served as a hotbed for Zionism, it was one of a host of social, political, and economic institutions that the Zionist movement would found or adopt over the years in its systematic endeavors to build the infrastructure for a new society and a viable Jewish homeland, from scratch.

The State of Health in the Baron's Agricultural Settlements[12]

In 1882, in the wake of pogroms in Russia, the first Zionist settlers (members of the Lovers of Zion movement, a harbinger of the Zionist movement) came to Eretz Israel and established agricultural villages. Between the years 1882 and 1884 the first seven Zionist settlements were founded—four in Judea southeast of Jaffa, one in Samara on the central coastal plain, and two in the Galilee to the north, a total of 480 inhabitants.[13] Most of the immigrants who founded the villages were Orthodox Jews who had received a traditional Jewish education and maintained a devout religious lifestyle. In Eastern Europe they had engaged in petty trade or were tradesmen or minor public officials in the Jewish community and had arrived in Eretz Israel equipped with meager financial means. Moreover, most came from urban environments and lacked any agricultural experience. They were married and for the most part middle-aged, and brought their families with them. Two small groups were an exception to the rule within the population of the villages: a handful of young, single, nonreligious pioneers from Russia with meager financial means but a broad secular education and socialist leanings who belonged to the Bilu movement; and a small number of educated and liberal-minded young people from among the founders of the village of Rishon le-Zion. Most of the villages were culturally and ethnically homogeneous; the founders or the overwhelming majority of inhabitants came from the same country in Europe.

A short time after founding their settlements, the villagers realized that they could not support themselves independently and needed the regular support of a patron of means in order to prevail. At the beginning of 1883, village representatives turned to the Baron Edmond de Rothschild requesting his assistance and financial help. Rothschild responded favorably to the request. Thus began the Baron's comprehensive support system for the villages that had been established by the First Aliyah (1882–1903).

The village lands were registered in the name of the Baron in return for financial backing. A group of administrators—the Baron's clerks—were appointed and employed by the Baron, and charged with training the settlers as agriculturists, overseeing their operation and providing for their needs in agriculture, health, and education.

Thus, doctors, pharmacists, and paramedics were hired to treat the villagers, sick rooms were built, and significant funds were invested in fighting malaria, which took a heavy toll among the settlers. The physicians, paramedics, and pharmacists were community employees whose salaries were paid by the Baron de Rothschild. In addition to medical care, the medical staff was responsible for sanitation in the village and conducted regular house visits to instruct and oversee domestic hygiene. Most of the sick were cared for by the doctor or the paramedic who assisted the physician. In complex cases, the patient was sent to the hospital in either Jaffa or Jerusalem, and in special cases of need (on doctor's recommendation) sick settlers were even sent for medical treatment abroad or convalescence in the mountains of Lebanon. The Baron took great pains to maintain a high level of medical service among the doctors he hired, and did not hesitate to dismiss physicians who did not measure up to professional standards.

The most common illness among the villagers was malaria of all kinds, and particularly swamp malaria. According to epidemiologist Zvi Saliternik malaria was the most important common, endemic disease among all contagious diseases in the country during the period of Ottoman rule, and there was not one settlement free of it.[14] Dr. Hillel Yafe's records also report that most of the inhabitants of the villages, farmers and laborers alike, suffered from malaria. In the village of Hadera, malaria affected more than half the inhabitants of the village and endangered its very existence as a community. Only toward the turn of the century, on the initiative of Dr. Yafe and with the backing of the Rothschild family, was an active campaign to eradicate the source of the disease undertaken: draining swamps, planting Eucalyptus trees, spraying breeding places with kerosene, and regularly distributing quinine to settlers. Turkish authorities did not generally take steps to prevent the spread of the disease, except for quarantine of areas struck by epidemic outbreaks of disease and partial inoculation of the population against smallpox. After visiting the country in 1887 Emanuel Vensiani reported to the Baron Hirsch—another renowned Jewish philanthropist—that "the Land simply devours its inhabitants."[15] Zvi Saliternik wrote in his comprehensive work on the war against malaria in Eretz Israel that malaria epidemics decimated the population of entire villages due to the lack of suitable medical services.[16]

Medical Assistance in the Baron's Villages

Up until 1884, most medical care in the villages was provided by paramedics hired by the Baron's chief administrator, in accordance with on-site needs. The paramedic lived in one place, and was required by contract to visit each of the villages once or twice a week, and make special unscheduled trips in special pressing cases. In order to obtain medications, the settlers had to travel to Safed, Haifa, or Jaffa, as there were no apothecary services in the villages themselves.

The three main villages—Rosh Pina in the north, Zichron Yaakov in the Sharon, and Rishon le-Zion in the south—were established between the years 1884 and 1887. With the backing of the Baron de Rothschild, regular on-site medical services, including a pharmacy and a paramedic-pharmacist in residence, were provided for. Those in charge of medical service continued to live in a nearby city, working part-time for the Baron, but from this point on they were certified physicians.

Unlike other professionals, doctors and pharmacists were required to obtain certification from Turkish authorities. From time to time, inspections were carried out at medical institutions and fines were levied on apothecaries whose pharmacists were not certified. In 1887, the Baron began appointing district physicians who resided in the three major villages, each being responsible for the smaller villages in their vicinity. By the end of the first decade, when the number of inhabitants in the Baron's villages reached nineteen-hundred inhabitants, Rothschild decided to establish a hospital in the main villages—in Rishon le-Zion in 1889, and Zichron Yaakov in 1890. The apothecaries in the main villages were improved, equipment was purchased, and the value of the medications dispensed was substantial. The staff generally included women settlers who served as paid midwives, and women who engaged in nursing hospitalized patients. In the smaller villages, small local apothecaries were opened where pharmacists or pharmacist's assistants were employed, as well as paid midwives from among the inhabitants. The pharmacists in the smaller settlements operated under the supervision of the district doctor, who also served as a traveling physician, visiting each settlement once or twice a week. In more isolated settlements, some settlers sought medical assistance from Arab doctors living in the vicinity, such as Dr. Mijallah Majdida in Marjai'un (today a city in southern Lebanon) who for years provided treatment to Jewish residents of the village of Metula in the Upper Galilee.

Over time, clerks salaried by the Baron joined the medical staff of the Baron's villages until in certain places their number exceeded the number of medical staff. Dr. Yafe who served as director of the hospital in Zichron Yaakov from 1893 wrote in his diary: "I was astounded by the number of clerks in the hospital as well. Fourteen beds and nine clerks, besides the doctor."[17]

Yafe believed that the Baron's functionaries would intervene in the work of the physician, providing permits for hospitalization in Jerusalem hospitals and coverage of medical treatment abroad for close cronies, referrals that were not based on objective criteria of medical urgency. The Baron's officials permitted the doctors to practice on the side elsewhere, in situations not under the Baron's patronage, thus contributing to improvement of conditions in the Yishuv in general. In other Jewish settlements not among the Baron's villages, local pharmacies were also set up in the 1890s, and medications distributed gratis in district pharmacies under Rothschild's patronage. Moreover, in 1887, the Baron ordered that the physicians treat without fee all Arabs who came to the Jewish village clinics, and pharmacies were ordered to provide medications without payment, as well.

The level of medicine in the main villages was on such a high plane that according to historian R. Aaronson "There were many ill who came from Jerusalem to receive medical care at the hands of the village doctor."[18]

Yossi Ben-Artzi, a scholar of the first Jewish agricultural villages, wrote that the clinic and pharmacy were an integral part of the public building complex of the community. Such a situation was extraordinary even for Europe, where it was very rare to find medical services in traditional rural communities. In Arab villages in Eretz Israel and in settlements in Eretz Israel established by the Templers such services were totally absent. . The standard of living and the level of sanitation and medicine that the Jewish settlers demanded led to the development of health services as a core component in the structure of public institutions in the Jewish agricultural villages. Among the thirty villages established between the advent of modern Zionism in 1882 and the outbreak of the First World War in 1914, Ben-Artzi found no less than eighteen buildings that served as health institutions (clinics, pharmacies, and hospitals), compared to five libraries and twelve structures devoted to administration of the local governing committee and the Baron's officials.[19] Only the number of schools and synagogues was greater than the number of health facilities.

The state of independent settlers (some two thousand inhabitants) and Jewish laborers (approximately five hundred) in Jewish settlements not under the patronage of the Baron de Rothschild was quiet different. The cost of a doctor visit beyond the Baron's villages was very dear, generally five to ten francs, although there were cases where the fee demanded reached fifty francs, more than the average monthly wage of a Jewish laborer. Furthermore, a laborer sick for ten consecutive days was erased from the "Clerk's Register," making him ineligible for further work. As a result, laborers were forced to return to work before they were fully recovered. Discrimination in providing medical aid sparked much resentment and countless conflicts broke out between the settlers and laborers as a result. In order to receive medical care, most of the laborers were forced to turn to the Shaar Zion Hospital in Jaffa, which provided them and their families with medical services at a reduced rate. Discrimination in medical services in the villages was one of the primary factors leading to the growth of alternative medical services for workers: the workers' health funds

The exception to the rule were the laborers in the village of Rechovot, a community not under the patronage of the Baron. The Jewish workers received comprehensive welfare assistance via the Minucha ve-Nachala Society (home and rest) founded by the community. Members of Minucha ve-Nachla aspired to make employment of Jewish laborers economically feasible.[20] Consequently, they took steps to ensure suitable living conditions for their workers, providing housing, a kitchen, and medical services at the expense of the community as a whole, thus allowing the workers to sustain themselves on the low wages they received without impairing their productivity at work.

The Cholera Epidemic and Economic Crisis at the Close of the First Aliyah

In the year 1900, Rothschild transferred responsibility for his villages in Eretz Israel to the Jewish Colonial Association (JCA). At the time, there were 3,800 inhabitants in the Baron's villages and another 1,310 Jews in agricultural settlements that did not enjoy Rothschild's patronage.[21] From the outset, JCA took steps to cut back the number of functionaries in the villages, dismiss laborers as an economy move, and strengthen the economic base of the villages through credit and flexible budgets for farmers, while demanding that the settlers take responsibility for their own affairs and move towards mixed farming to enhance long-term sustainability. At the same time, JCA cut back on health and education services that in the past had been paid for out of the Baron's pocket. The inhabitants were informed they would have to finance these services on their own. The settlements in the Galilee were forced to make do with one doctor located at Rosh Pina and a pharmacist retained "on a small salary"[22] who were expected to supervise the heath of the communities.

The years 1901–1903 were particularly difficult for Jewish settlements in Eretz Israel. Of the population of some 55,000 Jews, 5,000 lived in agricultural settlements.[23] In addition to the shock of the transfer in patronage, there were many natural disasters to boot. In 1901 a fierce drought worsened economic conditions. Many Jewish laborers were dismissed and the farmers went over to employing primarily Arab workers whose wage demands were lower. A year later, in 1902, a cholera epidemic broke out, putting the efficiency of the Jewish medical network to the test. Some 20,000 people in the country died in the epidemic. The worst hit were Arab areas—Gaza and the Arab community of Jaffa.[24] Jerusalem, Jaffa, and the Jewish agricultural settlements were put under quarantine by Turkish authorities; train and ship movements were halted; schools were closed; and commerce came to a standstill. The closure of maritime activity put tremendous economic pressure on the Yishuv. In Jerusalem a joint health committee comprised of both Ashkenazi and Sfardi Jews was formed to extend medical and economic aid and prevent the spread of the epidemic. Thanks to their work, the number of casualties among the Jerusalem Jewish community was small. Similar action on the part of the governing committee of Jews in Jaffa also kept the number of casualties down. But despite the relatively small number of victims among the Yishuv many Jews fled abroad due to fear of the epidemic. The economic straits of the Yishuv made it difficult to care for those hit by the epidemic. The *Ha'hashkafa* newspaper described the situation thus:

> From week to week, many of our brethren leave our country and travel to distant [lands] and [abandon their] family…here in terrible straits and they almost die of famine.[25]

Agricultural work and commerce ceased as well, and after years of self-sufficiency, it was necessary to import flour and grain. On top of the cholera epidemic, in 1903 a cattle disease of epidemic proportions annihilated most of the herds in the villages, exacerbating the economic crisis and generating widespread famine. Dr. Yafe wrote:

> The cholera is devastating in Jaffa and the [Arab] hamlets. In some villages half of the population has been lost….In Jaffa between the 16th of October and the 5th of November, 300 souls succumbed. Among the Jews there were 22 cases of the disease, of which 8 cases died….On the other hand, poverty and want have amplified….People whose livelihoods are from day labor have remained without any means….A rapid assistance service has been formed in cases of cholera. Remedies and all that is needed to support the sick and convalescing are provided gratis. Resources, I am sorry to say, are dwindling and shortages are widespread.[26]

Despite the difficult health status of the Yishuv in general, and during the 1903 epidemic in particular, the question of medical assistance needed by the New Yishuv was not the subject of discussion in Zionist congresses. Even Dr. Yafe himself—at the time, head of the Zionist Federation's branch in Eretz Israel—did not report the Yishuv's serious health problems to the Zionist Congress; instead, Yafe informed the Baron de Rothschild in Paris, and afterwards the JCA. Perhaps he surmised that only they would have the financial means to help.

Attempts by the Jewish workers to organize in the face of the 1903 crisis were unsuccessful. Their call upon the JCA and Baron de Rothschild to solve the crisis by helping the workers establish their own settlements came up against a stone wall. Even the intervention of influential Zionist figures such as the leaders of the Lovers of Zion—Achad Ha'am and Menachem Ussiskin—were to no avail. In the summer of 1903, Ussiskin tried to organize a country-wide organization, and an "executive committee" was elected for the entire Yishuv led by Dr. Yafe, but this attempt also failed, primarily due to the crisis within the Zionist movement, sparked by controversy over the Uganda Plan.

Such was the situation in Eretz Israel when the first members of the Second Aliyah began to arrive, toward the close of 1903.

2

The Workers' Health Fund: Ideology and Beginnings, 1903-1914

The First Health Funds of the Workers

The Health Status of Second Aliyah Workers

In December 1903 the first group of survivors of the Kishnev Pogrom,[1] together with members of the Jewish Defense Group from Hommel[2] in Russia arrived in Jaffa. Their arrival signaled the beginning of the Second Aliyah. The Second Aliyah, the second major wave of Jewish immigration spurred by modern Zionism, continued until the outbreak of the First World War in 1914 and brought a total of some thirty-thousand persons to Eretz Israel.[3] Most of the members of the Second Aliyah were absorbed within the Jewish community in Jerusalem and in the new urban sector, first in Haifa and Jaffa, later in Tel Aviv.[4] A small number of immigrants turned to Jewish agricultural villages, purchased land, and were absorbed by the veteran settlements established by the First Aliyah. Only a small number—some 1500 to 2500 young Zionists with socialist leanings—sought work as agricultural laborers in the villages of the First Aliyah.[5] Zeev Tzachor, an historian of the Second Aliyah, believes that members of the Second Aliyah came to Eretz Israel out of sense of crisis. They were lonely, lacking in central organization, without a clear direction or guiding ideal, although their spiritual baggage included socialist thinking combined with new ideas of national regeneration of the Jewish People in Eretz Israel. Y. Gorny, in a sociological and demographic survey of the same group, finds that the members of the Second Aliya had clear common denominators: They hailed for the most part from southern Russia; most (65%) were secular Jews, unattached and in their twenties who came unaccompanied, without an occupation or an economic base. Approximately 30% had a high school education and the rest had received a traditional Jewish education. The educational level of the women was, on the average, higher than that of the men, but the latter had a better mastery of Hebrew.[6]

Soon after their arrival, it became evident to the new immigrants that the ideological gap between them and the settlers from the First Aliyah made it difficult to integrate as agricultural workers into the villages. Most members of the First Aliyah maintained a religious (i.e., orthodox) lifestyle and had no objection to financial assistance from abroad, and employed Arab laborers; their national-Zionist aspirations were limited to purchasing land and establishing settlements. The socialist visions that members of the Second Aliyah brought with them were foreign to the veterans, and generated opposition. The veterans looked with disfavor on the secular lifestyle of Second Aliyah pioneers. They were not swayed by demands that everyone speak Hebrew and rejected the newcomers' labor-Zionist ideology that championed a "conquest of labor"—an ideal that would spell total abandonment of cheap Arab labor in their villages—and placement of all agricultural work in the hands of Jewish laborers. They were particularly irked by the harsh criticism leveled at them by members of the Second Aliyah as if they, the farmers, were getting rich at the Baron's expense. They were incensed by charges of "Levantine" (shallow) thinking and claimed they had repudiated the Zionist idea by not opposing the Uganda Scheme at the 1903 convention of the World Zionist movement. The farmers countered the charges, saying that economic realities forced them to employ Arab workers, and that it was neither feasible nor moral to eject Arab employees—a move, they argued, that would only generate hatred for the Jews. These arguments did not impress members of the Second Aliyah. Soon conflicts erupted over this issue, and a deep rift developed between the two groups; the members of the Second Aliyah in the villages found themselves both socially isolated and denied work by their Jewish brethren. In 1906 the split between Jewish laborers and Jewish farmers reached a crisis stage: In Petach Tikva[7] the village governing committee declared a "boycott" of the Jewish laborers and demanded that community members not employ them, nor rent them housing. These difficulties were amplified by other difficulties. A harsh climate, shabby living conditions, arduous labor, and poor nutrition all had an adverse effect on the health of the young pioneers. Many fell ill and died from neglect, lack of care, and deficient or improper medical care.

In the larger villages such as Rishon le Zion and Rechovot, the laborers received only partial medical aid. Even then, care was contingent on the goodwill of JCA functionaries and the village-governing committees. Such dependence weighed heavily on the minds of the workers who viewed medical aid based on charity and compassion as running contrary to their social principles and aspirations for independence. The village governing committees did not consider it their duty to extend medical aid to a worker who fell ill. The Petach Tikva charter stipulated that a person in need of a doctor was required to pay if the individual was not a resident of the village, and if one did not have the means, the person would be denied medical care:

> And there was a case of a Hebrew laborer who became sick in Petach Tikva and he did not have two *bishlikim* [coins], and the doctor sent him away saying that a [doctor's] visit is not an duty, but an option.[8]

The social conflicts between members of the Second Aliyah and their employers only worsened the situation. Members of the Second Aliyah from Petach Tikva related that during the farmers' "boycott" of the Jewish workers, the village physician, Dr. Stein, was forbidden to assist the wife of one of the workers, but nevertheless delivered her baby. The midwife heeded the committee's orders, but it was revealed:

> Stein—a member of Bilu-a Zionist movement, who had always treated the workers well (and declined receipt of payment for visiting them) announced to the committee that he would not comply with their directive.[9]

In the farms operating under the management of the Jewish Colonization Association (JCA), there was no regular medical care for workers, and the controversy over medical aid was a factor in countless disputes between laborers and the farm manager. Yaakov Ori, a laborer who belonged to the Second Aliyah, related in his memoirs that those who cared for the sick on the farm were engaged in agricultural posts, and medical care was pitifully meager: "Quinine tablets and towels soaked in water in light cases, or remnants of sheets brought from there—from home, in serious cases."[10]

Because most of the sick laborers were single and had no kin to take care of them, the laborers began to organize on their own to assist one another when they fell sick. Neta Goldberg (Harpaz), another laborer, related in his memoirs that "as if by itself" the traditional Jewish institution of "linat tzedek" was revived—a framework familiar to the pioneers from the Jewish shtetls (townships) in the Diaspora from which most of them came. The healthy took turns staying with ill comrades during the day, and if the condition of the sick was particularly dire, they stayed by their bedsides even at night:

> Thus we began a bit in the manner of the things in the Diaspora. When a comrade got sick, we—the group members who dealt with worker affairs on a voluntary basis, took care that a sick comrade would be visited and cared for, before they knew or thought about treatment at the hands of a doctor and remedies.[11]

FIRST ATTEMPTS TO ORGANIZE HEALTH SERVICES FOR WORKERS

In their search for avenues to ease distress in cases of illness, the workers of Petach Tikva established a "linat zedek" society. Medical equipment (thermometer, cupping glasses and so forth) could be pawned from the village governing committee, but only after a long wait in line, for the laborers were considered "outsiders" in the village. In Rechovot one of the workers founded a mutual aid society for the sick entitled "Linah," designed to put visits and aid to the sick on a regular footing. Both workers and members of the village participated in the Linah Society. When many laborers migrated to the Galilee, they also establish a system to provide visits to the sick.

Historian Zeev Tzachor says that organization in groups to fill functional needs was a pattern distinctive to the Second Aliyah as a vehicle for coping with the harsh realities in Eretz Israel without relinquishing their unique worldview and mission. The pioneers were unwilling to integrate into existing frameworks, disassociated themselves from their employers among the villagers, refused to receive assistance of any kind as a matter of charity, fiercely protected their autonomy, and created organizational tools for themselves to solve their own burning problems, such as social isolation, the shortage of food, difficulties in the workplace, and inadequate housing. Organization began spontaneously but haltingly as a local social initiative, and then slowly expanded to operate on a regional basis. Afterwards a leadership sprang up and with it—organization on the political level, manifested in the establishment of two workers' parties.

The first attempts to create an organized and comprehensive medical framework that would care for the needs of workers were in the villages in Samaria (Zichron Yaakov and Hadera)—an endeavor spearheaded by Dr. Hillel Yafe. Yafe's ties with members of the Second Aliyah began during the days when the doctor had served as director of the Jaffa hospital (1901–1904). Yafe was in the habit of devoting half his time to visits to the villages in Judea to care for sick workers and advise them how to protect their health and prevent attacks of malaria. As part of this effort, he even published a pamphlet in Hebrew entitled *Protecting One's Health in Eretz Israel* (c. 1904?). Even after he returned to the hospital in Zichron Yaakov in 1904, Yafe took it upon himself (voluntarily) to attend to the health of Jewish workers in Samaria, and continued to visit the villages on a regular basis. He arranged for the hospital kitchen in Zichron Yaakov to serve as a kitchen for the clinic and the workers as well, allowing them to use the hospital services and install a bathtub for bathing on the premises. Dr. Yafe organized orderly lodgings for the workers in abandoned buildings and provided them with wood sleeping pallets (a dear commodity at the time). Due to a shortage of auxiliary medical staff among groups of workers—and particularly paramedics, he initiated local training for female members of the Second Aliyah, bringing them in to work in the hospital and teaching them first aid so that in the future the women could assist when new settlements would be established by groups of workers.

One of Yafe's most important endeavors was his initiative to institutionalize a working arrangement between the hospital and the workers in Hadera (1909). He offered the workers of Hadera hospital services in Zichron Yaakov in return for a yearly lump sum. The arrangement ensured that medical services would be provided as an entitlement, not out of mercy, and would allow all workers in Hadera (including the unemployed) access to medical care they needed. Yafe even initiated establishment of a "Mutual Responsibility Fund

Against Epidemics" that in essence was the first step toward establishment of a health fund for workers based on the principle of mutual aid.

THE WORKERS' PARTIES AND ORGANIZATION OF MEDICAL AID ORGANIZATION

The Hapoel Hatzair (The Young Worker) and Poalei Zion (The Zion Worker) parties established in 1905 encompassed three-hundred members each—only a small portion of the Jewish laborers in Eretz Israel.[12] Hapoel Hatzair aspired to realize Zionist ideals and protection of the workers' interests in Eretz Israel.

Concern for workers' interests was manifested in the opening of communal kitchens, organizing mutual loan funds, operating laundries and labor exchanges, and fostering mastery of Hebrew through establishment of evening classes and libraries. Poalei Zion saw themselves as the bearers of the legacy of the Poalei Zion party established in Russia in 1897. At the beginning, Poalei Zion was a Zionist-Marxist party whose aim was to create a Jewish proletariat that one day would take part in a worldwide class war. Despite their differences, the two parties were united in their desire to build the foundation for a Jewish working class in Eretz Israel. Both rejected private settlements based on individual landowners and upheld manual work (primarily in agriculture as salaried employees) as a personal goal and a collective Zionist objective (i.e., not to be an employer and "exploiter" of others' labor).

The object of discord between the two parties was the Workers of Eretz Israel Fund, established in 1909 by the World Covenant of Poalei Zion to work on behalf of workers in Eretz Israel. The money in the fund was collected in the Diaspora. Members of Hapoel Hatzair and apolitical workers were angered on both administrative and ideological grounds—protesting that Poalei Zion held the purse strings, while they also disapproved of funding their activities on donations from the Diaspora and the charity of others.

In 1907 the first organizational steps were taken by the workers' parties to ease hardships tied to lack of medical aid. Eliyahu Monchik, a member of Hapoel Hatzair whose mother served as housekeeper of the Shaar Zion Hospital in Jaffa, secured the agreement of Shimon Rokeach, director of the hospital, for admission of workers for hospitalization without payment. At the same time, Monchik opened a makeshift clinic for workers in the washroom of the Hapoel Hatzair office, inviting Avraham Kosovsky, a laborer from Petach Tikva and a paramedic by profession, to extend aid to those in need. The washroom clinic was sparsely equipped—a thermometer, some bandages, cod liver oil, and quinine, but its primary significance was that it provided the workers with an "address" in time of need. Within a short time, the Poalei Zion party also opened a clinic for its own members. The funding for the two clinics hinged on donations, and was only able to ease the plight of the workers to a very limited extent. Monchik wrote in a critical vein of the divisive nature of these first endeavors:

> The advent of medical aid in Eretz Israel was [marked by] splitting limited forces and meager donations. A pair of clinics, and they were founded voluntarily by the political parties in the country.[13]

Throughout this period, the issue of medical assistance—lack of services and the high cost of existing services—remained on the agenda of the workers. In practice, however, attempts to actually do something to rectify the situation were few and far between (and for the most part unsuccessful). Already in Hapoel Hatzair's "program blueprints" dated the Hebrew month of Av 1906 (July–August) the health issue of workers was studied and a recommendation made to establish "funds to assist the sick and unemployed." Two years later, in the protocols of the Hapoel Hatzair governing council convened early in the summer 1908, the need for a loan fund and health fund was again mentioned, but in a less "theoretical light." This time it was noted that "on the first, we have 500 francs and the second there is also a certain sum in cash and it's possible to begin actualizing this in practice."

A year later, at the Hapoel Hatzair conference held in early summer 1909, the issue of workers' unemployment, hunger, and disease was again raised. Records of the gathering reported:

> [T]ears flowed from the eyes of many who took part in the conference, upon hearing these dreadful and heartfelt stories. All are voicing the nettling question: From whence shall my help come?[14]

The party newspaper *Hapoel Hatzair* published caustic reports in a similar vein the same year:

> While all over the world, it is customary that even criminals sentenced to life, even they are not withheld medical aid, and here—in regard to Hebrew workers…[they] are treated in a extraordinarily cruel manner.[15]

In reports from its Sixth Convention in October 1910, Poalei Zion urged that the initial work of the Eretz Israel Workers' Fund be taken as the vehicle for broad-based arrangement of masses of workers in Eretz Israel, "through creation of…workers' clubs, medical aid, loans and so forth, through support of these institutions that already exist."[16]

Nevertheless, the two workers' parties and the unaffiliated laborers recognized the necessity of a separate institution that would provide medical aid to laborers. But this was not sufficient to bring about immediate establishment of such a body. According to the worker Yaakov Ori, there were even many opponents to the idea. The Poalei Zion party held that care of the sick should be one of the functions of the Eretz Israel Workers' Fund, affiliated with the party, while Hapoel Hatzair viewed the establishment of a health fund as a form of "secession" from the community-at-large, arguing:

> [It is] something that in itself is undesirable, and doesn't even benefit the workers because it can't prevail solely on its own meager means and maintain health institutions and clerks.[17]

Some workers feared that an institution established to assist only workers would lead to a split within the Jewish community. "[E]veryone needs assistance, and one should not differentiate between one sick person and another."[18]

Some held that the state of the Jewish laborer in Eretz Israel was a matter for Jewish workers in the Diaspora. Others remained apathetic about the entire issue. Yaakov Ori addressed the "large number of 'doubters and questioners,'" asking: "Can we do it? Do we have enough strength to bear this mission on our shoulders?"

> [T]he most enthusiastic on behalf of establishment of an institution for health matters of the working public and

> advocates of immediate action were the unaffiliated workers [i.e., who were not bound by any political considerations of any kind].

Unaffiliated workers from the Second Aliyah frowned on the competition between the two labor parties and internal struggles within each of them. They sought to invest their efforts in actions whose primary impact would be improvement in the lives and welfare of the agricultural worker. It was against this backdrop that nonpartisan federations of agricultural workers were established in Judea and the Galilee in 1911. The primary mission of the federations was to improve the circumstances of agricultural workers on farms (Kinneret, Ben-Shemen, and Hulda), organize the agricultural workers in the Jewish villages in a group framework, play an active role in "settlement work" of the Zionist movement's national institutions, and establish bodies dedicated to mutual aid such as kitchens, laundries, and "health funds." The federations struck a cord with the working public, and within a short time of their founding they had already enrolled a membership of five hundred laborers. The agricultural federations in Judea and the Galilee were, in essence, the foundation upon which the Federation of Labor would emerge after the close of the First World War.

THE ESTABLISHMENT OF THE JUDEA AGRICULTURAL WORKERS' FEDERATION

In May 1911, soon after the establishment of the federation in the Galilee (Passover, April 1911), and a short time prior to the establishment of the federation in Judea (June 1911), one of the workers, Baruch Freiber, lost a hand in a work accident while attending to a pump at a well in a Petach Tikva citrus grove. Freiber noted the effect:

> This accident underscored to the working public the health problem in all its acuteness, tipping the scales among all the doubters and the apathetic as to the need for organizing medical aid and ensuring the sustenance of workers in time of illness.[19]

The amputation of Baruch Freiber's arm galvanized the working public that convened its first convention (June 1911) in the village of Ein-Ganim near Petach Tikva to establish the Judea Workers' Federation.

The members discussed the accident extensively, and decided to pursue a comprehensive solution to the issue of medical aid for workers that would be fitting to the declared objectives of the nascent organization. In the final (fourth) clause on the convention's agenda it was resolved that deliberations should commence as to:

> ensuring the sustenance of the laborer who was injured at work in the grove (next to the motor)...and it is resolved that addressing the question will be referred to the Federation committee that is to be elected.

In the wake of the convention, arrangements were made with Shaar Zion (Zion Gate) Community Hospital in Jaffa to provide hospitalization services for members. The hospital committed itself "to take in without delay any worker that became ill," while the Judea Workers' Committee took upon itself to underwrite the cost of group hospitalization. Under the agreement, the hospital allocated two beds for hospitalization of workers and "a four-bed room for sick workers who had been cured at this facility but whose health was still shaky and could not yet return to their arduous labors."[20]

The decisions of the First Convention of the Judean Workers' Federation aroused differences of opinion among members of the Federation's executive committee on matters of practice. Consequently, it was decided to convene another convention in Petach Tikva in December 1911. Berl Katznelson, head of the unaffiliated workers and one of the founders of the Galilee Workers' Federation, who had begun working in Judea in late 1911, joined the initiators of the second convention. Katznelson supported the idea of a health fund for workers and was convinced that those who should establish such a framework were the workers' federations themselves. Workers, friends of Katznelson, reported that already in his first year in the country while at Ein-Ganim (1909), Katznelson envisioned the idea "that it was time to establish a health fund for workers, first for the laborers in Petach Tikva, and then for all the workers in Eretz Israel."[21] He was calling upon the participants to "broaden the boundaries" and go beyond the framework of merely creating a labor union—to be active in cultural affairs, education, and mutual aid among laborers—"to create a health fund."

On 18 December 1911, the Second Convention of the Judea Agricultural Workers' Federation convened in Petach Tikva, and passed a resolution stating: "The convention recognizes the necessity of creating a health fund through membership dues of workers in Eretz Israel."

Katznelson's motion to finance the fund's activities on members' savings, based on the principle of mutual guarantees and mutual aid, was passed. Afterwards, a Health Fund Committee was elected—based not on party affiliation, but rather along geographic lines or workplace. The health fund, however, was not at the top of the convention's agenda, and when the first Federation's executive committee reported to the convention on its activities, the subject was mentioned only briefly: "The committee engaged in negotiations with the hospital in Jaffa that there should be the possibility of bringing in every sick worker, without delay, and the matter is almost closed."

Actually, there had not been any progress toward getting the health fund up and running, and this reference by the committee was only a reiteration of the agreement with Shaar Zion Hospital about which they had already spoken six months earlier at the first convention. In general discussion following convention reports, Katznelson pressed for giving health a higher priority: "[M]ore attention should be given to the living conditions of the workers. Mutual aid is needed and it can't be delayed."

It seems that despite the need and the relative importance of a health fund in the eyes of the workers, nobody could be found who would take responsibility for actualizing the decision. No serious or extensive discussion of the health fund question was conducted at either the first convention or the second. In retrospect, the decision to establish a health fund was almost a parenthetical "fluke of fate." Moreover, without the pressure of Katznelson, the resolution might not have been adopted at all.[22] Other than the decision to establish a health fund, the Second Convention discussed other matters that at the time were deemed more important in the eyes of the laborers—for instance, the Eretz Israel Workers' Fund and "expanding the boundaries" of the organization's mission beyond unionism. Yet, in retrospect Anita Shapira says:

> From a practical standpoint this was the most important decision taken by the Convention. Under the conditions of self-neglect and poverty in which the laborers of the Second Aliyah lived, the establishment a health fund was an historic turn.[23]

A short time after the decision failed to establish a health fund in Judea, similar resolutions were passed at meetings of delegates of laborers in the Galilee (13–14th January 1912), and at a convention of laborers in Samaria (July 1912). In Samaria a five-member health fund committee was appointed to organize "staying overnight with the sick" and a health fund.

The reaction of the workers to the decision to establish health funds was mixed. The party newspaper *He'achdut* wrote:

> Ben-Shemen was one of the nimble in the matter of a health fund. Right after the meeting—the meeting of the Judea Worker's Committee, there was an assembly of workers in Ben-Shemen about the health fund. The members were apathetic to this important project, and now it has been decided to begin orderly action on this matter under discussion.[24]

Neta Harpaz, a worker and later a scholar of labor history in Israel, noted the crux of hard-line opponents:

> There were members who on principle believed that assistance to a comrade at a time of illness was patterned similar to the halukah [living "dispensation"][25] upon which the veteran community [i.e., the Old Yishuv] founded its existence—and they refused to accept such a form of assistance.[26]

The decision to establish a health fund was difficult and was delayed for quite a long time, but actual organization was all the more complex and drawn out. A memorandum sent by the Judea federation's executive committee (in July 1912) declared the first practical steps in this direction: "collection of membership dues in the health fund of half a bishlik a month [0.14 pounds] and creation of a reserve fund of 600 francs [33 pounds]."

According to Baruch Freiber, half a bishlik (coin) was a fourth or a third of the daily wage of a Jewish laborer. Since most didn't work a regular workweek, the levy was not an insignificant amount. The memorandum closed with an exhortation to all the workers: "[E]veryone must participate in aiding the sick and [in such a case] all the sum needed will be collected in one year and assistance to the sick can be initiated."

This sum was earmarked as the fiscal foundations for operating the fund. Two weeks later, members of all the local committees of the Judea Workers' Federation convened in Rechovot in general assembly. Katznelson drafted the text for a charter, based on the principles that:

> 1. Membership would be open to laborers and self-employed craftsmen;
> 2. Every member would pay a one-franc registration fee and half a bishlik a month membership dues;
> 3. Each member would be dutybound to participate personally in caring for the sick at night or would arrange to send another person in his stead.

A status report published in the newspaper *He'achdut* under the headline "Concerning the Health Fund" describes the state of the project at this time—the summer of 1912—six months after the resolution to establish a health fund was adopted:

> In Ben-Shemen there are 35 participants in the health fund and the attitude of the members is positive, money has been collected to the amount of 46.5 francs. In Petach Tikva 40 francs have been collected. In Rechovot no action has been taken because most of the workers are guarding the vineyards. Only at the close of the season will activity begin. In Rishon le-Zion and in Beer Yaakov the workers change and therefore nothing has been done. In Hulda, where the workers are apathetic to all the institutions, [the workers] demonstrated a positive attitude toward this institution in particular. The attitude of laborers in Jaffa is unclear. From the account of the delegates in the agricultural villages it has become clear that the attitude of workers to this institution is generally positive and already a fourth of the sum needed has been collected. There is room, therefore, for optimism that development will be good for this institution in the future.[27]

Despite the positive tone of the article and the positive attitude of the workers toward the establishment of a health fund, monies were not collected at the required pace, and the need for medical assistance became all the more urgent with the arrival of new workers from the Diaspora. Consequently, it was decided to convene a founding convention of the health fund in Jaffa, with the participation of delegates from all Judea farms and villages and the Laborers' Club in Jaffa.

THE FOUNDING CONVENTION OF THE HEALTH FUND OF THE JUDEA WORKERS' FEDERATION

The primary question on the agenda of the convention was how to organize the fund and mobilize the funding that was still missing. In his opening remarks, Meir Rotberg from the Ben-Shemen farm defined the role of the fund as "care for transporting a sick member and his hospitalization in the hospital in Jaffa or in Jerusalem; assistance to a member recovering from illness, particularly those with families."[28]

The fund was to be founded on "mutual aid" and its efforts were to assist both the member's family during his illness and also the sick in their recuperation.

In order to mobilize the missing funding, Rotberg recommended setting a "health fund day" when the day's wages of all would be channeled to meet the funds needs. The motion generated controversy among convention delegates. Those opposed argued that the distressed state of laborers in Eretz Israel made it impossible to demand a day's wages, while others moved to make do with membership dues or mobilize the needed backing from the organization of raffles, balls, and donations. Rotberg, however, rejected these motions on principle because such activities would involve participation of nonmembers. In his opinion, the workers themselves should establish an institution founded on mutual assistance among laborers, solely by their own means. As for the proposition to conduct a "health fund day," Rotberg claimed that "a day such as this would unify the membership" and would be an expression of identification with the project on the part of the working public. Another participant, David Bader, moved to raise the scope of the fund from six hundred to a thousand francs, and other than membership dues, to accept donations from members. In the end, it was resolved by a majority vote to collect six hundred francs by Hanukah (in December) and declare the Jewish holiday of Tu b'Shvat (Jewish Arbor Day in March) as "Health Fund Day," when the daily wages of all members would be donated toward the workings of the health fund.

The convention discussed the proposed health fund charter drafted by Katznelson and passed it provisionally, planning to discuss the ordinances in detail at the next convention of the organization, after bringing the details of the proposal to the rank-and-file in the workplace. Three members from Petach Tikva and two from Jaffa were elected to serve as the health fund steering committee.

INITIAL DIFFICULTIES IN REALIZING THE IDEA

Even after the first health fund convention, there were was no signs of actualization. David Pochas, who had been appointed by the first health fund convention to organize administration, wrote of the apathy he encountered among local committees and laxity in collecting funds. Even the decision to hold a "Health Fund Day" `on Tu b'Shvat was not fully carried out. Nevertheless, the labor newspapers reported that thirty-two francs had been collected in Ruchama farm and sixty francs in Ben-Shemen, and most of the workers in Rechovot had dedicated their daily wages to the health fund (except for the Yemenite Jews among the workers, who were excused due to their dire financial straits).

The fourth convention of the Judea Workers' Federation held in Ben-Shemen (December 1912) raised the issue of the health fund again and elected a new committee. The new committee published a call for support, and even succeeded in collecting seven hundred francs. At Passover in the spring of 1913, the newly elected health fund committee planned to convene a second convention of the health fund in Petach Tikva to discuss two issues: "working out the charter plan"—based on Katznelson's draft that had been sent to all branches, as a basis for discussion among the rank-and-file—and "working out a plan for operating the fund…one delegate for every 15 members."

In the end, a second convention was convened in Jaffa in early summer 1913. Besides the delegates from the agricultural villages and national farms, members of the provisionary office of the health fund and delegates from the steering committee of the Judean Workers' Federation participated in the convention, as well as representatives of the Workers' Club in Jaffa, and Dr. Sherman, representative of the Hebrew Medical Federation (founded in Jaffa a short time prior to the convention of January 1912 by the Yishuv's medical community).

Thus, the Judean Workers' Health Fund was the first institution in which laborers from the city and agricultural villages participated together. At the convention, members formulated a short-term working program that settled organizational questions and defined sources of income. A detailed charter of the health fund was passed. The ordinances adopted were published in Jaffa in 1913 and contained the foundations of the fund and criteria of eligibility for membership. The decisions and the ordinance clauses set forth by the founders suggest their view of the character mutual aid should take.

THE CHARTER OF THE FEDERATION HEALTH FUND

The ordinances and the main resolutions of the "Health Fund of the Federation of Agricultural Workers in Judea"[29] as they were ratified by delegates to the Second Convention held in Jaffa in early summer 1913 were as follows:

- The health fund of Judean workers was founded and operates on the basis of mutual aid of its members.
- Workers and craftsman who themselves labor [i.e., were holders of supervisory or management posts barred from membership] are eligible for acceptance as members.
- Each member is obligated to participate by himself in activities of spending nights at the bedside of the sick, or sending another person in his stead.
- A sick member will receive the services of a doctor, medication and lodging, and where necessary also hospitalization.
- All those in the member's family enjoy his rights, even if there is only one worker in the family.
- For laborers who are newcomers to the country and haven't yet had a chance to become members of the fund, the fund will assist them just as it does its members in all respects during their first two months in the country. Workers who have been in the country two months and have not yet fulfilled their obligation to the fund will not be able to enjoy its privileges. In outstanding cases, the fund has the authority to grant them assistance.

The Fund's charter was a practical expression of the ideal of mutual aid—one of the ideological pillars of the Second Aliyah. Particularly outstanding was the requirement that a member actively participate in tending to the sick at night—a core morale-lifter among sick workers, who for the most part had left family in Europe, had come unaccompanied, and were still single and without any other familial support system. Even prior to the establishment of the fund, the custom of "linat zedek"—attending to the sick at night—had proven to be one of the most effective vehicles for assisting unaccompanied sick comrades. Ironically, making such an act obligatory reflected the adoption of a traditional Jewish mitzvah or religious commandment concerning care of the sick that had been an integral part of Jewish community life in the Diaspora for generations—patterns from which the pioneers sought so desperately to disassociate themselves when they chose to leave home and became Zionist pioneers in Eretz Israel. Integration of this obligation in the organizational framework of the health fund sprang from deep and very "Jewish" sources.

The original health fund ordinances did not encompass a practical plan for the establishment of institutional frameworks such as sick rooms or clinics; their sole purpose was to set forth the codes for a form of group medical insurance. Even clauses dealing with sick leave and convalescence were not included in the ordinances. But it is noteworthy that even at this early stage, it was decided to extend coverage to the families of members and new immigrant laborers.

Although the idea of a health fund was born in a village setting and was formulated by agricultural workers, there was no discrimination whatsoever between urban and rural workers in the ordinances. The founders sought to establish a joint project that would encompass all the Jewish working public. The only stipulation was that the applicant be someone who labored rather than someone who managed others. Criteria for membership remained a point of controversy—destined to be discussed time and again and the subject of disputes over principles throughout the history of Kupat Holim as it emerged and developed. It was against this background that the second convention raised the question of the status of the Yemenite[30] workers in the agricultural villages, particularly in Petach Tikva and Hadera. Delegates adopted a resolution calling for establishment of a clinic for the Yemenites, funded by registration fees of members and monthly dues. The delegates at the second convention also adopted a resolution that obliged all health fund branches and their members "to participate with devotion in all endeavors that would be done to rectify the dire health status of the Yemenite workers."

The health fund's ordinances were tailored to the needs of the workers at the time, but their importance goes beyond their time. For many years, these ordinances served as the organizational base upon which the fund operated, but, all the more important, they also constituted the ideological underpinnings upon which the health fund as an institution grew, until Kupat Holim became an organization of tremendous power.

THE FIRST WORKING PLAN

Along with adoption of the ordinances, the convention also formulated a working plan for the health fund for the short-term:

> ...to organize in the cities of Jaffa and Jerusalem [adjacent to worker-operated institutions] committees that will maintain a strong tie with the health fund office and assist it in admission of sick patients, negotiation with the hospital administration and so forth...to speak-up and make contracts with the doctors and hospitals...to maintain contact with the doctors in the agricultural villages and with the village medical aid committees...in every place, to arrange lodgings for the sick according to local conditions...in villages with many laborers to try and rent a room to be designated for the sick, at least in times when illness became rampant. To support a nurse (or paramedic) on a regular or temporary basis (according to the needs for medical care at this or that site or time)...to conduct affairs with the Eretz Israel Office and representatives of the settlement organizations in order to determine the duty of the farms and the organization toward their workers in arranging medical aid...to endeavor to unify all the existing private health funds among the workers for cooperative operation.[31]

Unlike the first proposal of ordinances, which focused solely on operating principles and financial questions, this broad-based action program had a practical format—dealing with establishment of committees in the cities, preparation of sick rooms, establishment of ties with doctors and heads of the agricultural villages for concrete medical aid, collaboration with hospitals, arrangements for workers on the national farms, and educational work and guidance in enhancing levels of sanitation.

As for organizational issues, it was resolved that the fund's resources would come from the following: registration fees, monthly payments and donations from members, organization of lectures, celebrations and so forth among the workers, and monies collected through wages donated from the annual "Health Fund Day." In short, all sources of income came from one source: the workers themselves.

The majority of laborers believed that they should not accept any budget from the Eretz Israel Office in Jaffa, the local arm of the World Zionist Federation, holding that acceptance of assistance would be a form of charity degrading to the dignity of the workers. They believed they must fend for themselves. Only at a later stage—from 1921 onward—did they begin to accept the idea that employees and settlement organizations should bear responsibility—moral and financial—for the health of the workers.

ORGANIZATION OF BRANCHES AND ESTABLISHMENT OF OTHER WORKERS' FUNDS

After arrangements for financing the venture were hammered out, practical plans for establishing branches were drawn up and put into action. Local branches were set up, designed to treat members of the fund in their places of residence and work. It was decided that a committee would be chosen to manage each branch and would include a member of the local workers' committee as a representative of the public. The health fund management would be elected at the general convention, and one of the members would serve as a representative of the Judea Workers' Federation on the management team. Each branch would be required to send a detailed monthly report on its activities, expenditures and income, together with 75% of all monies collected. The remaining 25% of the dues stayed in the local branch's fund. If expenditures at the local branch exceeded this amount, the local branch received additional funding from the head office on a temporary or regular basis according to need. It seems that a general budget did not exist. Control of funds was in the hands of the head management, and only at its discretion were additional funds dispensed to branches in need.

Three aspects of organization stand out:

First a representative of the public—that is, of recipients of the service, the sick—participated in management of the local branch of the health fund, thus, granting the "clients" a position where they could influence the nature and quality of the service they received.

Second, a representative of the Judea Workers' Federation sat on the local governing board and at the national management level. This close tie between the health fund and the workers' organizations would typify Kupat Holim's organization from its beginnings through the first forty years of the state of Israel, until enactment of the National Compulsory Health Insurance Law in 1995 that ended the stipulation that members of the health fund had to be members of the General Federation of Labor. At the time, this arrangement enhanced the voice of the agricultural workers' federation in the workings of the health fund, but for decades following the establishment of the state, it also bolstered the Federation of Labor's membership rosters and allowed the Federation to funnel health fund capital to pursue other agendas, beyond health care.

Third, there was a total absence of health professionals—doctors, pharmacists, paramedics and nurses—in management posts and positions of influence in both local branches and the head office. The professional organization of physicians in Eretz Israel—the Hebrew Medical Federation founded during the same period—was not a partner in crystallization and organization of the health fund. The chairperson of the Hebrew Medical Federation, Dr. Sherman, while participating in the founding convention of the health fund, was present solely in an advisory capacity, without any authority or ability to influence the way the fund was to be organized.

In short, from its beginnings, the health fund was an organization of laborers, for laborers, and managed solely by laborers. Even when physicians began to serve in the health fund at the end of the First World War, doctors did not enjoy any special standing above that of other salaried staff. This relationship continued even after the establishment of the state of Israel.

The Judean Workers' Health Fund became operational in 1913, eighteen months after the original decision to establish it (December 1911), and was the first health fund in Eretz Israel.

From the outset, the fund had seven branches and 150 members, almost all of them agricultural workers. The Galilee Workers' Health Fund agreed upon at a convention of agricultural workers in the Galilee in January 1912 began to operate only at the end of 1915. In the interim, workers in the Galilee receive medical aid from the Judean Workers' Health Fund. The health fund for workers in Samaria inaugurated their operation only in 1916—at first in collaboration with the Judea Worker's Health Fund, later as an independent organization. Another health fund is cited in only one place, and that parenthetically, during the fourth convention of Judean Workers' Federation in 1914, when it was reported that members of Hashomer, a small, clandestine organization of guardsman, designed to protect Jews and Jewish property against Arab marauders, had a separate health fund of their own. There is no further evidence of this fund's existence.

WORK ORGANIZATION OF THE FIRST STAGE OF OPERATION, 1913-1914

Toward the close of 1913, the first office of the Judean Workers' Health Fund was opened in the village of Ein-Ganin, under the management of the worker Yitzhak Izakovich, the first secretary of the fund. Izakovich worked during the day as a laborer, conducting the fund's administrative work in the evenings, on a volunteer basis. The secretary conducted correspondence, wrote memorandums, and reguarly visited the branches. In each branch an elected committee coordinated the fund's activities on-site. The secretary was responsible for visiting the committees, urging them to be active, and for collecting monies mobilized on the annual Health Fund Day. The primary authority invested in the secretary on a practical level was dispersion of the "pitka"—the chit or note written and signed by the secretary that enabled a member to turn to a physician or buy medicines at a reduced price. The chit was given to the worker at the member's request and granted solely at the discretion of the secretary. The secretary's frequent visits at branches made it possible for sick workers to receive referrals to the doctor in their place of work or residence, and eliminated the necessity of wasting time and money in going to the health fund's head office in Ein-Ganim. If the visit of the secretary was delayed, it was possible to obtain a referral to a doctor through the auspices of a third party—a fellow worker visiting Ein-Ganim who could deliver the chit to the sick applicant, or by writing Izakovich, who would find a way to pass the chit on to the sick worker. This arrangement set in motion a system by which services were brought to the ill person rather than the sick seeking out services—a pattern that was destined to became a core feature of the Kupat Holim system, almost an "entitlement" in the eyes of its members.

The first activity of the health fund was a contractual arrangement on a group basis with the Hebrew Medical Federation in Jaffa and with Dr. Sherman, who was engaged by the fund in an advisory capacity. The agreement stipulated that sick workers who turned to a physician who was a member of the Hebrew Medical Federation "via health fund chits" would be charged 50% of the doctor's regular fee, and the remainder would be covered by the fund. A similar arrangement was made between the health fund and pharmacies in Jaffa and Jerusalem. Izakovich revealed that the organization had a very "personal" touch:

> At the time, almost everyone was considered a member of the health fund, those who paid and those who didn't pay….According to the ordinances, the maintenance of a sick person during hospitalization was given as a loan, and the person was duty-bound to pay it back to the fund, but we were not sticklers in this matter, and those who had reimbursed [the fund], and those who didn't have didn't reimburse [the fund].[32]

Izakovich stressed that the operation of the health fund hung on the forcefulness of the secretary in collecting monies and transfer payments that had been promised to doctors, according to the chits he issued. Had he not paid the doctors, the physicians would have ceased to provide medical aid to sick workers, he noted.

Yaakov Ori, one of the heads of the health fund, added:

> Sometimes [the secretary] was "saved" by the destitute state of the sick person who lacked the means to get from his place of residence to the doctor, but in practice, this was also taken care of, and transportation costs also fell on the shoulders of the "manager."[33]

Despite the fund's promising beginnings, Izakovich encountered many difficulties in collecting monies and increasing the membership roster. The primary stumbling block was the financial straits of the workers, disputes between the workers' parties that commanded most of the public attention and pushed the health funds onto the sidelines, and lack of ideological clarity about the nature of the fund's work—whether it was a charitable venture, a relief organization based on subsidization, or a mutual aid system. In a letter sent to the branch committees of the fund a short time after the 1913 health fund convention, Izakovich called upon laborers to stop being apathetic and to take action to establish "this precious matter much-needed by us." In a letter a month later, Izakovich noted that "for various reasons of which you are aware, the work of the health fund had ceased of late." In another letter, he requested the recipient's assistance in organizing the Hadera branch of the health fund, revealing that "already twice [the worker Bader] has called for a meeting about the health fund and no one has come. He is the only one left on the health fund committee and [it is] impossible to work [this way], and the disputes between the parties delay things."[34]

The role of the Eretz Israel Workers' Fund was a subject of dispute among the workers' parties and within the Judea Workers' Federation even after the third convention of the Judean workers. The main focus of controversy was the workers' labor exchange that operated under the auspices of the Eretz Israel Workers' Fund. Members of the Federation viewed this body as a rival to their own work exchange. The dispute had a negative impact on the health fund. In early 1914, Izakovich called upon the workers via the labor press, and again in a personal appeal in writing, to cease being apathetic and work on behalf of expansion of the health fund's operation.

At the outset of 1914, the number of young Zionist pioneers immigrating to Eretz Israel increased, and there was somewhat of an improvement in the relations between the workers' federations and the workers' parties. The directorate of the Judea Workers' Federation elected by the third convention succeeded in breaking the stalemate over the health fund, but this was not enough. The feud over this question was finally resolved at the fourth convention held in December 1914—a gathering attended by all Federation members regardless of party affiliation. The resolution passed by the convention requiring all members of the Federation to also be members of the health fund[35] brought about an improvement in the state of the health fund. Yet, in practice, the resolution requiring dual membership was not applied, there being no person or machinery at the time capable of enforcing the decision, and no clear roster of Federation members. The issue of obligatory membership remained on the agenda of the working public for years to come, and fierce disagreements over this issue were not settled until 1937 when reciprocal membership in both organizations—the General Federation of Labor and the General Health Fund (Kupat Holim)—became a reality. Even after

1937, this issue continued to occupy the two organizations. In essence, disputes over dual membership were settled only by a "divorce" imposed in circumstances beyond the control[36] of the pair—a government "bail-out" of the two debt-ridden organizations in 1992, a period beyond the scope of this volume.

ORGANIZATION OF MEDICAL WORK

A short time after the Fourth Convention of the Judea workers, the health fund redoubled its efforts to enlist additional members. In Petach Tikva a sick room was established adjacent to the workers' living quarters and a paramedic was charged with maintenance and care of the sick until their recovery. Those in need of specialized care were sent to the Shaar Zion Hospital in Jaffa, and payment for hospitalization was covered by the health fund's yearly subscription for group services. In a similar manner, paramedics were appointed and operated other branches of the health fund in collaboration with the Eretz Israel Office. Soon after establishment of a sick room in Petach Tikva, a health fund office was also opened in Jaffa for urban laborers under the management of the worker Yaakov Aphter, a member of the Hapoel Hatzair movement's leadership. In years that followed, Aphter and Izakovich coordinated the activities of the health fund, serving as the primary address for assistance among sick Jewish laborers throughout the country.

Compared to the previous system where the sick were sent to doctors, the establishment of on-site sick rooms near the dwellings of laborers was a vast improvement. This was the first attempt to cope with the special character of disease among workers in the Jewish agricultural villages—the prevalence of malaria, typhus, and intestinal diseases that required ongoing supervision and regular adequate nutrition, two components that were generally missing from the lives of the workers. Distance and the cost of travel (by wagon) and lack of regular transportation services to the hospitals, and an almost chronic shortage of beds in the hospitals were all factors in the decision to establish on-site sick rooms.

Moreover, sick rooms lent themselves to the mode of operation that Izakovich championed, based on a belief that the health fund should bring services to the laborer, not vice versa, and that the health fund should provide health services of its own, not merely be an insuring agent. The establishment of a sick room in Petach Tikva and afterwards in other locations made it possible to provide care-hospitalization to a larger number of individuals. Moreover, this move transferred responsibility for care of the sick directly onto the shoulders of the health fund. Consequently, the health fund began to initiate establishment of sick rooms, fund their operation with the assistance of the Eretz Israel Office, and hire professional personnel (in most cases paramedics) to staff the sick rooms. This was a divergence in principles from the original idea of a health fund as first envisioned—that the fund would serve solely as an insuring body, leaving responsibility for seeking medical aid from external service-providers up to the member-insuree. The establishment of sick rooms and provision of medical service on-site became a binding precedent from this point forward.

The establishment of sick rooms for agricultural works in their place of work or residence underscores the significant difference between the health fund model that emerged in Eretz Israel, and the health funds that appeared in the world in urban proletarian centers and adjacent to hospitals, in the wake of the industrial revolution. Kupat Holim emerged in a rural setting. The village with its particular health needs continues to be the primary model for medical operations of Kupat Holim everywhere in the country, urban or rural, to this day. At the time, small clinics were established in agricultural villages and in working-class neighborhoods so that every sick person could turn to the clinic closest to his or her home, eliminating the necessity of traveling and waiting in long lines. The small neighborhood clinic network also encouraged establishment of a personal tie between patient and physician.

In August 1914, just when it appeared that the health fund had finally "taken-off," the outbreak of the First World War confronted the health funds with an existential challenge: Justifying their existence as the primary institution caring for the health of workers.

Ultimately, circumstances led to amalgamation of the various workers' health funds into a united body—the General Health Fund or Kupat Holim, a process that will be examined in upcoming chapters. At this juncture, however, it is fitting to pause to examine, in a wider perspective, the organizational and ideological pattern of the Israeli system that emerged in the formative years of Kupat Holim prior to unification of the regional workers' health funds. After all, the health fund model did not emerge in a cultural void. The second part of this chapter seeks to present the behavior of the founders against the backdrop of circumstances in both the Jewish world and the world-as-a-whole, examining the ideological currents and social patterns that were afoot, at the time the Kupat Holim concept was first taking shape.

The Health Fund: The Concept

The model of health fund for workers that crystallized among members of the Second Aliyah stood on three main ideas: a general fund as the defining principle for the organizational framework; mutual aid as the moral basis for the fund's operation; and health insurance reflecting the social ideals championed by the workers of the Second Aliyah.

What were the wellsprings for the idea of a health fund for workers? Was this a unique idea, formulated and crystallized by members of the Second Aliyah in order to alleviate the distress of their living conditions and health under arduous circumstances? Or, was the establishment of the health fund part and parcel of a worldwide phenomena—the growth of health insurance for the proletariat around the world that began in Europe toward the close of the nineteenth century?

Mutual assistance is a principle at the core of the health fund's operation throughout its history, but where did it originate? Was the wellspring the traditional Jewish values and patterns of community organization that had sustained Jewish communities throughout the world in the past? Or was it the strategic principle, "there is strength in numbers," upon which forerunners to labor unions such as guilds and other occupational brotherhoods founded "sick funds" at the close of the Middle Ages?

Health Funds in Jewish Tradition

The Hebrew term for a health fund—*kupat holim*—draws on vocabulary and traditions that are deep-seated in Jewish culture. The first mention of a "kupat" in the sense of a "kupat tzdaka"—a charity or alms box for financial assistance[37]—can be found in the Mishneh, the first part of the Talmud that contains rabbinical interpretation of the Bible: "He who has…will not take from the kupa."[38]

The word *kupa* may have been borrowed from the Latin "cupa"—or box, coffer, basket, and so forth. The medieval Jewish philosopher Maimonides also mentions the expression "kupat tzdaka" when he spoke of the vessel where the beadle in the synagogue stored money collected from the residents of the city to maintain the poor, and from which money was allocated to the indigent every Friday so they could prepare for the Sabbath.

Over the years, the term kupa became a cornerstone of social welfare in Jewish communities—a tool that was part and parcel of Jewish life. Communities managed kupot for the poor, for brides, for orphans, to support men who devoted their lives to studying the Torah in Talmudic academies (yishivot), to support the Jewish community in Eretz Israel, and to aid the sick.

Care for the sick was considered a mitzvah or a holy commandment—a pillar in *Halacha*, or Jewish Law. The obligation to visit the sick encompassed all members of the community regardless of status, and the mitzvah included care, feeding, washing and attending to the sick. To a great extent fulfillment of this religious commandment served as a kind of substitute institution to the public hospital. Major rabbinical thinkers such as Maimonides and Moshe Ben Nachman-RAMBAN viewed this mitzvah as a cardinal commandment. Bikur Holim and Linat Tzedek Societies dedicated respectively to visiting the sick and tending to the sick at night were cornerstones of Jewish community life from the Middle Ages onward. These two institutions were the primary source of medical assistance within the community for over a thousand years—up to the mid-eighteenth century.

Researcher Meir Balaban noted that the ordinances of the Krakow community in Poland in 1595 included a kupat holim or health fund. Yehoshua Lebowitz and Shmuel Kottek describe in their scholarly work similar community services for providing a physician in Jewish communities in central Europe in the seventeenth century. Philipsborn reports similar medical services in Berlin's Jewish community in 1703. A Jewish health fund on a broader scale—beyond local institutions—was inaugurated in Eastern Europe in 1912 by the AZA (an acrostic in Russian for "The Association for Preservation of the Health of the Jews"). According to the founders, since every ethnic group had its own particular health needs, and there should be a health system that attends to the health of its members. In 1922 AZA—together with TAZ, a health organization that operated primarily amongst the Jewish communities in Poland—founded a world federation to organize health services for Jews. AZA-TAZ's activity spread to cover all of Europe, and was particularly marked between the two world wars in Romania, Latvia, Poland, Germany, and France. At the time, a separate health fund run by the Bund party was also active in Russia.

At the close of the nineteenth century, following mass immigration of Jews from Eastern Europe to Western Europe and the United States, Jewish health funds sprung up in immigrant neighborhoods on a landsmanschaft basis—groups based on a common place of origin in Europe. Organization by *landsmanschafts* was common among Jewish immigrant communities, particularly for practical reasons of common language, shared cultural patterns and customs, and communal and personal bonds. At the beginning of the 1930s during the Great Depression, predominantly Jewish trade unions also founded health funds for their members. Health funds for Jewish laborers also arose in England and Holland.

CONCEPTS OF MUTUAL AID IN HEALTH SERVICES

The first accounts of mutual medical aid in Eretz Israel appeared at the time of the Second Temple among members of the Essenes sects (145 B.C.–75 A.D.) who dwelled in the area of Ein Gedi, an oasis overlooking the Dead Sea. Shmuel Kottek and Chaim Harpaz note in their works that the Essenes community as a whole was responsible for medical care for the sick. Special attention was also given to care of the elderly. Medications and physicians' fees were borne by the community as a whole:

> [I]f a person among them will become ill, he will be maintained in his illness from the wealth of the community and besides this, all will serve him with much devotion and care for his well-being.[39]

References to mutual aid among workers can also be found among guilds in the Middle Ages in Europe. The guilds took care of members struck by illness or injured in work accidents. According to their charters, apprentices received medical care at the expense of their masters. In the fourteenth century, guilds of apprentices were organized on a similar basis with assistance funds; medical aid was extended as a loan and was expected to be repaid after the apprentice returned to work. Haim Harpaz notes that from the fifteenth century on, one can find groups of young Jews who also operated on a mutual aid basis, providing medical aid and burial services for their members. Most were single, and married members were accepted only with special approval. In 1560, for instance, the Single Workers' Society in the city of Lucerne in Switzerland set forth in its charter the following stipulations:

> Any member who falls ill or is disabled will receive if he needs it, the sum of 3.5 penny per day. With his return to health and his place of work, he must return the money. Should his disability continue and should his needs grow and increase, he should be allowed to continue to borrow money against collateral. If he will die, the Society will recoup its losses from his assets.[40]

With the growth of cities during the Renaissance and the rise in the number of unemployed and paupers, laws arose to address the need for medical aid to the poor. In 1601, under the reign of Elizabeth I in England, the first Poor Laws were passed. However, eligibility was problematic because of the humiliation inherent in the law—both the language of the law that viewed the poor as backward laggards and a burden upon society, and requirements that applicants substantiate their poverty to receive an allowance. Over time, broad groups of workers organized to establish mutual aid associations designed to provide medical aid in time of need. In 1685, the Quakers' Friendly Society was formed, and other similar organizations in its wake. Due to the large number of such societies—in 1825 there were a million—the British parliament legislated a law in 1793 that dealt with mutual aid associations. Some societies provided payment for sick leave, annuities for the elderly and allotments to families who had lost their breadwinner. But many difficulties obstructed smooth operation of these operations—particularly lack of consistency in payment of membership dues, the absence of any government backing, and meager endowments, factors that limited their effectiveness on the practical level.

Renewed impetus in the concept of health insurance came with the growth of new economic thought in Europe at the advent of a new era. In 1697, Daniel Defoe claimed in his book "Essay of Projects" that all workers and craftspersons should insure themselves against illness or injury through mutual aid societies; Defoe called for the establishment of a large fund based on compulsory payments that would cover medical care and hospitalization for workers. In 1786 John Ackland suggested a program of compulsory participation of the public in mutual aid clubs. Howes raised similar ideas in 1786, as did the Swiss historian and economist S. Sismondi (1773–1842).

The industrial revolution in the eighteenth century and the process of proletarization in its wake hastened and amplified the need for insurance on the basis of mutual aid. The ascendancy of unbridled capitalism gave rise to masses of workers employed under conditions of harsh exploitation. When the first unions were formed (mostly in England) one of their first activities was to address the need for medical assistance on the basis of mutual aid. The main weakness was that the system was founded on low wages of laborers and the kind of aid that could be given to members was very limited and did not provide a real solution. The solution needed was a social institution based on compulsory dues and subsidized by the state.

HEALTH INSURANCE IN THE MODERN AGE

Compulsory health insurance for workers first appeared in Europe at the close of the nineteenth century. The idea was first raised by Bismarck, chancellor of Germany. In 1883, for political reasons—in order to weaken the Social Democrats—Bismarck inaugurated establishment of a state system of health insurance and pensions for laborers based on progressive dues. While the move was designed to sway public support among workers in favor of the German government, its roots were in a feudal outlook that the poor should put their personal safety in the hands of their masters—that is, Bismarck's autocratic government. This attitude became all the more valid following the collapse of Germany at the outset of the modern era.

The duty of nobles to care for the health of their workers and subjects existed as far back as the Roman Empire in the days of Julius Caesar. During the Middle Ages this view was further strengthened by the feudal system; although not anchored in any written or binding legislation, it was widely accepted by both masters and serfs as an unwritten law. In a number of known cases serfs demanded that their masters provide health services in keeping with this norm, and kings demanded that the nobles fulfill this duty to their subjects. A noble who did not fulfill his duties lost face and prestige in the eyes of his fellow nobles. The noble's liability for the health of his subjects continued up into the late Middle Ages, but with the rise of the cities, the power of feudal institutions waned and the duty of caring for the health of residents shifted from noblemen to the state and the community.

Justification of the states' "interference" in matters of economics and society was provided by the "father of economics"—Adam Smith (1731–1790). The Scottish economist, renowned for providing the foundations of *laissez faire* capitalism, nevertheless argued that in areas where free enterprise does not work for the social good, one should forego unfettered economics on behalf of social remediation. Thus, Smith favored government intervention in broad areas, even in opposition to a free enterprise system. While his writings deal primarily with agricultural society, his ideas caught on in urban and industrial Europe.

The spread of epidemics in European cities at the beginning of the nineteenth century due to overcrowding, poverty, and poor sanitation put pressure on authorities to intervene more in the lives of inhabitants. Such moves were founded on the concept that governments must control the economic and social system—not for the benefit of the individual as the socialists maintained, but as an imperative for ensuring the integrity of the state. Groups of laws and ordinances (Frankfort 1849; the Northern German Confederation 1866) regularized intervention of the regime in the life of the inhabitants. Enforcing sanitation extended all the way to regulation of conditions in the private domain—encompassing standards of cleanliness in households to prevent sources of contamination that could spark epidemics. Germany, the most far-reaching in terms of the scope of its public health focus, in 1876 founded the "National Office for Health" to supervise all health matters in the country. The Office publicized programs for inoculations and supervision of sanitation, and granted regional managers absolute legal authority to intervene in any activity that had a medical and health element. Similar governmental machinery operated in England, but its authority and ability to intervene in city life was limited due to differences in the nature of the regime.

According to Shryok in his study, *The Development of Modern Medicine*,[41] the willingness of the average German citizen to acquiesce to government interference in one's private life and follow ordinances and laws set by the government, as well as the structure of the Bismarck state which granted the chancellor broad powers, all played a part in the process that led to passage of the Health Insurance Law in Germany under Bismarck. It is important to stress that it was not the health of the individual that concerned the legislators who passed this landmark legislation, but rather that a political philosophy of the role of the government in matters of economics and society provided the legitimacy for such a step and paved the way for passage of such a comprehensive law.

Bismarck's initiative in legislating a health insurance law was a natural procession in the concept of the intervention of the state in the lives of its citizens, as put forth by Adam Smith, and the legal steps to fight sanitation hazards and prevent epidemics taken by the Germany city-states at the beginning of the century. A law regulating provision of health services to indigent workers was an economic-social tool in the war against poverty and maintenance of the health and well being of the state.

Bismarck passed laws that provided health insurance, the right to pensions, and compulsory insurance against work accidents. The laws were spurred by a belief in the right of the nation to intervene in social and economic matters, together with more immediate and partisan exigencies—winning the election by undermining the appeal of the Social-Democrats, who supported social legislation on behalf of the working public from the standpoint of human rights and entitlements, not as a governance tool for the benefit of the state. Bismarck killed two birds with one stone: he gained the admiration of the working public and he won the election. Legislation ensured the smooth flow of funding from workers and employers to underwrite health services through health funds, in distinction to past patterns of insuring agencies and private doctors or charitable organizations. Receipt of health services became an entitlement under law, thus workers were no longer dependent on charitable institutions, while the health status of laborers also greatly improved as a result of the law.

At the outset Bismarck's health plan encompassed only one "minority" group—laborers. Only in years to come was health insurance broadened to include other classes in society, and the center shifted from ensuring funding for health services for laborers to ensuring health services on an equalitarian basis to all citizens. In 1885 there were four million members (laborers) within the German health- insurance system whose monthly dues were deducted from their salaries at the source—entitling the worker to health services, pension and workers' compensation in case of accidents

Following Germany, similar legislation was passed in Austria (1888) and Sweden (1891), and by 1912 such laws had been enacted throughout Europe, with service provision based for the most part on voluntary mutual aid organizations that had operated prior to passage of the laws. According to the findings of Harpaz,[42] these bodies reorganized in stable frameworks that received official recognition, and the state supervised and granted subsidies and a host of dispensations in order to reinforce and broaden their activity. Most of the health funds functioned as insurance companies and did not provide medical aid of their own. They were tied to doctors who worked for them as independent agents (not salaried personnel), receiving remuneration by the number of patients they received, while insurees were free to choose their own physician.

It should be noted that the first health fund to organize under Bismarck's law was met with opposition among laborers on political grounds. The workers viewed his social legislation as solely a vehicle for gaining their support for Bismark's policies, which indeed was its purpose. Bismarck planned to use the law as a weapon against the socialists, but initially the workers' movement did not foresee the advantages that compulsory insurance carried.[43]

THE SECOND ALIYAH AND THE IDEA OF KUPAT HOLIM

Laborers from the Second Aliyah faced two main approaches toward the organization of medical services when they began establishing health funds for workers in Eretz Israel at the outset of the twentieth century. In the first (reflecting the traditional Jewish attitude they were familiar with from the Jewish shtetl or township in Eastern Europe where most of the Zionist pioneers had grown up) the community as a whole took responsibility for its sick and provided care through institutions such as "linat tzedek" and "bikur holim." In the second (modeled on the health funds that operated under Bismarck, and then spread to the rest of Europe) the government provided compulsory health insurance on a class basis (labor-socialist). .

The Second Aliyah workers, proponents of European socialism, were familiar with health organizations for workers in Europe and viewed them as a worthy model. The workers' press in Eretz Israel regularly carried in-depth reports about goings-on in labor movements around the world, including their health organizations. The newspaper *He'achdut*, for instance, reported in detail about the health fund established by the non-Zionist Jewish Bund party in Russia,[44] while *Hapoel Hatzair* told of the "Hebrew workers' health funds" in America and England, stressing that "the funds do not receive assistance from the government, and no one has the authority to intervene in their business."[45]

Despite their familiarity with health insurance in Europe, the first institution that members of the Second Aliyah established in Eretz Israel was a "linat tzedek" format—a solution that sprang from the traditional Jewish way of caring for the sick and the needy in the community, a solution that was well suited to the small-group situation in which the laborers lived. Only afterwards, when they came to the conclusion that this was not enough, did the founders seek other ways and new ideas for solving their distress in health matters. At this point, the members of the Second Aliyah turned to the idea of health funds as they had crystallized at the close of the nineteenth century in Europe, but they still did not abandon the institution of "linat zedek" that was a core element and not merely an appendage to the charters of the health funds for laborers that they had established.

Even if the European method manifested itself in the principles behind the health fund in Eretz Israel, from an *organizational* standpoint they were very different. The initiative for organization in Europe was based either on political considerations or affiliation, or a common occupation. The funds were large-scope urban frameworks with thousands of members. In many cases the organization enjoyed government support and was accompanied by legislation, following the growth of an urban proletariat of factory workers. In Eretz Israel, the initiative sprang forth from among agricultural workers who operated in small groups in a rural setting. Organization took place against the backdrop of the growth of the New Yishuv, without any governmental intervention by Ottoman authorities. The organization of the health fund among agricultural workers was, in its essence, an exception for its times compared to patterns of development of health insurance as they took shape in Europe.

A similar attempt was made at the end of the 1930s in the United States as part of Roosevelt's New Deal during the Great Depression. The federal government formulated a health insurance plan for rural populations whose economic straits made it impossible for farm families to pay for medical aid on a regular basis. The Farm Security Administration was a form of voluntary cooperative health insurance for rural regions: A member was required to pay monthly dues in order to obtain medical assistance, and contracts were signed with groups of local doctors who committed themselves to provide medical services for a reduced fee. The plan was based on the economic principle that a communal fund with many members paying regular dues would bring about a significant reduction in the cost of health services to its members, ultimately providing access to medical aid even for those of limited means. The architects of the FSA hoped that the plan would improve both the quality of living and the economic circumstances of farmers who joined the plan. Monthly payments to the physicians for services rendered were based on the number of members who had availed themselves of the doctors' services. Members who had difficulty keeping up monthly payments received free treatment at the expense of the fund. The plan also incorporated a team of ambulatory public health nurses who administered inoculations and educated patients in good hygiene and nutrition. At its height, the FSA incorporated some 600,000 members and operated in a third of the rural counties in the U.S. The program operated up until 1941 when the United States entered the Second World War, and was cancelled following improvements in the U.S. economy and the mobilization of many doctors into the military.

There were two major differences between the health fund in Eretz Israel and that of the FSA. First, the U.S. Government played a core role in organization of the plan, while in Eretz Israel the health funds were the fruit of independent enterprise. Second, the American plan invested much energy in preventive medicine, while the health fund in Eretz Israel in its beginnings dealt solely with curative medicine and care for members in cases of illness. Elements of preventive medicine such as education and inoculation became a part of the health fund's agenda only after the establishment of the state of Israel.

3

The Workers' Health Fund in the First World War

The Yishuv on the Eve of the First World War

At the beginning of August 1914, Germany declared war on Russia and the First World War broke out. Although Turkey had not yet entered the war, the impact was immediately felt in the Yishuv, at the time a community of some 85,000 Jews. The Yishuv was cut off from its principle wellsprings of financial support in Jewish communities in Europe, first and foremost in Russia, creating immediate economic pressure that was a source of growing concern. With a freeze on financial activity declared by the Turkish government, the situation further deteriorated, thrusting the New Yishuv in the cities and Jewish agricultural villages into serious economic crisis.

During the first two weeks of August 1914, Jews who were Ottoman subjects were required to pay an indemnity to receive exemptions from military service; the authorities requisitioned war materials such as vehicles and work animals, disrupting agricultural work. Jewish settlements were isolated from markets in Europe, bringing a halt to exports, for the most part, oranges and wine from the Jewish agricultural settlements. Not only were farmers severely hit but, as a consequence, countless Jewish laborers were also laid off and left without a source of livelihood. Reductions in agricultural activity left hundreds unemployed and thousands sought the assistance of charitable organizations which themselves were forced to close due to disruption of funding.

A week after the outbreak of the war, the mayor of Tel Aviv, Meir Dizengoff, convened a meeting to address how to cope with the growing crisis. The gathering moved to establish what was labeled a "Committee to Ease the Crisis" comprised of delegates from all strata in society. The Committee resolved to take all steps necessary to ease the straits of the settlers during the crisis, to seek solutions to daily hardships, and most important, to mobilize financial means.

Three months later on October 30, Turkey joined the war alongside Germany and Austria. With the declaration of war, the Ottoman regime abolished the capitulations—special status and privileges granted citizens of European nations and the United States by the Turks—that had served as an important component in the legal status of the Jewish community in the Eretz Israel. Members of the Jewish community were forced to choose between being deported as foreign nationals or accepting Ottoman citizenship, including the duty of military service in the Turkish army. Issues of basic essentials and mere physical survival became the central concern, due to deterioration of the economy.

Services providing medical aid to the Yishuv were badly hit from the outset of the crisis. The rupture of mail services and transfer of funding from abroad led to the closure of hospitals throughout the country. Most physicians were drafted into the army and sent to serve in the hospital in Gaza, leaving the burden of medical care for the new Yishuv on the shoulders of a handful of women doctors and female nurses who were not drafted due to their gender. The author and worker Moshe Smilansky recalls in his memoirs:

> From the outset of mobilization, almost all the Jewish doctors in Eretz Israel were taken into the army and in the first days male and female nurses volunteered for the army. Most of the mobilized physicians were Jews . . . .[1]

When Turkey entered the war, medications and medical equipment was confiscated, and all institutions and buildings previously enjoying privileged status under the auspices of foreign consulates that were now enemy nations (France, England and Russia) were commandeered for the Turkish war effort. This included many hospitals.

Dr. Moshe Sherman testified that in the summer of 1914, prior to Turkey's entrance into the war, German officers came to the country headed by General Von Kersenstein, in order to assist the Turks in their war with the British in Egypt.[2] The heads of the German army's medical corps sent to Eretz Israel were named Yunglas and Hoffman, the latter a German, born in Jerusalem. The pair planned to divide military hospitals on the front into three categories based on the religious affiliation of the casualities: Christian, Muslim, and Jewish soldiers. The Jewish soldiers were allocated the British mission hospital in Gaza that had been abandoned at the outset of the war. Thus, most of the Jewish doctors were drafted, —including Dr. Pochovsky, head of the Hebrew Medical Federation. In the course of the war, the special status of the Gaza hospital as one designated for Jewish soldiers was ultimately abolished, and the Jewish staff dispersed among various Turkish army units.

The female physicians left to care for the civilian population were Alexandra Belkind, Bat-sheva Yunis Gutmann, Tzila Berginsky and Chana Birchiyahu. Birchiyahu took over the position of her husband, Dr. Mordechi Birchiyahu (who had volunteered for service as a physician in the Turkish army) as physician to the Herzliya Gymnasium. In Jerusalem there were two additional female doctors—Helena Kegan and Miriam Nofach.

Organization of Kupat Holim at the Outset of the War

Already from the start, the crisis had an adverse effect on the health fund of the Judea workers, which was the only health fund operating in Eretz Israel at the time. Income from dues diminished, and there were physicians who declined to see sick members of the fund due to fear that they would not receive payment. Branch committees of the health fund—and primarily Yitzhak Izakovich and Yaakov Aphter, the fund's two secretaries—held that during the war and due to the sharp rise in disease in the country, the Judea Workers' Health Fund should be responsible for the entire Jewish working public, including those who were not members and had not been participating dues-paying members prior to the outbreak of the war. This decision was viewed as paramount—a watershed decision even at the time, not only in retrospect.

In the days preceding the war, Izakovich and Aphter strove to establish the fund on a membership of dues-paying workers and opposed the widespread attitude within the organization that the health fund should provide services to "those who pay and those who don't pay" as was common in the early days. Registration and dues payment as a matter of principle was one of the reasons the membership had not grown in the Fund's first year of operation. Yet, at this juncture, in light of the war situation, the fund opted to abolish all limitations on acceptance of new members and took upon itself responsibility for *all* the working public. Thus its status underwent a fundamental transformation—from a tiny local organization serving a small membership only, to a broad-based public institution that cared for the working public-at-large, whose public duties preceded its own narrower interests as an organization (operational arraignments, economic feasibility and its own founding ordinances, which limited eligibility for services to registered paying members). It seems that this decision was a tremendous booster in improving the image of the fund in the eyes of the workers and the public-at-large. At the same time, the decision was a source of economic hardship that was destined to follow Kupat Holim, and the Israeli health system as a whole, to this day.

The Committee to Ease the Crisis, and Medical Assistance

In order to implement this goal, the Judea Workers' Health Fund needed financial resources it could not sustain in its present form. On August 22, two weeks after the establishment of the Committee to Ease the Crisis, the Fund convened a special council comprised of delegates from the its branches (Jaffa, Petach Tikva, Nes Ziona, Ben-Shemen, and Hadera) and representatives of the Eretz Israel Office, the labor parties, the physicians, and the Shaar Zion Hospital in Jaffa. The council approved a decision that extended medical aid to the working public as a whole, including laborers who were not members of the fund. To do so, it was resolved that workers' settlements, communes, and workers' communal kitchens should set aside a percentage of their income—with the consent of the workers' committees—to fund the operation. The council approached all the labor organizations and requested that they extend credit to the fund "until the crisis would pass" in order to allow it to continue operation. In return the Judea Worker's Federation promised that:

> The fund takes upon itself to pay its debts immediately after the grave situation will pass. The Judea Workers' Federation will serve as a guarantor for the fund on behalf of the workers' committees.[3]

At the same time, the council turned to the medical community and requested that they extend medical aid to sick workers, care for them without demanding immediate payment, and lower their fees. In return, the health fund obligated itself to "keep an account and refund their wages when the crisis had passed." The Medical Federation (whose official title was "The Hebrew Medical Society in Eretz Israel") consented to the Judea Workers' Health Fund's appeal and convened a general meeting two days later on August 24 at which the professional organization of physicians resolved that:

> [The Hebrew Medical Federation] finds it fitting that doctors will aid the workers during present grave times and will extend medical aid to workers who turn to them under the auspices of the health fund, with billing delayed until the crisis will past and will be reimbursed for visits at a rate of only half the conventional fee.[4]

All this was contingent on the sick person's bringing with him a written referral note from the health fund. Similar arrangements were made with pharmacists and with the privately-run kitchens catering to workers. The representative of the Eretz Israel Office (the agronomist Akiva Ettinger) also responded favorably to the Judea Workers' Health Fund's request to extend credit to the sum of nine-hundred francs. When the monies were exhausted, the health fund received additional funding from American aid that began to arrive in the country with the entrance of Turkey into the war— an arrangement mediated by Henry Morgenthau, the American ambassador in Kushta (Constantinople). These were the first steps towards assuring medical assistance to the working public during the war.

Probably the willingness of doctors and pharmacists to respond favorably to the Judea Workers' Health Fund's request was taken on the assumption that the war would be short-lived. No one expected it would last four years. Nevertheless, the arrangement was honored throughout the war, allowing the fund to survive and continue its operations. In retrospect, it is evident that these decisions were a decisive factor in the development of the Judea Workers' Health Fund. The "national" scope of responsibility—as a public institution that took upon itself to address the health needs not only of workers, but also of other groups (craftspersons, government employees, and others) in time of crisis—was what brought about the rapid, broad-based growth of the organization. The health fund that entered the war as a small, weak local organization fighting for its life was transformed into a core institution of the Yishuv by the end of the war.

In the first year of the war (1915), seven hundred individuals sought the assistance of the Judea Workers' Health Fund—an average of sixty a month. Shaar Zion Hospital reported one thousand hospitalization days of workers in the first four months of the war.[5] Unemployment, poor nutrition, and substandard living conditions all aggravated the prevalence of illness among the working public. Most of the sick suffered from malaria, dysentery, and typhus. In the second year of the war (1916), the number of patients seeking medical assistance through the fund's auspices almost doubled, reaching 120 persons per month. In Tel Aviv, the number of inhabitants in need of a doctor tripled compared to the previous year.[6] In the fledgling independent communal settlements (kvutzot, kibutzim) and the national farms where there was work and nutrition was better (particularly in the Galilee, where the Galilee Workers' Health Fund had begun to operate), the number of sick was significantly lower.

Yaakov Aphter, secretary of the Judea Workers' Health Fund in Jaffa, noted in his reports that the workers appreciated the work of the fund, and this was reflected in their willing payment of dues.[7] Within the framework of American aid to the Yishuv in Eretz Israel during the first years of the war, a percentage of the aid was channeled towards creating jobs for workers and orderly payment of their salaries so they could survive. A regular source of income also allowed the workers to pay dues to the health fund. The broad-based responsibility that the Fund took upon itself was also reflected in other areas during the war years. Sick workers, primarily those just released from the hospital, were entitled to a period of convalescence, receiving a loan to cover the recuperation period "in order to allow the sick to get well and begin to return to work." When it became difficult to find people to fill the duty of staying with the sick at night, the Fund paid from its own resources for "lodging and supervision" in hotels for unattached sick workers for whom no room was available at the hospital but who needed to be taken care of at night. In the face of widespread distress, the prior arrangement with the hospitals—reserving a certain number of beds for sick workers—was suspended, and the sick were hospitalized on a "first come, first served" basis. In most of the Jewish agricultural villages, sick rooms were established where paramedics and nurses tended to the sick. Medications were purchased through the auspices of Dr. Arthur Rupin, head of the Eretz Israel Office, who had been deported due to his Zionist ectivity, and resided in Kushta. Bandaging, sheets, towels, and so forth were collected from among the workers.

Those laborers mobilized for government work far from their places of residence had special needs that the Fund sought to meet. For instance, it organized sick rooms as well as shower and laundry rooms for groups of laborers from Samaria who were sent to Beersheva in order to maintain decent hygiene and prevent the outbreak of disease. The Health Fund sent doctors to conduct visits in such work camps and evacuated seriously ill to sick rooms in nearby Jewish agricultural villages or to the hospital in Jaffa. The workers Yaakov Aphter and Avraham Hartzfeld conducted regular periodic tours among concentrations of laborers to monitor conditions and organize medical assistance. Yaakov Aphter even went on foot from Jaffa to Petach Tikva, visiting concentrations of laborers along the way, assessing their health status, and distributing quinine to stave off malaria. Hartzfeld went as far afield as Beer-sheva in order to assess the scope of typhus among the laborers and take appropriate steps to provide them with medical services, even arranging for receipt of medical assistance from the doctor of a German unit posted between Gaza and Beer-sheva.

Financial Hardships

The primary problem facing the Judea Workers' Health Fund during the war years was lack of funding. The fiscal straits forced the Fund to take a decision that went against their principles regarding receipt of financial assistance—a move tantamount to charity, a form of assistance the workers had refused to accept prior to the war. The decision fell immediately following the outbreak of the war in a special meeting of the council convene by the Judea Workers' Health Fund office on August 22, 1914, which resolved "to approach all the relevant institutions to 'cover' the health fund until the war will pass."

Thus, collaboration with the Eretz Israel Office was inaugurated. Dr. Tahon, a representative of the office, reported regularly to Yaakov Aphter concerning the health situation in various localities and provided allocation of funding to cover the operation of the health fund from American aid. Intermediate financing was procured through a "loan from the Benevolent Fund" obtained from the Rishon le Zion (governing) committee.

An ongoing struggle to obtain funding led to clashes and pressure on the working public. Yitzhak Izakovich turned to the branch committees of the health fund, demanding that chits for referrals to the Jaffa hospital be withheld from those who did not settle their dues-paying in an acceptable fashion, and warning that a sick person who lacked a referral note would be turned away. Izakovich demanded regular reports on the status of dues collection, registration of members, and outlays at the branch level in order to monitor the general financial state of the health fund, tighten the ties with branch offices, and "rescind the rights of those workers who intentionally dodge fulfilling their duties to the Fund."[8] In a letter to laborers in Hulda, Yaakov Aphter wrote:

> We address you now with a request to first of all bring in all the sums accounting from the "Work Day" decided upon of late and also regular payment of the monthly dues—a bishlik—to the Health Fund. If you are unable to bring in all the sum in cash (not in paper) pay half in money and half in script, and the main thing is to fulfill immediately our request, because [our] distress is very great.[9]

Similar letters were frequently sent to local committees of the health fund throughout the war.

Two issues were raised time and again in Judea Workers' Health Fund correspondence during the war years: Stricter maintenance of procedures in granting referral notes for medical care, and the direct tie between the member and his branch. Insistence on the former was motivated primarily by financial considerations, for the chits served as the basis upon which service providers were paid by the fund. However, there was a broader significance: The chit was given only to those registered as members of the Judea Workers' Health Fund. Many asked to enroll, including individuals who were not laborers. Consequently, referral notes were the catalyst for the marked growth in the scope of the health fund's membership. This fact became an important factor at the close of the war: The demand that all services and referrals be issued to a member solely via his or her local branch was an organizational tool. The constant movement of workers from place to place during the war made it hard to administer recording referrals and doctors visits in the health fund office, and therefore workers were required to receive services solely through the branches where they were registered, or according to instructions of the branch at their places of work. The success of this method led to its adoption as a standard procedure even after the close of the war.

But despite the demand to maintain some semblance of order and organization in the workings of the health fund, the personal tie with the membership was maintained. This is reflected in countless letters written by laborers to Yaakov Aphter requesting his assistance in easing their distress. Thus Chiyuta Bussel from Petach Tikva wrote:

> Shalom Aphter!
> I am writing to you by moonlight and the lines jump in front of me, it is hard to describe the current situation among us. All of us are half-sick….You must expedite whoever needs to arrange things because if things continue this way for some period of time—we'll all go crazy….We are sending a young woman to Jaffa—Miriam Greenblatt. If you can admit her to the hospital—great, if not—she must be given the necessary means until she can [re-]gain her strength. You should know that she is young and refuse to receive assistance and we talked to her heart-to-heart…."[10]

Nachum Sneh from among the Samarian workers wrote:

> Advise us how we can ensure quinine in foreseeable time for the Samarian workers. [Is it] feasible to obtain some sort of loan for this purpose? Can you help us in some way on this matter?[11]

Many laborers turned to Aphter to request that he help them with their financial matters, arrange loans for them, order special medications for them, help their friends in times of crisis, or assist them in paying for the burial of their comrades—committing themselves to fulfill their duties to the health fund and pay their debts when their circumstance would improve. Thus, in essence, the Judea Workers' Health Fund served as an address for the distress of workers in general, and not only in health matters. From Yaakov Aphter's correspondence from that period, it becomes evident that members of the Judea Workers' Health Fund office staff read every letter and strove to assist as much as possible. The image of the Health Fund, as reflected in the letters of laborers, is of an organization one could depend upon for assistance at every turn.

The struggle between the need to organize the work of the fund and collect dues, and the need to provide medical assistance to all was central to the character of the Judea Workers' Health Fund throughout this very trying period. The struggles and tensions that were part and parcel of the war years also affected relationships between Izakovich and Aphter. Harsh exchanges of correspondence concerning overstepping of authority (from Izakovich to Aphter), threats to resign (by Izakovich), publicity in the press (by Aphter) and accusation of organizational mismanagement (Izakovich against Aphter) were raised more than once in correspondence from the period. Personality conflicts between the moderate and cautious Izakovich anxious to maintain order and organization, and the forceful Aphter who was in the habit of putting actions before decision-making, working more on instinct than careful calculation, only further aggravated the clash between the two men. After the war, Izakovich left his post as the secretary of the Judea Workers' Health Fund and administration of the fund remained solely in the hands of Aphter and Hartzfeld.

Workers' Health Funds in the Galilee and Samaria

The operation and organization of the Judea Workers' Health Fund at the outset of the First World War acted as a catalyst for the establishment of a similar framework under the auspices of the fledgling federation of laborers in the Galilee—at the time an organization encompassing some 350–400 members.[12] In general, the laborers in the Galilee were better off at the outbreak of the war than their comrades in Judea; the former had regular jobs and the farms, primarily family-owned, produced products for the local market and were thus not dependent on European markets made inaccessible by the war.

The decision to establish a health fund for Jewish laborers in the Galilee had been taken early in 1912, but for a host of reasons actualization of the resolution had been delayed. At the Fifth Convention of the Galilee Workers' Federation at Kinneret farm in the fall of 1915, Eliezer Yafe, the secretary of the organization, detailed the chronic difficulties he had encountered in operating a health fund in the Galilee:

> To organize a health fund in the Galilee has been attempted many times without success. Approximately two years ago, a small amount was collected for this purpose but more was laid-out than was collected and the business came to a halt. Up until the past year, a need for a health fund was not particularly felt, because most of the workers were regular employees on the farms, however in the [past] year the number of workers without work and a regular place have increased, and when one of them is sick, there is no one to care for him except himself. Of late a lot of workers from Judea have come to convalesce at the Tiberas hot springs or have simply arrived and gotten sick before they have had a chance to get organized. We must help these ones, for who [can] if not us?...Besides a central health fund in the Galilee, the need to arrange a health fund in each and every place is greatly felt. There are laborers who are sick for not short periods. They can't work, their expenses are great and thus they sink into burdensome deficits without any ability to get out of them.[13]

Yafe called for a collective of workers to raise the sums that the workers were paying to the communal kitchen, and to allocate monies for operating a health fund from the general account in order to appoint a person responsible for caring for the sick.

The core figure in renewal of the Galilee Workers' Health Fund's operation was Berl Katznelson, who went up to the Galilee at the outset of 1915. Berl Katznelson had been an instrumental figure in the decision to establish the Judea Workers' Health Fund, and upon arriving in the Galilee learned of the gap in health services between communities of workers in the Galilee and in Judea. Soon afterwards, he girded himself to work towards establishment of a health fund for workers in the Galilee. In a letter to Yaakov Aphter, on the eve of the convention of Galilee workers during Sukkot 1915, he wrote:

> In the Galilee they are about to found a health fund. It would be most desirable to send with someone a few copies of the ordinances folder if they still exist, and if not—a few copies of "Hapoel Hatzair" [the newspaper] in which the ordinances [S.S. the charter] were published. There is hope that if the matter will be started here (S.S. at the convention)—the matter will grow and come alive.[14]

At the close of 1915 as the crisis worsened due to the war, the Galilee Workers' Health Fund began to take shape and commenced operations. Berl Katznelson, however, was not satisfied with this feat and called for amalgamation of the health funds—a move that was delayed only due to the war, and only raised again when hostilities were drawing to a close.

A short time after the Galilee Workers' Health Fund began to operate, the Samaria Workers' Federation began to reorganize under the leadership of three workers: Shmuel Yavnieli, David Remez, and Nachum Sneh. The Samarian workers had already resolved to found a regional health fund of their own in 1912, but up until 1916 had received medical services from the Judea Workers' Health Fund. Due to the war, economic distress, and transportation problems, the Samarian workers—some two hundred in all—decided in 1916 to organize on a separate footing and realize the four-year old decision to establish their own health fund. Nachum Sneh was assisted in this endeavor by Yaakov Aphter from the office of the Judean Workers' Health Fund in Jaffa and Dr. Hillel Yafe, director of the hospital in

Zichron Yaakov who had in the past had played a positive role in advancing health matters among Samarian workers. With their assistance, Nachum Sneh organized the work of the Samaria Workers' Health Fund, together with the Zichron Yaakov Hospital.

Collaboration among the Workers' Health Funds

With the establishment of regional health funds in the Galilee and Samaria as well, a country-wide constellation of health services for workers was formed under the auspices of their respective agricultural workers' federations. The three health funds operated in a fully collaborative fashion, free of competition, providing good services for sick workers and making the health of the membership their top priority. The close cooperation diminished the relative importance of the branches, and sick workers received care at the closest location, wherever they happened to be at that time, regardless of which fund the individual was enrolled in. While there is no detailed documentation of how this reciprocal relationship was administered, the correspondence of branch secretaries indicates that a system existed for "balancing out" debits for services rendered among the three health funds.

Cooperation, balancing of accounts, and mutual assistance were underlying principles in the organization of *Hamashbir*, an institution established by the Galilee workers in 1916 that within a short time became responsible for supply of foodstuffs at reasonable prices to the entire working public in the country. Similar to the health funds, Hamashbir served the public-at-large during the war years—teachers, clerks, and craftspeople, not only laborers alone. Due to expansion of the scope of their operations, the two organizations—Hamashbir and the health funds—commanded an important economic position in the Yishuv at the end of the war.

On 28 March 1917, Turkish authorities deported the entire Jewish population of Tel Aviv and Jaffa to the interior of the country in anticipation of a British offensive. Most went to the Lower Galilee and some to the villages of Kfar Saba and Zichron Yaakov, where they received care and lodging thanks to the work of Dr. Hillel Yafe. Attempts were made to find funding to feed thousands of deportees who had been left homeless and bereft of any means of supporting themselves. Yafe wrote a report on the health situation among concentrations of deportees in Kfar Saba and Zichron Yaakov—telling of a 20% increase in the mortality rate, a drop in the birth rate, and the spread of typhus epidemics. Within weeks, three hundred died from the epidemic among the deportees in Kfar Saba. Yafe described the intensive work of the "Assistance Committee" and the health funds in preventing the spread of the epidemic "while Arab hamlets in our vicinity were obliterated in this epidemic." Yafe called the year 1917 "a bad nightmare in the eyes of its immigrants and diseases."

The close cooperation among labor organizations (political parties, Hamashbir, and the health funds) is even more marked against the backdrop of the crisis sparked by deportation. The leadership role of worker organizations in alleviating the distress of the Jewish civilian population during the war years stands in stark contrast with the performance of other sectors in society. Members of the Old Yishuv and the First Aliyah conspicuously failed to address hardships generated by the war. Historian Zeev Tzachor believes that the cooperation exhibited among worker-affiliated bodies during the crisis years was what generated recognition of the need for a unified presence founded on amassing road-based support—a "general federation of labor."[15]

In the spring of 1917, a short time after the deportation, representatives of the labor federations met at Kinneret in order to prepare a convention that would culminate in amalgamation of the three labor federations into one body. Due to controversies among the workers' parties, the convention was convened only a year later. The agenda of "the preparatory committee of workers in Eretz Israel" was to discuss amalgamation of the regional health funds into one united body.

The idea of merging the health funds was not new or out of the ordinary. It was an integral part of the general idea of amalgamating the workers' federations—an objective that Berl Katznelson had championed since 1914. Four years earlier, when Katznelson penned the ordinances of the Judea Workers' Health Fund charter, he wrote that "efforts should be taken to unite all the existing private health funds among the workers for cooperative operation."[16]

In order to carry out the unification of the health funds, the preparatory convention elected a four-person "collective general health fund committee"—Eliezer Yafe, Shmuel Yavnieli, Elimeleh Levin, and Yitzhak Yardena'i. Already in the first deliberations on the form the new organization should take, members of the committee addressed questions that were destined to occupy the heads of Kupat Holim for years to come: What would be the economic base of the united health fund in light of the fiscal problems encountered to date, and could the working public carry the organization on its own shoulders alone? While it was clear that there was a need for a health fund, the question remained—whether it was feasible and sustainable? No clear-cut answer was forthcoming. In closing the deliberations Eliezer Yafe concluded:

> One moment of sorrow, when a person sees himself as lost, is weighted against a deficit of thousands of francs. The reason for the deficit—lack of management. Not that there is no need for institutions, but we must come to a verdict—how to arrange them. Our "echo" must be—to base our institutions in such a way that sick workers will not be left abandoned, that they will obtain within our institutions the assistance they need. We must be accompanied by the recognition that we must take care of our sick comrades: Those that do not have friends...should find us to be their friend, their helpmate.[17]

Despite the need, the planned incorporation of the labor federations did not materialize, and the issue of a united health fund was postponed to a later date.

In November 1917, Great Britain published the Balfour Declaration.[18] In December the British army liberated Jerusalem and in the summer of 1918 concluded the occupation of all of Eretz Israel—bringing an end to hundreds of years of Turkish rule. The Jewish community of Eretz Israel received the British with joy and viewed them as genuine saviors. The war years had left a denuded population: Out of 85,000 Jews prior to the war, 57,000 were left—for the most part hungry and destitute, some homeless. While anxious about the future, the community also harbored hopes for a better life. Thus, the period of British control of Eretz Israel was ushered in under expectations of a genuine turn for the better.

4

Health Services in Eretz Israel in the Nineteenth Century

The Health System in Eretz Israel Under British Military Government

In late 1917, after issuance of the Balfour Declaration and following the conquest of the southern part of Eretz Israel by the British army, the political and economic situation of the Yishuv as a whole took a turn for the better. New ideas and agents of change swept the country with new outlooks and initiatives that had a great impact on the Jewish Yishuv. The workers' health funds were also influenced by these changes. Hadassah (The American Zionist Women Organization) came to the aid of the Yishuv, and from this point forth, left its stamp on the development of health services in Eretz Israel.

Hadassah Medical Federation

The state of the Yishuv at the close of the First World War was extremely bad. Out of 85,000 Jews at the outbreak of the war, only about 57,000 remained—the others having fallen victim to deportations, disease, and hunger. The survivors suffered from frail health, physically and psychologically. The Committee of Delegates of the World Zionist Federation headed by Chaim Weizmann, visiting Eretz Israel in 1918 with British approval and encouragement, surveyed the poor health status of the Jewish community and took steps to extend medical aid to rehabilitate the existing Yishuv and reorganize its health institutions. The task was placed in the hands of the American Zionist Federation, which in turn gave responsibility to the Zionist Women's Organization, "Hadassah."

There were several reasons why American Zionists came to the rescue of the Yishuv. First, the Committee of Delegates was perturbed by the plans of the International Red Cross to initiate broad-based work in Eretz Israel under the auspices of the British Foreign Office. They feared that under the guise of humanitarian work, bodies with interests and agendas beyond medicine would penetrate the country. This fear was based on experience in the past, and there had already been cases of Christian missionary bodies that had taken advantage of the need for medical assistance to proselytize among members of the Yishuv. Second, at this time Judge Louis Brandeis, leader of American Zionism, was actively seeking to unseat and replace Chaim Weizmann as head of the World Zionist Movement. Thus, Brandeis urged American Zionists to mount a political offensive to establish the hegemony of American Zionism by demanding an active role in matters in Eretz Israel. Brandeis even visited the country himself. Stirred by the harsh circumstances of the Jewish community, Brandeis upon his return worked to mobilize funding to obtain the medical aid needed by the Yishuv. Third, from a practical standpoint, only the Jewish community in America had the means to fund medical assistance to the Yishuv, for it was this Jewish community alone that had not been indirectly hurt by the war and whose economic state after the war was strong. There was no real option other than to place the mission of providing medical aid in the hands of Hadassah.

Hadassah in Eretz Israel and Its Attitude Toward the Yishuv's Medical Institutions

The beginnings of Hadassah were in the Daughters of Zion Society, a society of Jewish Zionist women founded in New York in the year 1912 by fifteen women headed by Henrietta Szold. The society saw its mission as "encouraging Jewish institutions and projects in Eretz Israel and strengthening Jewish ideals." Already in 1913, two nurses were sent to Eretz Israel under the auspices of the Daughters of Zion, funded by the Strauss family, in order to establish a center for providing medical care and guidance to Jewish mothers in Jerusalem. The pair remained in Jerusalem until the outbreak of the First World War, when they were forced to return to the United States.

When the Daughters of Zion Society joined the American Zionist Federation, it changed its name to "Hadassah—The Women's Zionist Organization of America." Henrietta Szold stressed that the organization did not intend to engage in charity work in Eretz Israel:

> No charity! We are going to Eretz Israel equipped with experience in philanthropic-social work of American Jewish women; our intention is to bring to Eretz Israel the achievements of American medicine....If we can bring order to this country of chaos, no one can accuse us of being a charity organization.[1]

Carol Kutcher in her work on the formative years of Hadassah[2] claims that more than philanthropy stood behind Hadassah's willingness to provide medical assistance to the Yishuv. Kutcher holds that Zionist women, like their compatriots in church groups, the Salvation Army, and organizations of American Christian women, sought a platform for broad-based public activity by women. In the first year of the Society, prior to the First World War, the American Zionist Federation had declined to grant them membership because they were women. But, with the development of the women's rights movement in America and the growth of women's organizations during the First World War, attitudes changed and the Daughters of Zion became part of the American Zionist Federation. However, even after they were accepted as a member organization, Hadassah women had been unable to engage in the kind of activity they sought. The political frameworks of the American Zionist Federation remained closed to them as women, and their status lacked any real power. Thus, philanthropic-social activity in Eretz Israel was a lifesaver for the organization in terms of a raison d'être and a domain for building a base of influence, while at the same time offering a acceptable way for the American Zionist Federation to keep Hadassah women far removed from the organization's power centers. The health arena in Eretz Israel was what finally provided Hadassah women with a Zionist international mission that carried public prestige and political clout.

Donald Miller has also examined Hadassah's formative years[3] He views the organization of Zionist women as part of a broader social movement that gave birth to a host of women's organizations in the United States at the close of the nineteenth century (for instance, the Suffragettes) and that reached its zenith during the First World War. The Jewish activists, like their Christian women colleagues, were for the most part members of the middle class and college graduates. Since Jewish women were not welcome in Christian women's organizations, they were forced to establish their own parallel organizational frameworks along the lines of the Christian organizations. The activity of Jewish women's organizations was part and parcel of the process of their integration into American society as a whole.

At the end of the First World War, when the state of health of the Jewish community in Eretz Israel became known, Hadassah women mobilized to address the need with medical assistance.

On the 11 June 1918, the American Zionist Medical Aid Unit set forth for Eretz Israel with a compliment of forty-four doctors, dentists, pharmacists, paramedics, and nurses, plus a sanitation engineer and administrative and medical organizational staff, all headed by Dr. Max Rubinow. The Unit was equipped with over $25,000 in medical equipment and a budget of $400,000 to cover operation costs, half underwritten by the JOINT.[4] From the day of their arrival in August 1918, the Medical Unit struggled with burning health issues, and only towards the end of the year, in November 1918, did the Unit finally have time to attend to opening hospitals in urban centers. The Unit renewed operation of the Rothschild Hospital in Jerusalem, which was transferred to the authority of Hadassah, and served as the central hospital for the Medical Unit in Eretz Israel under the name Rothschild-Hadassah Hospital. Shaar Zion Hospital in Jaffa, which had been closed since the end of the war, was also reopened, and hospitals were founded in Tiberias and Haifa and a special sanatorium for TB patients in Safed. Adjacent to each hospital, clinics and laboratories were established, including dentistry clinics (although these were closed within a year due to lack of funding). First steps were taken towards establishment of a nursing school adjacent to the Rothschild Hospital in order to train health personnel to extend the Unit's activity into rural areas, organize a war on malaria, and expand activities into the field of sanitation and preventive medicine. British authorities welcomed the work of the Medical Unit, and at the end of March 1919, proposed that the Committee of Delegates headed by Dr.

Rubinow accept management of all public health matters of the Jewish community within the framework of the "Health Unit of the Committee of Delegates"—a move that in the minds of Mandate authorities would allow separation of the health services of the Yishuv from the Public Health Unit of the British army, preventing frictions. Dr. Rubinow rejected the proposal, however, and stood by his position that the Medical Unit should remain autonomous, under American management, independent in its operations and initiatives, and refuse to accept sole responsibility for the heath of the Yishuv. In Rubinow's estimation, if the Unit were made responsible for all health matters of the Yishuv, its independence would be impaired, and it would have been transformed into an Eretz Israel institution, subject to the authority of the Mandate government.

The Yishuv and its institutions welcomed the Medical Unit and its endeavors, hoping that within a short time an improvement in the dire health status of the Yishuv would be felt. The workers' health funds and the professional organization of physicians in Eretz Israel were quick to establish ties with the Committee of Delegates and members of the Unit's staff to brief them on the state of health matters and establish an institutional framework for collaboration among all parties. Despite the readiness of all parties to cooperate, efforts to integrate health agencies in the country were unsuccessful. Collaboration between veteran physicians native to the country and physicians from the newly arrived Medical Unit were extremely strained. Dr. Hillel Yafe who had taken upon himself to help "acclimatize" his medical colleagues and brief them on conditions in the country said that members of the Unit were unreceptive to his input, abstained from inviting the Yishuv's doctors to partake in their health work, related to their local colleagues professionalism with disdain and arrogance, and made light of all that had been done to date in advancing the health of the Yishuv prior to their own arrival. The Americans, for their part, sought to maintain the high level of medicine and the professional standards they had brought with them from the United States, standards that were more advanced than the prevailing situation in the country. As a consequence, a common operational framework between the two organizations was not forged, and relations remained very formal. The workers' health funds in particular, which suffered from financial difficulties that prevented them from providing their members with adequate medical assistance, hoped to establish a collaborative relationship and gain assistance from the Medical Unit.

The American Zionist Medical Unit/Hadassah Hospitals

The First World War left the Yishuv in Eretz Israel without any active hospitalization system. During the war, the Jewish hospitals that had operated in Jerusalem and Jaffa were closed, their medical equipment and inventory of medicine were commandeered and turned over to the Turkish Army, and most of the doctors were drafted. At the end of the war, the Yishuv was left with empty hospital buildings with no equipment or suitable personnel to operate them.

The arrival of the American Zionist Medical Unit and its willingness to take upon itself organization of a health system for the Yishuv was an opportunity to rehabilitate the disposition of hospitalization and expand it in keeping with new health needs.

The community hospitals in Jerusalem—Shaari Tzedek, Misgav Ledach, and Bikur Holim—were reopened with the assistance of the Unit and contributions from abroad. Ownership of the Rothschild Hospital, the largest and most central facility, was transferred to the Unit and became its central hospital in Eretz Israel. In 1918, the Unit also opened a hospital in Jaffa in conjunction with the administration of the Shaar Zion Hospital that had operated in the city prior to the war. A year later, hospitals were opened in Safed and Tiberias. In 1922, after the Unit became the Hadassah Medical Federation, a hospital was also opened in Haifa. The number of Jewish patients admitted to Hadassah hospitals doubled within a year. The ratio of Jewish patients in Hadassah hospitals in 1918 was 4.8 per 100,000 inhabitants in the Yishuv; by 1919, it had grown to 7.2, and by 1923 to 8.6. Within a short time, Hadassah hospitals became the core and almost the only hospitalization service in the Yishuv. The Third Aliyah (the wave of immigration that began with the conquest of Eretz Israel by the British) brought approximately 70,000 new immigrants, and the Fourth Aliyah, beginning in 1924, brought approximately 150,000. Both spurred expansion and growth of hospitalization facilities. During this period, the number of Hadassah hospital beds tripled; during the corresponding period, the number of beds in government hospitals established by the Mandate government rose only by two-thirds.

In 1922, Hadassah had 5.4 beds per thousand inhabitants and a 90% occupancy rate. Occupancy in government hospitals during the corresponding year was 67% and in other Jewish hospitals in

Jerusalem, 76%, while occupancy in the mission hospital stood at only 49%. The number of Jewish patients that chose or were referred to non-Jewish hospitals was only 10%. In essence, provision of hospitalization services to the Yishuv in the first years of the 1920s fell squarely on the shoulders of Hadassah. This continued to be the case until 1938, with Hadassah's hospitals carrying the primary burden for hospitalization needs of the Yishuv throughout this period.[5]

Examination of the statistical records of Hadassah on the number of hospitalizations in its institutions in the 1920s and 1930s reveals that Hadassah cared for over 200,000 Jewish patients during this period—more than half the total number of hospitalizations in the Yishuv during these two decades; the remaining hospitalization services were provided by Jewish hospitals in Jerusalem; the General Health Fund's hospital in the Jezreel Valley (opened in 1930) and in Petach Tikva Beilenson (opened in 1936) and by a number of small private hospitals in the Tel Aviv and Haifa areas (with capacities of a only few dozen patients each). All told, throughout the 1920s and 1930s, only 5% of the Jewish patents received hospitalization services from Mandate government hospitals and only 10% from hospitals run by the mission. Therefore, it is understandable why Hadassah complained regularly about the great pressure facing its institutions, difficulties in immediate hospitalization of patents due to lack of beds and budgets, and bed-occupancy rates that in the latter part of the 1930s was 100%. In some areas such as Tel Aviv and the surrounding agricultural settlements, as well as the Galilee and among the agricultural villages of the Jezreel Valley, Hadassah hospitals were the only hospitalization service provider in the Yishuv until 1930. It is not surprising that this state of affairs led to dissatisfaction among some of the hospitalized, particularly those who were politically and culturally distanced from Hadassah, such as the labor organizations who spearheaded recurrent clashes with Hadassah over the scope and the procedures for providing Hadassah hospitalization services to Jewish laborers covered by Kupat Holim. These clashes were part and parcel of the texture of life in the Yishuv in Eretz Israel throughout the 1920s, and had a great impact on the relationship between Hadassah and Kupat Holim.

The Health Committee and Mandate Health Services

Towards the close of 1920, British military government was abolished and the first British High Commissioner of the Mandate government, Herbert Samuel, was appointed to the post. At the same time, a representative body of the Jewish community in Eretz Israel, the National Committee, was elected. Within the National Committee, a "health committee" was formulated, headed by Dr. Abraham Katznelson-Nissan, one of the leaders of Hapoel Hatzair party. During the First World War, Nissan had administered the Eretz Israel Office in Kushta (Constantinople), and in 1924 headed the health department of the Jewish Agency, as well as being a member of the National Committee. The National Committee's health committee was the organizational foundation upon which the Health Ministry of the state of Israel was ultimately established when the Yishuv achieved independence in 1948. At the time of its founding, the Yishuv's health committee was designed to be the central institution for health matters for the Yishuv. The value and importance of the health committee was in its being the only institution in the Yishuv that dealt with health needs of the Jewish community as a whole, while acting as a coordinating body for all other health institutions in the country, primarily between the Medical Unit (whose name was later changed to "Hadassah Medical Federation"), Kupat Holim, and the Hebrew Medical Federation. The Yishuv's health committee regularly supported the health funds on the grounds that they needed and were entitled to develop as an organized health body of the local Yishuv. This evaluation was expressed at the Twelfth Zionist Congress in Karlsbad in September 1921, when the issue of allocation of funding for health services was raised.

In 1920, Mandate authorities established a Public Health Department (its name was changed in 1923 to the Health Department). This department had already existed under British military government, administered by two government employees who were transferred from the military to the civilian settings, continuing to fulfill their functions. At the head of the department stood Colonel G. W. Herron, who had engaged in health issues in the Middle East for over two decades. He had begun his service with the British Medical Corps, and prior to serving in Eretz Israel had served as director of public health in Egypt. Herron was assisted by three deputies and a number of senior employees, including a sanitation engineer, a chemist, a bacteriologist, a medical entomologist, a stock manager, a supervisor of medications, and a public institutions inspector. The entire department had a staff of 75, including 42 medical clerks, 8 chief medical clerks, a medical team for the railroads, and staff for the British government's central medical laboratory in Haifa. The department fulfilled two primary functions: public health and lab services. At the main office the chief medical officer and sanitation engineer engaged in prevention of malaria and contagious diseases, and the labs conducted examination of lab material sent to them from throughout the country. The country was divided into four districts—Samaria & the Galilee, Jaffa, Jerusalem, and Haifa, each headed by a chief medical officer. Policy was based on the belief that Jews and Arabs were entitled to the same level of services. Moreover, in that the Jews enjoyed the services of the Medical Unit, financial backing from abroad, and established machinery for collecting money for health services from within the community, while the Arabs lacked all of these mechanisms, the Mandate government viewed it as their duty to concentrate their activity on the Arab sector and provide the Jews solely with "moral support," on the assumption that the Jewish community would provide itself with all the rest. Thus, British support for health services for the Yishuv was marginal. In essence, the Mandate provided health services for only 20% of the population-at-large (Jews and Arabs).[6]

Most of the Mandate government's energies were invested in the war against malaria. In September 1920, the High Commissioner appointed a regular advisory committee charged with providing advice. The committee encompassed representatives from other governmental departments and was headed by Colonel Herron, who had much experience in the war on malaria from his service in Egypt. In 1922, the advisory committee was granted official status, and its decisions made legally binding. According to an agreement between the Mandate government and the JOINT, which also engaged in providing health services to the Yishuv, $86,000 was transferred to the Mandate Health Office for this purpose.[7] However, in 1927 the JOINT's backing of the government's anti-malaria program was discontinued. The Hadassah Medical Unit, which up until 1927 dealt with malaria on its own, transferred responsibility for this matter to the government's Health Office, including budgeting from its own resources. This move won the organization the appreciation and respect of British health authorities, which subsequently gave the Unit preferable treatment compared to Kupat Holim.

Ongoing work was conducted primarily by the Department's medical officials: supervision of contagious diseases, inspection of sanitation in schools and government-owned structures, supervision of sanitation in villages, vaccinations, registration of births and deaths, issuance of burial permits, fumigation, attention to legal suits, and supervision of water and milk quality. Other than malaria and ongoing work, the Mandate's Health Department was also responsible for regular water supply to the cities, particularly Jerusalem. In addition, the Department supervised physicians, dentists, pharmacists, and midwives.

Government Hospitals and Clinics

By the end of 1922 the Mandate Government had eleven hospitals, nineteen clinics, and nine stations for treating contagious diseases where the public (Jews and Arabs) received minimal medical services.[8]

The chief function of government hospitals in the larger centers was to provide medical treatment for government officers and employees, police and gendarmes, prisoners, railway laborers, school children, and the poor of the local population.

The department of health was responsible for isolation and treatment of all infectious cases in hospital facilities.

Government hospitals with "infectious annexes" were situated in Jerusalem, Jaffa, Haifa, Ramlah, Acre, Nablus, Tul Keram, Ramallah, Beersheva, and Gaza.

Casualty and epidemic posts (without permanent staff) were located in major Arab cities such as Hebron, Jenin, and Nazareth.

The duties of the hospital medical officers—a position which existed only in larger centers—consisted of hospital and out-patient clinical work, medical examination and treatment of school children, attendance to medical needs of prison and police personnel, first aid lectures for police and department of health staff, and work on medical boards. In certain centers such as Tul Karem, Beersheva, and Ramallah, the medical officer also carried out hospital duties.

Medical instruments in all the hospitals were brought up to a standard, allowing performance of most general surgical operations;

the larger hospitals were supplied with the more specialized medical instrumentation.

The nursing staff for the 372 authorized hospital beds in the eleven government hospitals consisted of six head nurses, twelve staff nurses, and sixty-one student nurses.

The compliment of six head nurses was completed by the arrival of two nursing sisters from England. The appointment of British nursing sisters as matrons of the larger hospitals led to a marked improvement in the quality of applicants for student nurse positions, and enabled the facilities to grant nursing certificates after completion of a three-year course of training since hospitals with British matrons in charge faced a much lower dropout rate than was the case before their arrival. Supply of proper nurses' uniforms in government facilities also contributed to raising nursing standards.

Three hospitals had adjacent clinical laboratories and the hospitals' medical officers directed and supervised operations from the government's central lab. Ophthalmic work in the hospitals was considerably expanded in early 1922; this was both the outcome of ophthalmic treatment administered at the schools to the school population and referral by school medical officers to hospitals for children in need of operative treatment. Improvement in the supply of ophthalmic instruments and special training for medical officers at the mobile ophthalmic hospital and by the director of ophthalmic hospitals in Egypt made it possible to expand this type of care.

By 1922 an x-ray unit was installed at Haifa hospital, and a qualified operator with some experience of x-ray work was fully trained in Cairo.

In June 1922 a maternity ward was opened in Jerusalem at the Government Children's Hospital. The funds for its equipment were drawn from monies collected as a gift from Palestine to the British Royal Family.

The annual average number of admissions to government hospitals during the years 1919–1922 was close to 6,000 patients.

Government Clinics

Just as government hospitals were designed primarily to treat infectious diseases, government clinics were intended primarily to treat those classes of patients for whom the government was directly responsible (e.g., government employees and school children suffering from eye diseases, malaria, or contagious conditions). They also served as vaccination centers, as observation posts for new arrivals placed under quarantine, and venues for the meetings of district medical boards.

The large clinics had sections that dealt with special branches of medicine (in Jerusalem, for example, there were children's venereal and ophthalmic units). The government's policy was to develop these special units in as many places as possible, particularly medical treatment tied to infant welfare and ophthalmic work to eradicate communicable eye diseases.

Attendance at government clinics at the beginning of the 1920s was in the vicinity of 15,500 patients annually. No special staff was provided for government clinics. In places where the clinic was associated with a hospital, the hospital medical officer and the nurses operated the clinic; at other locations, the town's medical officer was in charge.

The scope of Mandate health services remained the same throughout British control of Eretz Israel, without any significant change for better or for worse until termination of the British Mandate in 1948.

The principles underlying Mandatory Health Department policies were simple: To care for British personnel serving in Eretz Israel, protect British interests in health matters, improve to some extent health services of the natives, and focus preventive medicine on preventing the outbreak and spread of epidemics—while allocating no more than 2% of the Mandate's budget to health services.

British concentration on enhancement of the status of the Arab community, with little investment in the Jewish sector, was particularly marked in the number of physicians and medical services provided by the Mandate government to the Yishuv, compared to those provided by the Yishuv itself. For instance, Mandate health authorities held that the appropriate doctor-population ratio per capita should be 1:4000, while the Jewish community enjoyed a ratio of 1:700. In respond to charges that the Jewish community was discriminated against in allocation of government resources, authorities responded:

> The demands of the Jews are greater than [those] of the Arabs in general in the stage development they are in at the

> present moment...and [in] any case, equality in care and medical equipment is not possible.[9]

Throughout the entire Mandate period, the government did not waver from this general principle, despite bitterness and protest within the Jewish sector. Most of the charges were leveled at the director, Colonel Herron, who was accused of disliking Jews, discriminating against the Yishuv on purpose, and creating unnecessary difficulties for Jewish health institutions. In actuality, it seems that Colonel Herron was merely faithfully carrying out British Mandate policy—that is, doing the minimum necessary and not an inch more.[10]

Health and Politics: The Workers' Health Funds, 1918–1920

After the First World War ended, the workers' federations were able to return to their old task of uniting their endeavors, including merging the three workers' health funds operating in Judea, Samaria, and the Galilee. Merger of the health funds was not a separate issue, but rather was the outgrowth of unification of the workers' federations into one body. It was clear to all that whatever decision fell concerning amalgamation of the federations would apply to the federations' health funds, as well. The idea of uniting the workers' federations was first discussed on a practical level at the preliminary convention held at Kinneret farm during the spring of 1917. At the time the idea generated a storm, due to differences of opinion over how to unite while both workers' parties feared unification would weaken their power. Disagreement and competition continued for another two years over the pros and cons of unification. Only during Purim 1919 (March) did a general convention of laborers in Eretz Israel convene in Petach Tikva with the objective of establishing a general workers' organization to be called Achdut Haavodah (the Workers' Union). The convention, however, did not succeed in bringing together all the faction in one body. Due to ideological reservations, members of Hapoel Hatzair decided to remain in a separate framework, preventing a complete merger. The other representatives of the workers (Poalei Zion), the unaffiliated workers, and three members of the Hapoel Hatzair party unified to form Achdut Haavodah. Thus two political parties-federations emerged from the convention—Hapoel Hatzair and Achdut Haavodah.

The amalgamation and the political schism among workers in Eretz Israel had an immediate impact on the health funds. Preparations to merge all the health funds were suspended, and the secretaries of the funds and their members who had taken an active part in the "amalgamation convention" split and regrouped along the new party lines and could no longer continue to operate in tandem as regional bodies. The health funds, embroiled by no fault of their own in political struggles and alignments, were disbanded as a result of the convention and reorganized as two country-wide health funds along political rather than geographic lines: the Hapoel Hatzair Mutual Health Fund and the Achdut Haavodah Health Fund (also called the Eretz Israel Workers' Health Fund). From this point forward, the health of workers was placed in the hands of the political system.

Ironically, the unification convention served as a catalyst for competition between the workers' health funds that had not existed prior to unification. While rivalry increased as a result of growing competition between the two political parties, the same rivalry had an upside: The two health funds actively competed for membership, doubling the size of their rosters, and opened sick rooms and central clinics in Jaffa and Jerusalem and clinics for the Yemenites in Petach Tikva and Rechovot. All were aware that every new member of the health fund was a new member for the party, and vice versa. Medical assistance became a political instrument. The struggle was primarily over new immigrants, members of the Hechalutz movement who began arriving at this time; each fund offered the newcomers free medical insurance during the first four months in the country, and continued coverage even if the newcomer became unemployed. In an article published in *Contras*, the newspaper of Achdut Haavodah, one of the new immigrants wrote:

> I didn't expect to see here what we saw in the first minutes upon first setting foot on the shore. We felt very affronted when we disembarked the ship and were surrounded by agents of the parties....We came to Eretz Israel for new lives and here we encounter the same life from which we sought refuge.[11]

Dr. Yaakov Norman wrote in the newspaper *Hapoel Hatzair*:

> It is hard for a person standing on the sidelines to understand why the quarrel between the parties go all the way to the patient and the hospital and how a laborer who has just come, who has not yet decided which of the parties he will give his support, and which of the funds to turn to, should behave? Perhaps he should form a third health fund, a fund of the unaffiliated?[12]

The Competition Between the Health Funds and Expansion of Service

The close tie between the parties and the health funds was also anchored in the organizational framework of the funds. The funds were administered by two national secretaries appointed by their respective parties: Avraham Hartzfeld from Achdut Haavodah and Yaakov Aphter from Hapoel Hatzair, who in the past had jointly headed the Judea Workers' Health Fund. The Hapoel Hatzair Health Fund's office reserved a job post for a party delegate, and the first clause of its charter stipulated that "members of the party are eligible as members of the health fund."[13] The Achdut Haavodah Health Fund's ordinances stipulated that all party members of Achdut Haavodah were *required* to be members of the health fund. The close ties between party and health fund were manifested outwardly during this period, and continued through the Mandate period, and even after the establishment of the state of Israel.

Competition between the two health funds was manifested not only in party ties, but also in the terms of medical coverage. A clear example is the ordinances of the Achdut Haavodah Health Fund, founded in Jaffa in May 1919. Despite the fund's difficult financial straits in the wake of the war, and despite the fact that in the past laborers were required to pay for doctor's visits (at a reduced rate for fund members), now the Achdut Haavodah Health Fund offered medical care to members and their families gratis, from visits to clinics to hospitalization and convalescence. The Achdut Haavodah Health Fund took this step in order to compete with the Hapoel Hatzair Health Fund that was smaller and provided medical assistance at reduced rates, and "was allied with doctors, pharmacies and hospitals in the agricultural villages and cities and gained regular discounts on curative fees."[14]

The mandatory tie between federation-party and medical services had a marked advantage for the health funds. In the past, the health funds had to work at mobilizing members, while now membership came automatically through party affiliation. The number of members grew significantly, and with it the scope of the fund's operation and its revenue. The parties also profited from this arrangement, for laborers—particularly new immigrants—who were in need of and sought out a source of medical coverage upon their arrival were thus "attracted" to the party as well, enhancing party membership. (Prior to linkage of party membership and health coverage, most of the laborers were unaffiliated.)

There is no mention of relations between the two health funds in the reports that accompany their operations. The two funds operated as separate entities from institutional and budgetary standpoints to the extent of totally ignoring each other's existence. When Dr. Rubinow, head of the Medical Unit, demanded that the Hapoel Hatzair Health Fund send its patients to the convalescence facility of Achdut Haavodah in Jerusalem—at the time the only convalescence facility in the country—Hapoel Hatzair members rejected the demand, until "they be given a representative on the management of the institution." Negotiations on this issue, between Achdut Haavodah and Hapoel Hatzair were not direct, but were conducted through the auspices of Dr. Rubinow, a reflection of hard feelings prevailing between the two funds. In another instance, the treasurer of the Committee of Delegates wrote:

> Regarding the principle of collaboration between the two health funds it appears there is a misunderstanding between us and them....[W]e hoped that the two workers' parties would be able to work shoulder-to-shoulder on a neutral basis. If the two parties will oppose working in collaboration on principle, we won't force them to do so.[15]

Health fund records show that the Committee of Delegates and the Hadassah Medical Unit maintained separate accounts for the two health funds, and separate agreements governed hospitalization of members of the two funds in Hadassah hospitals, apparently due to the tense relations between the two funds.

In an article published in *Hapoel Hatzair* under the headline "The Question of the Health Fund," the author noted:

> Demands for unification from above [S.S. from Dr. Rubinow] were a source of anger among the managers of both health funds. Their opinion is that the health fund is a party institution, like the labor exchange, and as long as a modus for cooperative work has not been found, it is entirely impossible to unite the health funds.[16]

Henrietta Szold noted in a letter:

> In the trying days of 1920–1921, when roads were paved[17] in the [Jezreel] Valley and the north of Eretz Israel…two health funds existed, a special one for each of the workers' federations, that received part of the work. Each federation demanded from Hadassah separate hospital services, and when the road was divided into segments by kilometers, they demanded medical aid for each segment. Hadassah cannot agree to this demand….[18]

In practice, Hadassah established one mobile medical service, and forced the two funds and all the laborers to use it jointly.

In 1920 the Achdut Haavodah Health Fund had forty branches with two thousand members (who together with their families, encompassed three thousand insurees), most of them salaried workers in the Jewish agricultural villages, including the Yemenite workers, and approximately 160 members of the Fortieth Eretz Israel Jewish Legion. Membership dues were the same for all, regardless of income. Consequently, the question of progressive dues raised at a later stage was not an issue. The Achdut Haavodah Health Fund's records show that in one year some 1,500 members visited its central clinic monthly. In the medical aid stations there were over 1000 visits a year—most malaria patients. And records show 200 persons were sent to twenty-five-day convalesces; 600 members received an average of ten days of economic assistance to sustain them during illnesses and 5 critically ill were sent abroad (to Egypt or to Vienna).[19] The overall picture from the Fund's records reflects a very comprehensive medical service.

Due to the competition, the two health funds operated a host of facilities—sick rooms, central clinics, a convalescence facility, and so forth—and so changing the character of the funds' work. Medical teams of nurses, paramedics, and pharmacists were hired, and the Achdut Haavodah Health Fund even hired the regular services of a doctor, Dr. Shabtai Malchin. The secretaries and branch committees continued to operate as in the past on a volunteer basis alongside their regular work, but medical responsibilities were transferred to medical teams, and referral notes for hospitalization were granted solely by Dr. Malchin or other physicians on a list of approved doctors. An increase in the number of sick rooms staffed by paramedics and nurses, and opening of central clinics in Jaffa and Jerusalem, enhanced services and reduced the number of workers hospitalized. The Committee of Delegates and the Medical Unit underwrote most of the budget for the health funds, demanding in return that procedures for referring laborers for hospitalization be strictly observed, thus contributing to reduction in the number of patients hospitalized and enhancement of ambulatory care.

Financing Difficulties in Operating the Workers' Health Funds

The budget of the Achdut Haavodah Health Fund in 1920 totaled 6,498 Egyptian pounds (about $2,000). Most of the revenue (80%) came from an American Special Aid Committee and only 15% from membership dues. Two hundred Egyptian pounds were budgeted by the Eretz Israel Workers' Fund towards operation of the convalescence facility in Jerusalem. Employer participation in the budget was minute—25 Egyptian pounds (.05% of the budget). The primary expenditure of the fund—40% of the overall budget—was channeled to sustain workers during illness and convalescence (mostly for malaria). Twenty-five percent of the budget was spent on operational costs of the branches (clinics) and salaries of medical staff—most of them nurses and paramedics. Less than 1% of the budget was used for doctor's visits.[20] Achdut Haavodah Health Fund records show that burial expenses were also covered, and the health fund also invested in maintenance of a library for workers in the Shaar Zion Hospital in Jaffa (the initiative of Berl Katznelson) and distribution of books and guides on hygiene. The budget also included payments to the Pasteur Institute in Jerusalem for rabies shots and, of course, payment of outstanding loans. Records indicate that the health funds enjoyed regular payment of dues by their membership because of methods used by the Zionist executive to support fledgling agricultural farms (kibbutzim). Health fund dues were deducted at the source before the subsidies were transferred to the cooperative communities accounts. Moreover,

> if there was a shortage, they simply deducted more from the budget given by the Zionist Executive to the farms. Thus, the status of individual members who had to pay 15 Egyptian grush(cent) a month, was not terrible for when they didn't have money to pay the monthly dues, they also received medical assistance because they received the money from another source.[21]

The Hapoel Hatzair Health Fund—like the party—was much smaller than the Achdut Haavodah Health Fund and operated primarily in the socialist-oriented independent agricultural sector of collective kibbutz and collective farm settlements. Reports submitted to the Committee of Delegates show the Hapoel Hatzair Health Fund had only twenty branches, whose budgets were covered for the most part by the Zionist Federation. Allocation of the budget was similar to Achdut Haavodah: 60% for sustaining sick members during illness, 15% for hospitalization.[22]

Financial records of the health funds in 1919–1920 (years marked by an ideological schism that further split the labor movement into warring camps, even tearing individual settlements asunder) reflect the principles that guided the funds' operation. The principle of mutual aid was fiercely maintained—that is, workers in the larger branches participated in covering assistance to comrades in small settlements. To ensure this, the budget was managed on a national level, and the funds strictly maintained equal services for each and every member—regardless of geographic location of personal economic circumstances. From this standpoint, the health funds of workers in Eretz Israel (and later the General Health Fund, Kupat Holim) differed from the model of social and medical insurance prevailing in Europe at the time. In Europe there were fluctuations in the level of medical services between residents of small communities and rural areas compared to residents of populated areas, and insurees from outlying areas were often forced to travel far afield to receive medical care.

Along with the principle of mutual aid, the funds also preserved the principle of on-site medical services—medical services "going to" workers rather than workers having to "seek" medical assistance. The two funds competed with one another, boasting of their ability to provide "better services, closer and more comprehensive to the worker, in the city and in the village." When Kupat Holim was finally founded on a merger of the two health funds, these two principles became founding principles of Kupat Holim's operation from the outset.

Financial records of the times reflect a third operational principle: money problems were not permitted to impair the quality of medical service provided to the worker. The secretaries were charged with finding suitable solutions, but were forbidden from curtailing medical aid as a matter of economy or "good management" by concentrating services in cities only—a move demanded by the support agencies, the Committee of Delegates and the Medical Unit. Thus, both funds began their operations with large budgetary deficits that for the most part stemmed from debts accrued during the First World War. They were able to operate due to outside funding provided by the Zionist Executive, the Committee of Delegates, and American aid. Outside aid became the primary source of funding for the health funds' day-to-day operations. In order to justify acceptance of American aid—although viewed as a form of philanthropy—the recipients claimed it was solely a temporary measure "until sanitation conditions in Eretz Israel improve," hoping that sooner or later the funds could sustain themselves without foreign aid.

The Beginning of the Parallel Tax (Mas Makbil)

One of the questions of principle raised at the end of the war was the question of employers participating in medical coverage for their employees. According to British law—the National Health Insurance Act of 1920—employers were required to participate in the cost of medical insurance for their employees.[23] In the formative years of the health funds in Eretz Israel (1911–1914), the Jewish workers objected to any funding from sources other than the working public, holding that the health funds should be run solely on self-capitalization. Now a change of attitude among the workers appeared, spurred for the most part by economic necessity when the membership realized they could not operate the health fund on independent sources only. The change of heart also emanated from moral justifications, in particular, the duty of national institutions of the Zionist movement to care for the health of the Jewish laborers whose lives and endeavors was the primary vehicle for Zionist realization. Furthermore, the change of attitude reflected exposure to enlightened social legislation current in the U.K. , following the occupation of Eretz Israel by the British.

The Hapoel Hatzair Health Fund's ordinances (1919) stipulated that the employer—whether a national farm, a cooperative settlement, a private farm, or private firm in the city or a rural village—must deposit a regular sum in the health fund to insure his employees (clauses 11 and 14). The amount varied from employer to employer depending on the scope of the service and the co-payment demanded by the health fund (clauses 12 and 14). If the employer provided first aid in the workplace independently, the sum paid to the health fund was smaller. The lowest fee was levied on the collective settlements—the Kibbutzim—under the assumption that they provided most medical assistance on-site, including food and lodging even when a laborer was ill, and the health fund only had to cover hospitalization (clause 12).[24] According to Yaakov Aphter, the national secretary of the Hapoel Hatzair Health Fund:

> The laborer and his family suffer from these conditions [malaria and poor sanitation] more than the rest of the Yishuv. The worker in this matter [suffers] from a double jeopardy: His material wealth is meager and the onslaught of disease upon him is greater. The farms and national farms should therefore bear part of the expense of medical assistance for the laborer working on them. This assistance is not given to the worker, rather to the farm where the worker is working, enabling [him] and making him healthy for settlement activity.[25]

In a memorandum sent to private employers at the beginning of 1920, the Hapoel Hatzair Health Fund wrote:

> You sir the recipient surly knows that in more or less developed countries three partners participate in arranging medical assistance: the worker himself, the provider of employment and the government. With us, there is no third party,

> and the Zionist Federation only fulfills a small part of this role, but the first two partners are the primary and the closest to the work, and must therefore bear most of the expense. And if the worker works under harsh sanitary and climatic conditions, if he sets aside 4-5% of his wages for the medical assistance fund, it is justified that the provider of employment will also enter a sum such as this to this fund. Up until now only one type of employer has participated in medical assistance,—the national farms and some of the private farms, but from this day forth it would be fitting that private providers of employment and all the private farms will participate in the arrangement of this kind of assistance, for it is time that the Yishuv in Eretz Israel will care for itself and provide all its own needs, and not lean solely on the assistance of our brethren abroad....We hope that you sir will accept our suggestion willingly and from this month hence will pay the bill presented [to you] by our representative...at the end of the each month for our comrades working for [sic] him during the month.[26]

At the same time, the Hapoel Hatzair Health Fund office also sent a memorandum to the branches calling upon them to collect the health fund dues from employers as well as from the laborers.

Response among employers was mixed. A farmer from one of the villages wrote in reply to the health fund that most of the farmers in the Galilee covered the care of their workers anyway, and therefore should not be asked to pay. Only a few farmers responded positively to the demand that they contribute a co-payment for heath insurance for their workers. The majority did not pay, not out of any objection in principle, but rather because of their own difficult financial straits. The secretary of the Yavniel village branch of the health fund recommended that the issue not be pursued.

A similar request to employers was issued by the Achdut Haavodah Health Fund, which argued: "The Fund's means should be the member's payments, participation by the work-provider and various plants where needed."[27]

The newspaper *Contras* wrote:

> We need to seek means to make insurance of workers mandatory also for work-providers and the government according to the model of European states. The insurance

> laws of England are rather liberal and suited to our purposes. We will need to pass this legally by the [British] government. Until we are able to do so, we will have to vigorously demand that the Zionist Federation fulfill its duty towards the working public in Eretz Israel.[28]

The demand that employers participate in underwriting medical assistance for their workers was founded on two pillars: the first, a broad moral, ideological, and Zionist principal that the Jewish laborer embodied, literally and figuratively, realization of Jewish settlement in Eretz Israel that was the fulfillment of Zionist aspirations; the second, a progressive sociopolitical philosophy reflecting enlightened social legislation in the world.

The first step taken by Kupat Holim after its establishment in 1921 was to demand that employers be required to participate in financing medical services by legislation, through a "parallel tax" to the health fund. Throughout the Mandate period, this demand—and difficulties in enforcing it in the absence of legislation—became a major source of dissension between Kupat Holim and employers in the economy in Eretz Israel, including economic enterprises established by the Federation of Labor.

5

The General Health Fund of Workers in Israel: Kupat Holim

Establishment of the General Health Fund

First years of operation (1920-1923)

In December 1920, at the general convention of workers convened in Haifa, the General Federation of Workers in Eretz Israel was founded. The decision to establish the Federation of Labor brought an end to a period of fragmentation and struggle between rival camps within the labor movement in Eretz Israel, and with it, the split into two workers' health funds. The Achdut Haavodah Health Fund and the Hapoel Hatzair Health Fund were amalgamated into one united general health fund—the General Health Fund, Kupat Holim.

The convention resolution stated:

> The General Federation unites all the laborers and workers in Eretz Israel who make their living by their own hands and do not exploit the labor of others, in order to organize all the settlement, economic and cultural matters of all workers in Eretz Israel, and build a Hebrew [Jewish] working society in Eretz Israel....[1]

The convention stipulated that the parties would continue to exist as separate entities and would be allowed to operate as separate bodies in the political arena. The resolutions detailed thirteen areas in which the Federation of Labor would operate. The first were "organization and development of agricultural farms and work branches in the village and the city, organization of labor battalions, groups for agriculture and industry."[2] Only the seventh ordinance dealt with "mutual aid," mentioning the health fund ("kupat holim, loans, and so forth").[3] The summary resolution passed by the convention stipulated:

> All the institutions dealing with matters within the areas of activity of the Federation existing now under the auspices of the parties in the country, will be transferred to the auspices of the General Federation of Labor.[4]

Bringing the unification about was to be the work of the "federation's council," an executive body elected by the convention.

Thus, in practice, the General Health Fund took form within the framework of the General Federation of Labor. The official name of the fund was "The General Health Fund of Hebrew Workers in Eretz Israel." However, the workers' themselves called the organization simply Kupat Holim. The federation council convened several weeks later to formulate the ordinances that would constitute Kupat Holim's charter, and appointed a governing council: Yaakov Aphter, Avraham Hartzfeld, Chaim Eretzyisraeli, Yosef Rabinovitz, and Mania Shochat.

A year later, in November 1921, the federation council resolved that "the Federation and its institutions will attend only to members of the federation who are card-carrying [members] and pay dues."[5] In the wake of the decision, it was stipulated in Kupat Holim's regulations that membership in the fund was open only to members of the Federation, and laborers who were not members of the Federation "would be admitted only with the approval of the executive committee."[6]

Historian Shabtai Tevet believes that the decision was taken at the initiative of and under pressure from David Ben-Gurion, who at the time was a member of the executive committee of the Federation of Labor, later appointed as the organization's secretary throughout its formative years:

> Ben-Gurion who went about building the Federation as a sort of workers' state, perceived

> Kupat Holim as the oldest Federation institution—a enforcement arm of the first order.... In his eyes, the value of Kupat Holim was tremendous as an arm for consolidating the authority of the executive committee.[7]

Tevet claims that in order to consolidate the power of Kupat Holim as an organizational instrument, Ben-Gurion demanded a precise census of Federation members, organization of card indexes and distribution of membership cards. This, Tevet believes, is the reason that Ben-Gurion commented a year later in November 1922: "Kupat Holim is the one institution that gives the Federation power."[8]

Tevet notes that Ben-Gurion did not hesitate in years to come to use the power of Kupat Holim to enforce the authority of the executive committee by threatening to withhold medical assistant to those who failed to pay dues. Ben-Gurion justified this, declaring: "We can't simply be generous. Kupat Holim is an institution of mutual assistance."[9]

Ben-Gurion knew that the power of Kupat Holim would grow as its medical services expanded, and the more it became an indispensable body, the more effective it would be as a political instrument in the hands of the executive committee. Consequently, he supported expansion and enhancement of Kupat Holim's services in its first years of operation. On the other hand, he made sure that Kupat Holim would not become *too* strong an organization, to the point of endangering the supremacy of the executive committee; he permitted the health fund to expand, short of the point where the executive committee was liable to loose control of its affairs.[10] Thus, for Ben-Gurion, Kupat Holim was first and foremost a power base and an organizational tool, and its value as a health organization was secondary—even marginal in his eyes.

ADMINISTRATION & ORGANIZATION OF KUPAT HOLIM

From the outset, Kupat Holim was perceived as an organizational instrument in the hands of the Federation of Labor, while playing a secondary role in national concerns such as aliyah, work, and settlement activity. This attitude was manifested in the resolutions passed at the founding convention of the Federation of Labor. The words of the worker Shmuel Yavnieli at the 1921 Haifa convention reflect this outlook. In one of his key speeches, Yavnieli spoke of the Federation's activities: "It is not a joint health fund only that it is our role to create today, rather [it is necessary] that we be an energizing power within Zionism…."[11]

Yavnieli related to the health fund "almost in the negative," which expressed the stature of the fund in the eyes of Federation activists over the years: a leading institution in terms of organizational importance, but secondary in terms of its original mission of medical assistance. Kupat Holim's management was not drawn from the most senior leaders in the labor movement, and the organization was not destined to serve as a springboard to senior government positions. Furthermore, Kupat Holim's budgets were regularly whittled down and channeled towards fulfilling more important goals of the Federation's and the nation's agenda. Moreover, the health fund was forced to constantly compete with other Federation institutions such as *Hamashbir* (provision of food and goods) and *Solel Boneh* (workers' building cooperative group) for its position within the Federation of Labor.

The Federation of Labor set up a complex system of appointments for managing its cooperative institutions. According to historian Zeev Tzachor, key personalities in the two parties were elected to the most important committees—usually four members from Achdut Haavodah and three from Hapoel Hatzair.[12] Because the number of party activists was small, each was forced to serve on several committees, and for the most part also served as party functionaries parallel to their posts in the Federation of Labor. Yaakov Aphter, for instance—the past secretary of the Hapoel Hatzair Health Fund—served concurrently as a member of the Federation's executive committee, as a member of the Kupat Holim directorate, as a member of the Agricultural directorate, and as a member of the central committee of his party. Thus, the managers of the health fund were overburdened by numerous responsibilities and found it hard to fulfill such a multiplicity of roles, particularly in terms of time needed to organize and run institutions properly. Aphter once revealed to his colleagues that "already three weeks he had delayed a trip related to operation of Kupat Holim because every evening he had a meeting in Tel Aviv."[13]

Even those engaged in the daily management of Federation institutions were chosen according to party affiliation—more often than not, thanks to personal ties with a member of the central committee of one of the parties. Moreover, in many cases party activists recommended themselves for posts without any connection with their practical capabilities. Consequently, many appointees failed at their posts. Turnover in jobs was rampant, impacting negatively on the quality of operations.

When it became clear that Kupat Holim was not operating properly, some members sought to propose a new procedure for filling management posts. But their suggestions were not very successful, and in the first year of Kupat Holim's operation under Federation of Labor auspices, the management changed hands time and again. The first director Yosef Rotberg resigned, charging that "I am not suitable for working in Kupat Holim,"[14] and Manya Shochat resigned from the management "because I am not able to work in this post and I cannot fathom the benefit of my work."[15] The executive committee appointed to manage Kupat Holim failed to convene, and there was, in essence, no one at the helm to address burning problems. The fund appeared to have ceased to function. A Federation of Labor activist described the state of Kupat Holim during its first year thus:

> The kitty is empty, pursued by its creditors, owing back wages to its only physician (Dr. Malchin), the only nurse (Sara Lishansky] and the only clerk (Ch. Pikarsky] who is in Tel Aviv, and there is a lack of ability to respond to the seriously ill whose health has been ruined by hard labor on the roads.…Yosef Rotberg who took upon himself the burden of management of this Fund was the worst off among all those holding posts in the Federation.…This fellow is always encircled by the sick, the disabled and the merely weak who come from the roads and from the villages, and they need basic medical treatment and reliable care.[16]

After Rotberg's resignation from management of Kupat Holim, Avraham Hartzfeld took it upon himself to run the institution in the interim, among his many other roles. The degree to which Kupat Holim's needs were pushed onto the sidelines is evident in the records and memoirs of Hartzfeld. In neither case are Kupat Holim matters mentioned, although other concerns Hartzfeld dealt with are recalled in detail.

Historian Idit Zartal wrote of conditions prevailing at the time:

> The Federation of Labor was given a "fetus" in terms of medical services the institution was able to provide its members and also from the standpoint of managerial organization. The Yishuv was not stable, the pioneers wandered from place to place, establishing temporary camps in the places where there were work opportunities, and were accompanied also by the health fund's mobile clinic, that is a tent with two beds and quinine. At times there was not even a nurse to administer the clinic, financial and administrative details [of the Fund] were registered in tiny microscopic script in a tiny notebook lodged permanently in the shirt pocket of Avraham Hartzfeld.[17]

In the summer of 1920, Yehoshua Chenkin initiated purchase of 50,000 dunam (approximately 12,500 acres) of land in the Jezreel Valley for Jewish settlement, and in the summer of 1921 the Zionist Congress in Karlsbad approved the funding needed to buy the land. The land purchase and the arrival of new socialist-oriented Zionist pioneers from the Third Aliyah spurred a new wave of Jewish settlement activity in Eretz Israel. In September 1921, members of the Second Aliyah established the cooperative village Nahalal, the first Jewish settlement in the Jezreel Valley. Ten days later the Labor Battalion set up camp in Ein-Harod (Harod fountain), and several months later in nearby Tel Yosef (Josef hill). The Valley filled with new Jewish settlers. The new settlement activity required Kupat Holim to reorganize itself on a more serious footing in terms of the strength of its administration.

In January 1922, the first Kupat Holim directorate was elected to replace Kupat Holim's council as the chief governing body of the health fund. The directorate was to be a three-person body with representatives of the two parties—two from Achdut Haavodah and one from Hapoel Hatzair. Y. Elbinger, past secretary of the Hapoel Hatzair Health Fund in the Galilee, proposed appointment of one head in place of a threesome, in order to economize on expenditures, but the two parties rejected the idea. Yosef Sprinzak, a member of the election committee, explained to Elbinger the rebuff, claiming:

"There is no alternative from adopting this lineup principle in an institution uniting two factions that were previously separate."

The worker Levi Venik was initially elected to represent Achdut Haavodah on the directorate, but was soon replaced by Yitzhak Kenivsky-Kenev, a member of Col. Trumpledor's followers at Tel Chai. Eliezer Perlson-Peri, a member of Hechalutz who had arrived with the Third Aliyah, was appointed as the Hapoel Hatzair representative on Kupat Holim's executive due to the organizational talents that he had manifested at the Hadera encampment of laborers, although Perlson-Peri was not a registered member of the party. The third member of the troika was Reuven Shenkar, a former member of the Labor Battalion, who became responsible for finances. Eliezer Perlson headed the executive and brought a semblance of order to the organization. As was custom of the day, Perlson mobilized several of his friends from the encampment of laborers in Hadera to work in Kupat Holim including Eliyahu Degani (later elected as member of Kupat Holim's directorate) and Moshe Soroka (who later became the treasurer of Kupat Holim and its administrative director).

Kupat Holim officially commenced operation in January 1921, but it was only in January 1922 that it began to function on a practical level. At the outset, the health fund had several thousand registered members and a deficit of four thousand Egyptian pounds (the legal tender at the time in Eretz Israel). However, health fund records were disorderly and one cannot be sure of the exact number of members and the exact budget at the time. Yitzhak Kenivsky-Kenev, a member of the first directorate, said that at the beginning of 1921, there were 3,200 members and within a year the rosters increased to some 5,700. Perlson, on the other hand, said that in 1922 there were 3,000 members in fourteen settlements, and since the number of children was not large, one could assume that the number of members was in the vicinity of 3,000. In her biography of Moshe Soroka, Idit Zartal wrote that in 1922 Kupat Holim had 4,000 members and within a year, 6,000, while Ben-Gurion cited 3,676 members in 1922 (out of 8,394 members of the Federation of Labor). According to Zartal, the Kupat Holim budget at the end of 1922 was 12,229 Egyptian pounds with a 4,000-pound deficit, but Ben-Gurion speaks of a 5,100 Egyptian pound deficit. The data as presented reflect not only the financial difficulties facing the health fund, but also the chaotic state of Kupat Holim in its first year.

Two facts stand out from this period. First, despite an obligatory ordinance passed by the Federation of Labor's council and anchored in Kupat Holim's own regulations, not all members of the Federation of Labor were members of the health fund. At the second convention of the Federation of Labor in 1923, it was stipulated that Kupat Holim and the Work Office (the Federation's labor exchange) would deal solely with card-carrying members of the Federation who had paid dues to the Federation of Labor. Nevertheless, there were members of the Federation of Labor who were not members of Kupat Holim, and the organization did not succeed in enforcing the rule. This issue remained on the agenda of the Federation of Labor as a bone of contention for some seventeen years, a subject of controversy at the Kupat Holim council in 1925, the second Kupat Holim convention in 1929, and the third Federation of Labor convention in 1927. Only in 1937 was membership in the Federation of Labor and Kupat Holim genuinely united through institution of a joint dues system, *Mas Achid* (see chapter 10).

Second, Kupat Holim suffered from a large deficit from the time it began operation. While at the second Federation of Labor convention, Ben-Gurion noted with pride that the rate of participation of workers in the Kupat Holim budget stood at 65%, in practice it was smaller. Only 57% of the budget came from dues. The remainder was covered by the Zionist executive and Hadassah (35%) and employers and other funding sources (5–8%). Backing from the Zionist movement and Hadassah was not automatic, however, and Kupat Holim had to fight again and again to receive funding. From its first years of operation, the health fund faced budgetary problems also due to the lack of clarity in fiscal relationships between the health fund and the Federation of Labor's executive committee. The executive committee had not yet received allocation of its own, and there was no set procedure for transferring funds regularly from the Federation institutions to cover the executive's needs, thus members of the executive committee would withdraw funds directly from the Kupat Holim account and use them for their own purposes, and even direct payments were drawn directly out of the Kupat Holim budget. This practice was a regular source of controversies and quarrels between the sides. Since the executive committee also suffered from a substantial fiscal deficit, in 1924 Ben-Gurion decided to transfer administration of money matters of the executive committee to Eliezer Perlson, who had recently been appointed head of Kupat Holim, with the hopes that this arrangement would settle the financial matters of the executive committee. Thus, the finances of both Kupat Holim and the executive committee of the Federation of Labor were handled by the same person. While Perlson's leadership brought about an improvement in balancing the budget of Kupat Holim, such an arrangement was not in the best interests of the health fund.

With the appointment of Eliezer Perlson as director of Kupat Holim, the fund finally began to run on a relatively smooth basis. His first step was to divide Kupat Holim into five districts—Jerusalem, Jaffa, Haifa, Tiberias, and Safed—each with its own permanent secretariat and regional office. Kupat Holim reached out to rural settlements, establishing sick rooms, reorganizing regular supply of medications, organizing dues according to orderly membership rosters, and appointing a director for each district. Work procedures in the districts were, in general, set according to on-site conditions and differed from district to district. Local initiatives and the individual talents of district managers impacted to a large extent on work procedures. Moshe Soroka, head of the Haifa district (including the Jezreel Valley), stood out as an able corporate leader. He established sick rooms, expanded the hospital in Kibbutz Ein-Harod in the Jezreel Valley, and formulated regular procedures for registration for membership and collection of dues.

Afterwards, Perlson focused on establishing channels for payment of membership dues and institution of joint dues (i.e., to both organizations in one payment). Because payment of dues to Kupat Holim was separate from dues to the Federation of Labor, Kupat Holim's directorate had the authority to change it at will. Yaakov Aphter suggested graduated dues be instituted in lieu of a set amount for all members. In order to encourage newcomers to join and enhance the principle of mutual assistance, he argued, the health fund should adopt a progressive system based on the laborer's income, while at the same time demanding that all providers of employment in the economy participate with a regular co-payment to Kupat Holim on behalf of their employees. His proposal was accepted by the second Federation of Labor convention, which resolved: "To seize all means necessary to demand all work-providers be required to pay parallel dues to Kupat Holim."

The goal was to mobilize co-payments from employers equal to the sum laid out by the insuree himself—thus the term "parallel tax." The demand that employers participate in coverage of Kupat Holim had a double significance for the Federation of Labor: On one hand, it was an ideological matter—that is, the belief that it is the duty of an employer to care for the hearth of his or her employees, as in Europe. On the other hand, it enhanced the status of the Federation beyond the working public—extending its authority to employers, not just laborers as Ben-Gurion had originally designed. An employer who failed to comply with the Federation of Labor's directive was liable to expose the business to sanctions and strikes. Of course, members of the Federation and the health fund also hoped participation of employers would reduce Kupat Holim's operating deficit and improve the balance of payments of the organization that also "fueled"` the Federation.

Participation of employers in ensuring the health of their employees was not something new. Even prior to the demand, there were many laborers who requested and received assistance from their employers in paying for medical insurance through Kupat Holim, but until this point participation on the part of the employer had been voluntary and provisional—a personal benefit granted as a matter of good will, not a social obligation required by all. First steps towards institution of the parallel tax was taken in 1921 by Eliezer Perlson, at the time secretary of the workers' committee in Hadera, and Eliyahu Degani, who dealt with medical matters in the labor encampment. Degani pressured the Jewish farmers in Hadera to sign a contract with the representatives of the Jewish laborers that stipulated: "For every day of work, the farmer will pay half a grush (cent) for a parallel tax."

Not all the farmers accepted the agreement willingly, but thanks to the persistence and pressure applied by Degani, the dues became a regular feature as long as an encampment existed in Hadera. A similar agreement was achieved in February 1921 with the Mandate's Roads Authority for payment of a parallel tax of 3% of the worker's wages for Kupat Holim services.

When Perlson was appointed director of Kupat Holim, he invited Degani to work with him side by side, and the two set about instituting an obligatory parallel tax throughout the country. Dues paid by workers was set at 3% of the employee's wages; therefore it was resolved that the parallel tax paid by employers should also be 3%. Payment entitled the employee to full rights of Kupat Holim: sick pay, insurance against work injuries (treatment and compensation), hospitalization, subsidence and travel expenses during illness, and sanitary supervision in the workplace. Despite the marked advantage of the parallel tax—for both workers and employers—employers were in no hurry to pay. In a report written by Reuven Shenkar to the executive committee of the Federation of Labor in mid-1923, Shenkar wrote:

> Despite all the decisions to date, we are not receiving parallel tax from the cooperatives and the contractor groups. You must employ all means and force the cooperatives to pay the parallel tax.[18]

Yitzhak Kenivsky-Kenev voiced similar sentiments concerning the scope of payment in the 1920s.

The scope of compliance with payment of the parallel tax was higher among the cooperative agricultural settlements established by the laborers—kibbutzim and farms—than in the private sector of the economy. In late 1923, the parallel tax constituted 21.7% of the overall income of Kupat Holim—5% from private employers and 16.7% from the cooperative farms. Relatively high compliance was tied to the economic support the agricultural farms received from the Zionist Federation that to a large extent allowed the farms to pay the parallel tax. In this respect, the cooperative farm was considered an employer just like any other "place of work." The Federation collected the parallel tax in a lump sum from subsidies earmarked to the farms, via the Agricultural directorate—a parent organization of the entire farming sector—prior to transfer of the funding to the farms themselves. Such control "at the source" gave the Federation of Labor a great deal of power. A cooperative that did not fulfill the Federation's demands was liable to face delays in transfer of subsidies. Thus, Kupat Holim ensured collection of the parallel tax on a regular basis, regardless of the financial state of the settlements.

Expansion of settlement activity in the Jezreel Valley and the organizational abilities of Perlson lead to the rapid expansion of Kupat Holim's activity. Health fund records from 1922 to 1923 reveal that within a year the number of physicians doubled from five to ten, the number of paramedics rose from twenty-three to thirty-five, and a central sick room was established in kibbutz Beit Alfa with twelve beds, in addition to the seven beds in the village of Balforia, and the hospital of the Labor Battalion in kibbutz Ein-Harod was expanded to a thirty-five-bed facility. In its infancy, the hospital was two huts established by the Battalion in 1920 and operated by members of Kibbutz Ein-Harod. At the close of 1923, responsibility was transferred to Kupat Holim, and the Ein-Harod facility became the central medical facility of Kupat Holim in the Jezreel Valley. The Ein-Harod Hospital was, in essence, the first permanent institution owned by Kupat Holim. The other sick rooms throughout the country were temporary affairs established on locations where encampments of workers were set up in areas hit by malaria, in both the Jezreel Valley and Samaria. When a malaria attack subsided, the size of the sick room was curtailed or the sick room was moved elsewhere, where needed.

The same year, the Central Office of Kupat Holim was set up in Tel Aviv. Adjacent to it, Kupat Holim's first clinic was opened, housed in two huts given to the fund by the Zionist executive. Reuven Shenkar, a member of the Kupat Holim central committee and the person responsible for the health fund's finances, orchestrated the supply of medications and basic needs from Hadassah storehouses in Jerusalem to the sick room. Shenkar related that allocation of medication was carried out in an original manner: "On the way back on the [Jezreel] Valley train I would throw the package [off the train] at the station for each point of settlement."[xix]

When the number of sick rooms in points of settlement grew, Kupat Holim organized for the first time to arrange convalescence facilities for its members (particularly for those regaining their health from malaria). Rooms were rented in hotels in Safed, Nazareth, near Jerusalem, and on the Carmel in Haifa, and Avraham Hartzfeld embarked on the establishment of the Arza Convalescence Home in the Jerusalem foothills to serve as a central convalescence facility for Kupat Holim.

At the outset of 1923, it seemed that Kupat Holim's activities had begun to function in an orderly fashion. However in mid–1923, the sense that the health fund had settled into a working routine was fractured by the kibbutz Ein-Harod affair, ultimately changing the face of Kupat Holim.

The Ein-Harod Affair: Kupat Holim as a Political Instrument

In 1921, a company of laborers from among the Trumpledor Work Battalion established a cooperative settlement of their own in kibbutz

Ein-Harod, in the Jezreel Valley. The group was comprised of members of the Third Aliyah, who were joined by a handful of members of the Second Aliyah—all of East European origins (for the most part Russia and Poland). Within a short time, two settlements were established in the Valley—kibbutz Ein-Harod and kibbutz Tel-Yosef. Yet, integration of the young members of the Third Aliyah together with the more veteran members of the Second Aliyah turned out to be a source of tension and disputes broke out among the leaders of the Battalion, particularly between Menachem Elkind and members of the Second Aliyah. Economic hardships added fuel to the fire, and heads of the Battalion were accused of appropriating funds earmarked for kibbutz Ein-Harod to cover the deficits of other companies in the Battalion. An inquiry committee was sent out. Failure of efforts to reach a compromise between the sides lead the executive committee of the Federation of Labor to split kibbutz Ein-Harod between those whose loyalties lay with the Battalion (who were to move to kibbutz Tel-Yosef) and those whose loyalties lay with the Federation of Labor (for the most part members of the Second Aliyah, who were to stay in kibbutz Ein-Harod). In the course of carrying out the split, members of the Battalion claimed that division should apply only to the common land holdings, and should not include equipment and livestock. During the clash, members of the Battalion in kibbutz Tel-Yosef seized the settlement's assets by force.

Ben-Gurion was greatly angered when he learned that kibbutz Ein-Harod had been left without any dairy cows and work animals. At his initiative and Hartzfeld's, the executive committee declared on 5 July 1921 that if within twenty-four hours members of the Battalion did not honor the directives of the division committee sent under the auspices of the Federation, all Federation of Labor institutions would sever all relationships with kibbutz Ein-Harod—including Kupat Holim. When the Battalion rejected the ultimatum, Ben-Gurion ordered on his own that all ties with the Battalion's settlement be ceased until further notice. The directive sent on June 10 to the Kupat Holim directorate stated:

> According to the decision of the executive committee in a meeting on June 5th, you must, like all the other Federation institutions, cease all ties with the Battalion's farm at Tel-Yosef until you receive

> from us other directives. Announce this immediately to all your branches in the country.[20]

The directive meant immediate stoppage of medical aide to members of kibbutz Tel-Yosef, including assistance provided by the hospital originally established by the Battalion, in kibbutz Ein-Harod. The fact that Kupat Holim was ordered to circulate the directive among its branches meant not only closure of on-site services, but that members of the Battalion would be prevented from seeking assistance at all Kupat Holim branches throughout the country.

Withdrawal of medical assistance from members of the Labor Battalion was a severe step. Members of the Battalion in kibbutz Tel-Yosef got around the directive through transfer of food from Hamashbir to kibbutz Tel-Yosef from other companies of the Battalion located elsewhere, but there was not substitute for Kupat Holim. The health status of the members of kibbutz Tel-Yosef, who suffered from poor nutrition, long bouts of malaria, and TB grew desperate. In the estimation of Dr. Ben-Zion Hirshovitz, the kibbutz Ein-Harod Hospital physician, the situation was unprecedented in severity:

> [W]hat brings about gloomy contemplation and apprehension of danger…if the current situation will continue for some time, only invalids and chronically sick will remain in the camp.[21]

Ben-Gurion's decision aroused anger and protest. Members of the Federation's own executive committee were angry at Ben-Gurion for carrying out the decision in practice without consulting them, for they viewed withdrawal of food and medical care as a threat that they did not plan on carrying out. Letters from throughout the country were sent to the executive committee protesting Ben-Gurion's step, particularly sanctions in the health domain. In Jerusalem representatives of fifteen labor groups signed a petition declaring that "The executive committee has no authority to withhold medical aid from members of the Federation, assistance given even to one's foes in the worst war."[22]

Eliezer Perlson had difficulty confronting Ben-Gurion in this matter. A year earlier Ben-Gurion had appointed him to deal with the finances of the executive committee in place of David Zakai, and had given Perlson free rein, confident that Perlson could extricate the executive committee from its economic hardships. Perlson found himself between the hammer and the anvil—between Ben-Gurion and Kupat Holim. He sought to mitigate the severity of the directive but did not dare oppose it openly. A day after Ben-Gurion's directive was received on June 11, the Kupat Holim directorate turned to the Federation of Labor's executive committee requesting clarifications:

> We request that you inform us if you intended is that we stop all medical assistance to them…or only part of the aid. Furthermore, in that patients from both collective settlements are at Ein-Harod [Hospital], it is hard to separate them. Please give directives in this matter, also. We request [that you] give the necessary orders soon, so that we be able to fulfill your orders in this letter.[23]

The tone of the letter testifies to Kupat Holim's hesitation and attempts to evade responsibility for withdrawal of medical aid, and an apparent attempt to attain further backing for such a step through explicit orders from the executive committee of the Federation of Labor. The difficulties in carrying out Ben-Gurion's orders should be taken at face value: the patients lay sick, side by side, and it would be difficult to separate them. Yet, in contrast to the indecisive tone of the letter as a whole, the closing sentence is far more resolute: "…so that we be able to fulfill your orders."

Whether this was a ploy designed to place any future blame for the consequences fully on the shoulders of the executive committee or whether it reflects the inferior status of Kupat Holim as a body subordinate to the will of the executive committee, without the ability to protest or resist, it is clear that the ties between Perlson and Ben-Gurion impacted on the response of Kupat Holim, even if it is hard to measure the degree.

The Federation's executive committee (not Ben-Gurion) disassociated itself at the outset from the order, and was influenced by the negative response of the working public. Quickly responding in a letter to the Kupat Holim directorate the very next day (June 12), the executive committee announced:

> Stoppage of ties does not mean removing members from the Federation, and therefore medical assistance to sick members is not cut off. It is obvious that assistance to the joint hospital con-

> tinues. Regarding your letter in detail, the executive committee will discuss and let you know its decision.[24]

Even prior to publication of the executive committee's stand, members of the Battalion in kibbutz Tel-Yosef and other Battalion companies elsewhere responded harshly to the Federation of Labor's move. A day after Ben-Gurion's directive, the Labor Battalion published a special issue of its paper in Eretz Israel and abroad—*Mechayeynu* (our lives)— in which it denounced the cruel decision and even published Dr. Ben-Zion Hershkovitz's account of the arduous health situation in kibbutz Tel-Yosef.

> The general assembly of members of the Tel-Yosef Company believes that the latest command of the executive committee of the Federation is an action that is totally underhanded…and there is no room for negotiations between Federation institutions and its members under threat to sever relations that means cessation of means of daily existence and medical aid.[25]

The members of the Battalion went on to denounce withdrawal of medical aid as "cruel" and "destructive" and purely politically motivated. Two days later, kibbutz Kfar Giladi announced it was severing its ties with the Federation as a demonstration of solidarity with Tel-Yosef, saying that from the kibbutz's standpoint the Federation could also suspend *their* medical assistance "just as you stopped them to such a malarial place as Tel-Yosef." Kibbutz Beit Alpha wrote to the executive committee that the cutoff was in total negation of Federation principles, while the Tel Aviv Workers' Council asked: "What right does the executive council have to use a seizure tactic against the working public?"

Ben-Gurion responded to the protests by condemning the protesters for "giving your moral support… to those who seized by force Federation assets and inventory belonging to another farm community." That is, Ben-Gurion had no moral scruples about withholding medical assistance to regain Federation property. Just the opposite: One should denounce those who opposed such a move for their "support for the theft of stolen property (equipment and farm animals)."

Five days after the order was issued, the executive committee convened a meeting without the presence of Ben-Gurion, in which the members of the executive expressed their sorrow at the rash decision, saying that there was no room for cancellation of medical services and annulling the decision. Nevertheless, although Ben-Gurion continued to hold that the use of Kupat Holim as a vehicle for political sanctions was justified, historian Shabtai Tevet believes that he learned from the episode. Following the Ein-Harod affair, Ben-Gurion was more prudent, refraining from openly using Kupat Holim for political purposes, while exploiting the principle of mutual assistance upon which Kupat Holim was founded as an indirect vehicle for enforcing Federation authority.

Throughout the Ein-Harod affair, Eliezer Perlson and the Kupat Holim directorate refrained from taking a stand. After the close of the affair at the end of the year (1923), Reuven Shenkar—a member of Kupat Holim's senior management— turned to the executive committee of the Federation of Labor demanding they publish a repudiation of what they viewed as defamation of Kupat Holim by the Labor Battalion. Shenkar claimed that the Battalion had blown the entire episode out of proportion and used the incident to attack the health fund due to prior financial disputes between the two bodies. At the same time, the Kupat Holim directorate published in its newsletter *Pinkas* a broad overview of the issue from the health funds' standpoint.

According to the Kupat Holim directorate's version of events, medical assistance to kibbutz Tel-Yosef was never cut off, even after Ben-Gurion's directive. Kupat Holim was vilified despite being innocent. Just the opposite, they claimed: the ones who had neglected the health of the workers were members of the Battalion itself, who had utilized funds from the Zionist movement earmarked for the hospital in kibbutz Ein-Harod for other purposes, while Kupat Holim had continued at the same time to support the hospital with equipment and medications. Kupat Holim also defended itself against claims spread by the Battalion that medical care had been denied members of the Battalion in Jerusalem:

> We know that members of the Battalion have spread and are spreading bogus stories among the working public about stoppage of medical care by Kupat Holim, that have led astray hundreds and

> thousands, and used this matter which never was as a tactical and political weapon in a war against the executive committee of the Federation. We protest with all our might against the Battalion's use of slanderous things concerning Kupat Holim as a target in its war on the Federation.[26]

In its rebuttal, the Kupat Holim directorate cited the directive of the executive committee from June 12 stipulating that medical assistance should *not* be withheld, and stressing: "[I]t is clear, based on the order of the executive committee that no order was given to any institution or branch of Kupat Holim about cutoff of assistance."

The claim that Kupat Holim refrained from taking any such a step due to a Federation executive committee directive testifies more than anything else to the consternation with which the health fund struggled, not knowing what to do with itself at the time—despite the opposite intentions of health fund staff in presenting their case in the aftermath.

Kupat Holim's behavior in the Ein-Harod episode reveals an organization that operated according to orders from others, ignoring the moral foundation of its own raison d'être—first and foremost the duty and responsibility to care for the health of the worker. Quite naturally, the version Kupat Holim chose to publish does not mention the letter sent to the executive committee by the Kupat Holim directorate on the June 11 requesting instructions on how to fulfill the orders they had been given. How would the health fund have responded had it had been told to carry out the withdrawal of medical aid in practice for an extended time? It is hard to know, but luckily Kupat Holim was not put to the test.

The clash of wills between the Labor Battalion and the Federation of Labor at Ein-Harod stamped Kupat Holim as an enforcement arm of the first degree in the hands of the executive committee of the Federation of Labor. It was not without reason that Ben-Gurion claimed, "Kupat Holim is the one institution that gives power to the Federation of Labor." This "role" was destined to accompany Kupat Holim for years to come. Kupat Holim emerged from the Ein-Harod episode as a loser on numerous counts: the workers' confidence in Kupat Holim was impaired; its stature as an organization that cared for the health of the worker everywhere and unconditionally was undermined; and from this point forward, Kupat Holim was viewed as a political-Federation institution, with all that such status entails.

In September 1923, Ben-Gurion left for Moscow, and the executive committee of the Federation of Labor concluded the division of assets and farm inventory between Ein-Harod and Tel-Yosef, bringing an end to the episode and restoring relations between the parties. In a letter to Ben-Gurion David Zakai wrote: "Between Ein-Harod and the Battalion there is peace, much peace."

THE EIN-HAROD HOSPITAL

Kupat Holim's ties with the Battalion and Tel-Yosef were not severed by the episode. Within a compromise agreement between Tel-Yosef and the Federation, it was agreed that Kupat Holim would continue to provide medical assistance to Tel-Yosef. It was also agreed to continue negotiations for the transfer of the of Battalion's hospital hut in Ein-Harod to the control of Kupat Holim. When Kupat Holim began to administer the hospital indirectly, the parties avoided the prospect of a dispute over ownership. At the beginning of July 1923, a meeting was convened between representatives of Ein-Harod and Eliezer Perlson. A member of kibbutz Ein-Harod reported a "suffocating atmosphere" in the hospital and demanded that Kupat Holim seek an immediate solution, on condition that "the personnel will be equal on both sides." Afterwards, the group discussed expansion of the hospital and funding of expenditures in the future. Perlson pointed out the fiscal limitation of Kupat Holim and demanded that members of the cooperative settlements contribute as well to maintenance of the hospital and its development, in addition to their payment of regular dues to Kupat Holim. The gathering unanimously passed a resolution that the hospital would be transferred within a short time to the authority of Kupat Holim. In another discussion devoted to financial arrangements, held several months later, it was resolved that any new arrangement concerning the hospital would be covered according to the following formula: a third would be carried by Kupat Holim, and two-thirds by Tel-Yosef and Ein-Harod (shared equally). The two communities would, in addition, enjoy preferential treatment in employment of their members at the institution.

At the outset of 1924, the hospital was officially transferred to Kupat Holim and became the first hospital in Eretz Israel belonging entirely to the health fund. Daniel Nadav, who researched the history of the Ein-Harod Hospital, wrote that transfer of the hospital to Kupat Holim held symbolic significance:

> It demonstrated the senior status of settlements and agriculture in the ideology and the actions of the labor movement. The establishment of the first hospital in the heart of an agricultural region in particular, was befitting of the Zionist and labor ideal of a renaissance through a return to nature and village life.[27]

A short time after Kupat Holim took over the hospital, two beds were added for women in labor. The allocation of beds as a "maternity ward" was essential, for most of the settlers lived in tents under severe conditions. In the case of difficult deliveries the women were transported to Haifa, but such travel was expensive and disrupted work on the farm. In 1925, the number of beds for women in labor was expanded to four, and in 1926 to seven. From this point forward, over 90% of all births in the Jezreel Valley were delivered at the Ein-Harod Hospital. The proximity of the hospital to a point of settlement eased medical supervision of women waiting to give birth, instruction for mothers and care of newborns, coordination of the war on malaria with the supply of quinine to residents of the area, and sanitary supervision of settlements. Reports on disease and mortality rates in these years (1924–1926) testify to the great improvement in health status of the residents and reduction in spread of epidemics—all due to the smooth operation of the hospital under the auspices of Kupat Holim.

6

According to Needs or According to Ability: Kupat Homlim, 1924-1930

From the beginning of 1924, when the Fourth Aliyah began to arrive in Eretz Israel, Kupat Holim had to address the central issue that was to accompany it throughout its history[1]: how to continue operation in the face of constant financial difficulties and a large deficit. Dealing with this challenge forced Kupat Holim to address core questions concerning its functioning.

Financing of Health Services: Who Should Pay for the Worker's Health?

Financing problems and difficulties underwriting the health fund accompanied Kupat Holim's operation almost from the outset. The small number of dues-paying members in the fund's first years (1911–1914), economic crisis during the First World War (1914–1918), the years of operation that preceded unification of the health funds within the framework of the Federation of Labor (1918–1921), and the period in which Kupat Holim reorganized in the wake of the merger of workers' health funds (1921–1923) all contributed to Kupat Holim's budgetary problems. Yet, there were expectations that once Kupat Holim began to operate on an orderly basis, with a genuine permanent management with organized work procedures, the number of members would grow and Kupat Holim would be able to support itself, even if assisted with a measure of outside support from other bodies such as the Zionist movement, Hadassah, the JOINT, and so forth.

At the outset of 1924, it became evident to Eliezer Perlson and members of the Kupat Holim directorate that their hopes had not been realized. Kupat Holim faced a harsh fiscal crisis that threatened its very existence. The heads of the fund were forced to struggle with the difficult question of finding sources of capitalization needed to continue Kupat Holim's operation. And what would become of the members, including entire settlements, that did not fulfill their duties of paying dues to the fund due to their own financial difficulties? Should medical assistance be withheld from those who did not pay? Should sick rooms be closed, paramedics fired, and doctors' visits to a kibbutz, farm, or workers' encampment cease under such circumstances? The question was particularly hard in light of the severe health status of the settlements, and the knowledge that withdrawal of medical assistance would exacerbate the situation, as the settlements and the workers had no other option for medical assistance available.

The question of assistance to the unemployed and new immigrants was also raised. Who should care for them and who should pay for their treatment? The question arose in all its poignancy in the wake of the wave of mass immigration that began in July of 1924: the Fourth Aliyah. The Fourth Aliyah continued to the end of 1926, bringing 55,000 new immigrants, most Eastern European Jews who arrived at a rate of 2,000 new immigrants a month.[2] Half were individuals of meager means, most of them Zionist pioneers who had received immigration certificates from British authorities under the expectation that they were assured work, for the Zionist executive had committed itself to be responsible for their livelihood during at least the first year. Due to the rapid increase in immigration and the character of the immigrants (pioneering laborers), membership in Kupat Holim witnessed a sharp increase. The membership rosters grew from 5,700 members (10,200 with family members) in 1922 to 6,600 members (15,000 with family members) in 1924. At the end of 1926 Kupat Holim rosters encompassed 15,364 members, covering 29,000 persons with family members.[3] Most were people of modest or no means, thus the increase in membership was not accompanied by an equal increase in revenues. In fact, Kenivsky-Kenev noted that revenue dropped by 30% per capita, primarily because a significant number of the Fourth Aliyah were heads of large families, not single persons as had been the case with previous waves of immigration, while membership dues were paid by the head of the family, regardless of the number of dependents. Furthermore, non-paying dependents included not only a member's spouse and offspring, but also his or her parents. Kupat Holim found itself facing serious organizational problems in both financing and providing services to its membership. Only the third convention of the Federation of Labor (1927) required spouses of members to register separately for membership in the fund, paying 50% of regular membership dues, with a small additional payment for coverage for the member's parents. A working spouse was required to pay full dues.

DIFFICULTIES COLLECTING DUES AND KUPAT HOLIM'S BUDGET DEFICIT

In mid 1924, Kupat Holim openly formulated a question of principle that would remain on its agenda to this day: Should the fund operate according to the fiscal abilities—that is, the dues of its members—or according to needs—the health of its members—when at the time costs were twice the revenue from dues? In an account of Kupat Holim's financial state in 1923, the fund's director, Eliezer Perlson, wrote: "The members' payments are about 50% of Kupat Holim's expenditures in assisting members."[4]

In a report of the fiscal status of the fund at the close of 1923, the Kupat Holim treasurer, Reuven Shenkar, wrote that out of the 25,000 Egyptian pounds laid out by the fund, only 57% was financed by membership dues, while the rest came from other sources. In addition, Kupat Holim carried the burden of a 7,500 Egyptian pound deficit.[5]

Kupat Holim's financial troubles were already evident in mid-1923 prior to the Fourth Aliyah, as preparations were being made to set the 1924 budget. Reuven Shenkar wrote in his report in June 1923 that

> The situation in Eretz Israel has turned for the worse. From all the regional offices we receive news of reductions in revenues, the number of sick in all places continues to rise, the hospitals are filled with our patients, tens of members wait in line for convalescence facilities, many members have become invalids and the situation has become more arduous.[6]

Shenkar pinpointed the primary factors for the fund's straits: outstanding debts, an operating deficit, lack of employment and with it reduction in payment of dues by members, and the refusal of many employers to pay the parallel tax. Shenkar stressed that

> If we won't receive a loan in the future, we will be forced to suspend part of our work…will not be able to arrange payment of promissory notes and will have to close a portion of our sick rooms.[7]

A July–August 1923 report by the Federation of Labor on the status of Kupat Holim also speaks of the severe economic straits of the fund. As to the source of Kupat Holim's troubles, the report spoke of

> [c]easeless wanderings of many kibbutzim….Most of the new immigrants almost automatically enter Kupat Holim and further burden all the more the situation of Kupat Holim….Lack of work has of late become a common phenomena on the state of Kupat Holim….Most providers of work dodge payment of the parallel tax to Kupat Holim….Lack of beds for the sick impacts negatively on the economic situation….Despite this situation, no Yishuv institution—not Hadassah and not the Zionist executive—has considered it necessary to itself carry the weight of responsibility for the health situation from these standpoints….Under such conditions only the local working public together with Kupat Holim is forced to take on its shoulder all the burden of medical assistance.[8]

Shenkar's reports and other correspondence at the close of 1923 and the beginning of 1924 repeatedly cite the arduous straits of Kupat Holim. In all, Shenkar reiterates the causes: lack of work, refusal of employers to pay the parallel tax, lack of beds in hospitals, and meager assistance from other Zionist institutions.

THE COOPERATIVE AGRICULTURAL SETTLEMENTS AND KUPAT HOLIM DUES

Many letters of complaint were sent to the Labor Battalion's companies concerning non-payment of dues that hindered Kupat Holim operations. Not only the Battalion, however, owed money to Kupat Holim. In a letter to the Zionist executive, Shenkar told of settlements that owed two years of back dues, debts to the magnitude of 2,000 Egyptian pounds. The kibbutzim Kinneret, Degania- B, Tel-Chai, Machanyim, and Ayelet Hashachar were among the primary guilty parties. Kupat Holim was entitled to withdraw medical services from a member who did not pay his or her debts for a period of more than six months, but there was no clause in the health fund's regulations governing negligence in paying debts by an entire cooperative settlement. What concerned Kupat Holim was primarily the moral question: Whether it was appropriate to withdraw medical services from an agricultural settlement comprised of dozens of members due to a financial debt, when it was clear to all what the ramifications of such a decision would be.

In July 1923, for the first time, the question of withholding medical assistance from cooperative settlements due to debts was raised by the Kupat Holim directorate. The directorate resolved that such settlements should be forewarned that if they did not arrange for settling their accounts, Kupat Holim would instruct its staff to leave the settlement and terminate medical services.

The Kupat Holim directorate even turned to the executive committee of the Federation of Labor requesting that a special session be convened to address Kupat Holim's situation. The Agricultural directorate, a roof organization under whose auspices the cooperatives operated, demanded a special discussion, demanding that the level of dues paid by the settlements be reduced, and higher dues paid by laborers in the cities whose economic situations were better. In October 1923, the executive committee published an announcement in *Briut HaOved* (The Worker's Health bulletin) of a "special council on Kupat Holim matters" (later termed a "convention") together with the Agricultural directorate and the executive committee of the Federation of Labor. On the agenda was the

> [a]rrangement of the settlements' old debts and collection of payments in the future. In addition

> the places where foreclosure or stoppage of assistance would be carried out should be determined. In the case of the latter, consent of the executive council is required.[9]

Two weeks latter, David Zakai, a member of the secretariat of the executive committee of Kupat Holim, sent a letter to the Kupat Holim directorate in which he expressed support for the decision to foreclose on assets and suspend medical assistance to cooperative settlements that refused to arrange payment of their outstanding debts to Kupat Holim.

Together with publication of the letter, David Zakai and Yitzhak Ben-Zvi, both members of the executive committee, sent warning letters and foreclosures to the kibbutzim Machanayim, Balforia, Kinneret, Kfar Giladi, Ayelet Hashachar, and Tel-Chai stressing that "for your part, there has not been the necessary efforts to schedule your debts to Kupat Holim."

The letter raised not only the matter of payment of the debt, but also the moral position of the settlement that had thrown off the mantle of responsibility vis-à-vis a fraternal Federation institution, Kupat Holim. A settlement that approached the Kupat Holim directorate and demonstrated a willingness to pay and requested rescheduling of its debts in keeping with its financial abilities generally received a positive response and payment was postponed or extended. A letter from the Kupat Holim directorate to the executive committee of the Federation of Labor (August 1923), concerning cooperative settlements with outstanding debts, stated:

> Taking into account the arduous circumstances of kibbutz Ein-Harod, kibbutz Tel-Yosef and kibbutz Beit Alpha we have resolved to negotiate with these settlements and assist them in better arranging assistance to these spots....We have seen our way to make it possible to add to these settlements a certain sum to ease the situation.[10]

Despite its difficult financial straits, Kupat Holim did not behave in an arbitrary manner with debt-ridden cooperative settlements, but always chose to seek cooperation and mutual understandings. This is reflected clearly in the case when the Labor Battalion's company in

Jerusalem ignored Kupat Holim's demand to settle its payments. Eliezer Perlson wrote to the Labor Battalion members in December 1923:

> We must draw your attention [to the fact] that this attitude towards a Federation institution undermines and destroys any institution and it would be worthwhile to finally take note of this....We think that continuation of this situation is total demoralization that endangers all the work of Kupat Holim, and within a week's time from today if this company will not arrange its payments, we believe it is necessary to cease all medical assistance to it, and for this we request your consent.[11]

Kupat Holim's demand to foreclose on funding and suspend medical assistance, with the consent of the Federation of Labor's executive committee, did not always go over well. The Labor Battalion in Jerusalem demanded arbitration with Kupat Holim in the wake of withdrawal of assistance to its members; kibbutz Beit, that settled temporarily near Nahalal, brought charges against the fund for demanding payment of debts despite the tough economic straits of the fledgling kibbutz. In March 1925, after failing to reach an agreement with Kupat Holim, the secretary of the kibbutz wrote the Federation of Labor's executive about the issue requesting support:

> As you know, our kibbutz has suffered for two years in Nahalal due to lack of work and therefore was not able to fully pay Kupat Holim dues during this period....Kupat Holim turned to us of late regarding liquidation of this debt and threatened us with cession of all assistance if we will not dispatch what is owned it....As you know our work situation does not permit us any possibility to even think today of paying debts such as this as long as we have not received new work....Therefore we request that you approach Kupat Holim and explain our situation to it so it will cease threatening us every time with cessation of medical assistance.[12]

The Federation executive committee charged with arbitrating the issue abstained from ruling on the matter. In a letter to Kupat Holim, the executive committee requested that Kupat Holim be considerate of the kibbutz's difficult finances, passing responsibility for a decision on to the Kupat Holim directorate.

Did Kupat Holim actually cut off medical assistance to the cooperative settlements as it had threatened to do? A letter from the executive committee of the Federation of Labor to the Kupat Holim directorate regarding kibbutz Beit dealt with this issue in detail:

> Ceasing medical assistance will impact badly on the health status of its members and we hope you will refrain from it, for you have not seized such vehicles as this towards other kibbutzim to date.[13]

It seems that in most cases, Kupat Holim did not implement its threats. The organization remained stuck between the anvil and the hammer. While the executive committee of the Federation of Labor permitted the health fund to employ all its power to increase collection of dues, it also took measures to link such a decision with its ramifications, that is, the complex significance of such a step as withholding medical care, thus influencing the way Kupat Holim responded in practice. Withholding medical aid to settlements because of outstanding debts had political significance as well, so the executive committee of the Federation of Labor was extremely prudent in taking such a step.

In October 1925, the Kupat Holim directorate announced to kibbutz Tel-Chai and kibbutz Kfar Giladi that medical assistance would be stopped due to ongoing debts dating back to 1923. This was not the first time that the Kupat Holim directorate threatened the two kibbutzim with a cut-off of medical services, but until this point there had been no attempts to carry out the threat. The fund finally took action, explaining the rationale:

> Such behavior by these collectives was liable to endanger the foundations for the fiscal existence of Kupat Holim, for what is permissible for kibbutz Kfar Giladi and kibbutz Tel-Chai is permissible for any other settlement site. We therefore request that the executive committee approve cessation of medical assistance to these collectives.[14]

When it became clear that Kupat Holim intended to follow through on its threat, members of kibbutz Tel-Chai and kibbutz Kfar Giladi took counter measures: They turned to Hadassah and requested it take responsibility for providing medical assistance to their settlements.

Feeling ran high in Kupat Holim. For the first time, a cooperative settlement had taken a political step that threatened the status of the fund. In an agitated letter to the executive committee, Shenkar requested that the Federation of Labor deal with the matter, closing his letter by asking rhetorically: "Have we indeed reached a [*sic*] Breakthrough such as this?"[15]

At the same time, Eliezer Perlson and Yitzhak Kenivsky-Kenev turned to Hadassah management to investigate who had initiated the appeal, Hadassah or the kibbutz. They feared that should Hadassah penetrate kibbutz Tel-Chai and kibbutz Kfar Giladi, it would undermine the status of Kupat Holim, and other cooperative settlements would seek to take similar steps in order to avoid payment of their debts to Kupat Holim. But Kupat Holim's fears were ungrounded. The entire episode emanated from an ideological schism that had developed during this period—between the Federation of Labor and the Labor Battalion in which whose members in kibbutz Tel-Chai and kibbutz Kfar Giladi were indirectly involved. The dispute continued until 1927, and was finally resolved when members of the Battalion left the kibbutzim, at which point the two kibbutzim placed themselves again under the authority of the Federation of Labor and Kupat Holim.

GROUP PAYMENTS AND ORGANIZATIONAL AUTHORITY

Historians Zeev Tzachor and Shabtai Tevet believe that there were Zionist leaders, particularly Ben-Gurion, who took advantage of the distress of the cooperative settlements and the threat to cut off medical assistance for political gain. After the Ein-Harod episode (see chapter 5), Ben-Gurion was reluctant to openly use medical aid as a cohesive political measure, and from that point on he employed mutual assistance at the base of Kupat Holim as a means of enforcing his authority. Thus, in February 1924, Ben-Gurion announced: "Assistance to those groups that cannot pay dues to Kupat Holim must be discontinued. We can't simply be generous. Kupat Holim is an institution of mutual assistance."[16]

In the dispute between kibbutz Kfar Giladi, kibbutz Tel-Chai, and Kupat Holim the heads of Kupat Holim and the executive committee headed by Ben-Gurion claimed that medical aid had been withheld due to outstanding debts, while the Labor Battalion's directorate claimed the step was really a political sanction designed to prevent unification of Tel-Chai and Kfar Giladi under Battalion leadership. Reading between the lines in the two episodes, it appears that that there is substance to the Battalion's accusations, and that the debts served merely as an excuse for political sanctions, although officially this could not be proven.

In other cases, mobilization of the power of Kupat Holim as an essential service was employed openly. The cooperative farm Nachlat Yehuda was a case in point. A letter of 11 August 1925 from the executive committee to Kupat Holim directorate ordered:

> The executive committee of the Federation of Labor has moved to cease all Federation relationships with the settlement Nachalat Yehuda due to the farm's lack of compliance with directives and resolutions of the Agricultural directorate and the executive committee. We request to begin immediately to liquidate your institutions in Nachalat Yehuda and to cease all aid to the farm for two weeks, from today.[17]

The dispute between Nachalat Yehuda and Kupat Holim focused on the economic distress of the farm, and the refusal of Kupat Holim to negotiate with each member separately. The fund demanded that the farm governing committee take responsibility for paying for every member of the farm without exception, and in such a case Kupat Holim would be willing to provide medical services and reschedule the farm's payments over an extended period.

In the controversy over Nachalat Yehuda, the principle question was whether Kupat Holim was justified in demanding that the cooperative settlements take responsibility vis-à-vis the health fund as a group, while laborers in the city were permitted to join Kupat Holim in an individual basis. Why should an entire farm be punished with withdrawal of medical assistance because a handful of members refused to pay their dues to Kupat Holim? The question of enforcing the authority of the fund over the cooperative settlements was raised time and again in years to come. Kupat Holim argued that from a fiscal standpoint, it could not maintain a clinic on-site if some members of a farm did not participate in its maintenance; if the farm governing committee could not ensure that all members paid their dues, medical assistance would be withheld on-site and the members of Nachalat Yehuda could receive medical services in Rishon le-Zion. Here as well the primary justification was the principle of "mutual assistance." The Federation's executive committee utilized the distress of Nachalat Yehuda and the farm's rejection of Kupat Holim's and the Agricultural directorate's demands in order to enforce its own authority over the farm.

The issue of withdrawal of medical assistance to settlements owing dues was discussed openly in the press, in letters from cooperative settlements against Kupat Holim, and reports on deliberations within the health fund on this issue. In September 1925, *Davar* published a complaint by farm Tivon concerning withdrawal of medical assistance and the great distress facing the farm. The members of Tivon viewed closure of the clinic as a criminal act and protested to the executive committee of the Federation of Labor. Because a large number of construction workers who were not members of the farm but resided in Tivon had been adversely affected by the dispute, Kupat Holim reopened the clinic, but services were provided to laborers only. Such selective provision of medical services only worsened the dispute. The Kupat Holim directorate responded unequivocally:

> Failure of the members for a year to fulfill their duties towards the medical institution, based on the principle of mutual assistance, strips them of all right to this assistance....[T]his is a necessity stemming from endurance of public interests and the very existence of medical assistance on the basis of reciprocity.[18]

In Tivon, as in Nachalat Yehuda, Kupat Holim demanded group liability of the farm as a whole for membership in the health fund and payment of dues. The ideological justification—the principle of mutual assistance—together with justifications based on economic feasibility served as a first-rate vehicle for enforcing organizational authority over settlements and indirectly enhancing membership rosters of Kupat Holim. But all attempts to broaden dues collection among the cooperative settlements and members of Kupat Holim, and all the ongoing conflicts over the cost of dues, did not solve the budgetary problems of Kupat Holim.

THE CRISIS OF THE FOURTH ALIYAH

In September 1925, three months prior to the special convention of the Kupat Holim council, the first signs of economic crisis began to appear in Eretz Israel. Brief items concerning the "economic situation" began to appear in the daily press and the newspapers often employed the word "crisis" to describe prevailing conditions. The number of unemployed steadily grew, accelerated growth in building construction that had typified 1924 diminished, and merchants and craftspersons tied to the construction industry closed their businesses and went bankrupt. Thousands of construction workers (most of them day laborers) were left without work. The flow of investment capital from abroad came to a stop, prices dropped, and bank credit was severely curtailed. Signs of economic crisis began to appear at the end of 1925, increasing in 1926 into one of the worse crises the Yishuv was to face during the entire period of the British Mandate over Eretz Israel.

Kupat Holim quickly felt the impact of the crisis. Due to continued immigration and the large number of unemployed, payment of dues by members shrunk. Kupat Holim regulations stipulated that unemployed members and their families would continue to receive health services even if they were unable to pay dues, thus creating a tremendous additional burden on the finances of Kupat Holim. The financial state of the health fund became all the more severe.

On 10 December 1925 the Kupat Holim council convened for the first time. Deliberations focused on the financial status of the health fund in light of the growing economic crisis. In media reports about the council, it was announced:

> The inability to clarify the basic questions in all their scope in the council of the Federation of Labor, requires us to seek another avenue for making our public a partner in solving the questions, in order

> that [the public] be able to influence the institution directly and take responsibility for its operations[19]

The central question on the council's agenda was how the fund should function—"according to need or according to ability"? However, because of the economic distress of Kupat Holim's insurees and the operational difficulties encountered by the fund, the council members refrained from taking a decisive stand or formulating practical solutions. In the closing resolutions, the council moved to make all efforts to increase Kupat Holim revenues and curtail expenditures, without setting any binding framework.

The participants proposed that the duty of dual membership in the Federation and Kupat Holim be enforced to bolster the rosters and increase revenues, to work towards bringing in members of Hapoel Hamizrachi into Kupat Holim, to increase the number of employers paying the parallel tax, and to approach the British Mandate government with a demand for legislation of a compulsory health insurance law that would be instituted through the auspices of Kupat Holim (see chapter 9). All agreed that expenditures must be curtailed, but without curtailing the scope of medical assistance rendered to members. Blame was leveled at the Zionist executive that had decreased its financial support of Kupat Holim, a move that had worsened the fund's deficit significantly. Part of the blame was also directed towards the Federation of Labor for declining to partake in finding a solution to Kupat Holim's difficulties. The only operative decision taken after a week of deliberations was to establish a regular council that would convene once every three months to discuss Kupat Holim's problems. No solution to resolve the health fund's fiscal problems was found.

Despite the determination of the 1925 Kupat Holim council to find a workable plan that would improve the fund's condition, realization remained a distant goal. One of the most trying years for the Yishuv was 1926. Unemployment among workers rose to 35%. Kupat Holim, that at the time encompassed a membership of 15,000, continued to cover 4,000 unemployed members—27%.[20] The fund's revenues shrunk, many cooperative settlements owed up to two years in back dues that Kupat Holim was unable to collect. The health fund sunk into debt, found itself unable to keep up with payment of interest, and faced foreclosure on its assets due to tardiness in payment of property taxes to the Mandate government.

In January 1926, when apprehension grew that Kupat Holim might face bankruptcy if sources of financial assistance were not found, the Kupat Holim directorate turned to the management of Bank Hapoalim (The Workers' Bank)—a sister Federation institution—to request assistance. In a report to the bank's management, Eliezer Perlson presented the financial state of the fund and analyzed the factors contributing to Kupat Holim's large deficit. Perlson stressed the imperative of a substantial investment in equipment:

> As it is known, Kupat Holim began working [with] almost no inventory. Expansion of operation and its improvement are impossible without inventory and [medical] instruments, [which] requires financial investment. For this purpose we have never received any monies from the Zionist executive from its regular budget, and due to this, the fiscal state of Kupat Holim has become so difficult....Investments have been to the sum of 11,167 Egyptian pounds that has been taken from [the fund's] turnover [working capital], whose absence is now felt in all its force.[21]

Perlson went on to explain why Kupat Holim could not use its assets as security to secure a regular loan, enumerating closure of credit lines from various institutions and the burden of high monthly payments on short-term loans that the fund had already been forced to take out. Kupat Holim viewed Bank Hapoalim as their last option. In his report, Perlson warned explicitly that without immediate assistance from the bank, the fund would be closed:

> We know that fulfilling our request is not easy for Bank Hapoalim, but we hope you will be willing to allow us get through this period of crisis until we will have the ability to find a radical solution to Kupat Holim's situation, and will not allow one of the most important institutions of the working public to be destroyed.[22]

Bank Hapoalim, however, did not answer Kupat Holim's plea, except in part, primarily because it too had been hard hit by the recession. In a March 1926 report to the executive committee of the Federation of Labor on the financial status of the fund, the Kupat Holim directorate noted that Bank Hapoalim had indeed taken it upon itself to liquidate a 3,000-pound loan given to Kupat Holim by the Anglo-Palestine Bank (today, Bank Leumi), but this action had led to closure of credit lines at *both* banks, and Kupat Holim's state remained as difficult as ever. The report spoke of difficulties releasing medications and instruments from customs, inability to purchase essential commodities, and the danger of closure of convalescence facilities. Even Hamashbir, a Federation institution, refrained from accepting promissory notes from Kupat Holim and closed its doors to the health fund. In the conclusion to the report, Perlson requested that the executive committee be mobilized to assist the health fund in obtaining further funding:

> The radical measures that could save Kupat Holim is obtaining 10,000 Egyptian pounds. We know for the moment the executive committee doesn't have the ability to obtain this amount right know, but you must help us vigorously and rapidly to seek sources to fill this amount…within a year and a half. Despite the fact that we explained the seriousness of the situation, the executive committee did not assist us in practice to save the situation.[23]

Kupat Holim's complaint had little effect. The economic crisis had undermined the health of the Federation of Labor just like the rest of the economy. Hamashbir and a host of cooperative industries also stood in danger of going bankrupt. The Federation sought to fight unemployment by expanding the number employed in public works, mobilizing funding to initiate work projects, providing work to laborers, and assisting the unemployed. Under such circumstances, the ability of the Federation to come to the aid of Kupat Holim, particularly when the main task was the war on unemployment and weathering the economic crisis, putting the health of the workers in a position of secondary importance.

THE FIRST KUPAT HOLIM INQUIRY COMMISSION (1926)

The arduous economic straits of Kupat Holim, and its numerous appeals to other institutions for economic assistance, prompted the Zionist executive under the leadership of Nachum Sokolov to come to Kupat Holim's aid. The Zionist executive, which had organized to assist in dealing with the economic crisis in Eretz Israel, was prepared to help Kupat Holim as well, but under the condition that there would be a comprehensive review of the fund's operation. At the close of 1926, the Zionist executive requested that the Yishuv's health committee establish an inquiry commission to examine the fiscal state of Kupat Holim. The members appointed to the commission were Dr. Feller (a statistician and member of the Zionist executive), Dr. Newak (head of the medical department of Kupat Holim), and Eliezer Bavli (treasurer of the Zionist executive). The members of the commission took upon themselves to conclude their work and submit an account to the Zionist executive and the Yishuv's health committee within twelves months. The commission dealt with two primary issues: The reasons for Kupat Holim's large deficit and ways to scale it down, and examination of Kupat Holim's organizational methods and the efficiency of the health fund's operation.

In April 1927, the commission published an interim report that focused on the fiscal issues. Members of the commission said that the primary reason for the deficit was large investments in buildings and equipment and care for a large number of unemployed and new immigrants. This deficit was accompanied by an operating deficit that had grown and during the first four years of the fund's operation. The report revealed:

> In the commission's opinion, it is essential to find a solution to cover all the debts. But taking into account that there is no possibility of obtaining such sums…the commission finds it proper to provide the amount needed immediately of 19,000 Egyptian pounds and to find a way to obtain this amount from the Zionist executive.[24]

The commission members also proposed that Kupat Holim put all its assets down as security on a long-term loan from Bank Hapoalim.

The commission's posture was surprising, for in the years 1924–1926 the Zionist executive had reduced the scope of its participation in Kupat Holim's budget, and now members of the inquiry commission, appointed by the Zionist executive itself, called upon the executive to take responsibility for covering most of the deficit that endangered the operation of Kupat Holim. The commission members noted in their conclusions that their recommendations were taken after conferring with members of the Zionist executive in Eretz Israel and London, and that they knew the importance of ensuring the continued operation of Kupat Holim.

The first Kupat Holim inquiry commission submitted its summary report to the Yishuv's health committee and the Zionist executive on 1 July 1927. Unlike the interim report that dealt primarily with the deficit and how to meet it, the summary report dealt largely with the organization of the fund and the efficiency of its operation. The members did not stop at a perfunctory overview. In order to fathom the source of the fund's economic difficulties in detail, members of the commission examined each district, seeking to pinpoint centers of waste and poor organization. This was the first serious examination of the work of Kupat Holim to be carried out from the time of its conception.

In its conclusion, the commission wrote:

> The Kupat Holim medical personnel is larger than the objective need and the ability of the institution....The [Kupat Holim] directorate does not take into account the need for fair and proportional allocation of expenditures in the districts according to their revenue....[T]he present method of cure via specialists is considered improper and exaggerated, in that in most instances general practitioners could treat the sick without the need for specialists.[25]

The commission also found that Kupat Holim was burdened by a higher-than-necessary number of employees engaged in administration and accounting.

From examination of the data submitted by the commission in their summary report, it becomes evident that there was an imbalance in allocation of budgets among the districts and lack of proportion between revenue from districts and their expenditures. In Jerusalem, for instance, revenue rose by 60% while expenditures rose by only 11%, while in Tel Aviv revenues rose by 50% and expenditures by 65% over the previous year. In the estimation of the commission, this was unjustified.

The commission wrote in its conclusions:

> It is essential to find a solution to cover the entire debt....The authority of the districts should be

> expanded even to the point of leaving the [Kupat Holim] directorate solely with core functions and supervision of districts....It is essential to seek a solution to the question of payment for the unemployed....The commission notes the need to curtail referral of patients to all sorts of medical assistance. The commission thinks that it is necessary to change the salary grade of the Federation that it believes [contributes to] lack of regularity in the budget and in general increases the cost of expenditures, and introduce in its place a [wage] scale according to post and place of work. [26]

In order to enhance the health fund's financial state, the commission proposed that a flexible salary scheme be adopted where workers would be employed according to need of each clinic and district separately, and not according to a uniform norm. The commission also called for "Reorganization of Kupat Holim...fiscal rehabilitation...decentralization of administrative work of Kupat Holim...and curtailment of administrative personnel."

In the commission's view, the fund's management was far too centralized and in order to economize their operation, the Kupat Holim directorate should share operative authority with the branches and limit its role to setting policy, supervision, and inspection.

In their summary, members of the commission added a piece of data and a conclusion that was not within the scope of their appointment, but which the members felt should be addressed:

> The Federation of Labor should do its duty vis-à-vis expansion of the number of Kupat Holim members, for it is known that a large number of Federation members are outside Kupat Holim.[27]

In fact this was a reiteration of the ongoing call of Kupat Holim to institute in practice the decision that required all members of the Federation of Labor to also be members of Kupat Holim. Up to this point, the Federation had refrained from demanding compliance with this decision out of fear that such a demand would lead to a reduction in membership in the Federation.

Despite harsh conclusions concerning flaws in Kupat Holim's operation, the commission stressed in its closing remarks the importance of Kupat Holim as an essential body, noting:

> The tremendous national and social value of Kupat Holim as a public health institution…already fulfilling a central role in work in the medical field in Eretz Israel, requires indeed material and moral assistance to the institution, and much vigilance for its needs on the part of all institutions responsible for health matters and settlement work in Eretz Israel.[28]

At the time this report was published, Kupat Holim encompassed 29,000 persons including members and their dependents—that is, 20 percent of the population of the Yishuv. Kupat Holim provided medical care primarily to laborers and agricultural settlements on the periphery, in areas that Hadassah's medical services did not reach. The fund cared for new immigrants and the unemployed and played an active role in ensuring medical assistance to agricultural settlements of all persuasions. The importance of Kupat Holim was clear to members of the Zionist executive and members of the commission, and the commission took pains to cite this clearly in its conclusions as the primary reason for its decision to extend assistance to the health fund and prevent its fall.

As for the fiscal difficulties facing Kupat Holim, the commission recommended that the Zionist movement in Eretz Israel cover the funds deficit within four years. Responsibility for liquidating past debts was tied to reorganization and implementation of a financial rehabilitation plan along the lines formulated by the commission. At a meeting convened on 11 July 1927, the Yishuv's health committee approved and adopted the inquiry commission's conclusions and arrangements for coverage of Kupat Holim's debts within four years, as recommended. The health committee's decision did not stipulate openly that coverage of the deficit hinged on implementation of the commission's recommendations, but the wording and scheduling of payment over four years underscored the tie between the two clauses.

In a letter of response sent in the name of the Kupat Holim directorate to Eliezer Bavli, treasurer of the Zionist executive and a member of the commission, Eliezer Perlson expressed the Kupat Holim directorate's agreement with most of the commission's findings. Perlson reinforced the commission's findings that most of the deficit stemmed from the overall economic distress prevailing in the Yishuv and large investments in equipment, buildings, and medications. His only reservations concerned areas that were not directly tied to Kupat Holim. Perlson believed that there was little chance that the Federation of Labor would act to realize the requirement that all its own members be members of Kupat Holim, primarily because a large portion of the Federation's membership received medical services gratis from Hadassah institutions. Perlson also questioned the willingness of the Zionist executive to pay the dues of the unemployed and called upon the Zionist executive to secure the participation of the Mandate government in supporting Kupat Holim's budget, for Kupat Holim had no means of doing so on its own. Despite his agreement with most of the commission's findings and recommendations, Perlson argued that Kupat Holim should not bear all the guilt for the severe economic crisis it faced, and that part of the responsibility was the Zionist executive's. In the past the Zionist executive had not been prepared to invest significant sums in Kupat Holim and to assist in covering its expenditures, and in Perlson's opinion this was one of the factors that had led to the crisis within the organization. In closing, Perlson expressed Kupat Holim's readiness to reorganize its work methods in accordance with the commission's recommendations, and requested the Zionist executive's assistance in carrying them out.

At the same time, Kupat Holim published a notice in the newspaper *Davar* on 25 May 1927 calling upon health fund members to take personal responsibility "to liquidate their debts and pay their dues punctually, for any delay or postponement in your payments endangers the existence of the institution."[29] *Davar* editorially announced that the inquiry commission had concluded its work, but did not disclose the details of its conclusions, and concluded:

> The Kupat Holim directorate discussed the details of the report and approved a whole series of proposals for implementation. The other suggestions that are not agreed with within the directorate will be raised for clarification within the authorized organization of the Federation of Labor, the executive committee and the Zionist executive.[30]

Later in the article, however, it becomes apparent that there were intentions to carry out the recommendations, without admitting so publicly:

> Regarding Kupat Holim's difficult fiscal situation, the fund's directorate resolved to curtail its work…including: reduction in medical and administrative personnel, reduction in expenditures at urban clinics, and so forth. [31]

At the same time, the health fund announced a dramatic change in the workings of the central clinic in Tel Aviv:

> Kupat Holim has resolved therefore to go over to a decentralized system in the order of its medical work in Tel Aviv and to introduce changes in the manner of providing assistance. In the main sectors of the city, branch clinics will be opened, and every member of Kupat Holim will have to go to the regional clinic closest to his neighborhood when sick. The assistance of a specialist will be given only on orders of the branch doctor.[32]

The fund explained that this change would enhance accessibility to the clinic within walking distance of the member's home.

> This method is employed all the time in the work of Kupat Holim outside the cities and has had good results in creating an ongoing tie between the physician and the patent. In the city as well, this method will ease things for the sick who will not need to drag themselves to the clinic and wait a long time.[33]

In retrospect, it is clear that this was the most important change in the operation of Kupat Holim. Weight was shifted from specialists to family medicine, from a central clinic to neighborhood-district clinics, as had been the case in agricultural settlements and neighborhoods outside the main cities. The "rural" model, that became the order of the day in the city and instituted in the wake of the inquiry committee's recommendations, was rapidly adopted and became the dominant operational pattern of Kupat Holim. It is employed to this day, with only small variations. The rural clinic and its intimate character remained the working model of Kupat Holim even during years that most of the fund's insurees were urban workers.

To what degree did Kupat Holim make strides in economizing and streamlining its operation? On the 20 June 1927, in a detailed article published in *Davar*, the Kupat Holim directorate detailed the steps it had taken: 10 percent cuts in salaries; curtailment of the work of doctors in nine points of settlement; reduction in the work of paramedics in fifteen other settlements; dismissal of six of thirty-one of the fund's administrative staff throughout the country (a 20 percent cutback in personnel); and cutbacks in all kinds of expenditures such as maintenance of the convalescence facility in the village of Motza. Together with institution of these cutbacks, the Kupat Holim directorate made a new suggestion: to establish a supervisory committee that would oversee the fund's operation.

The Kupat Holim directorate appointed four members who served, for all intents and purposes, as the fund's only operational management. Up to this point, there had been no other body that oversaw the tie between Kupat Holim's management and its members, or monitored the work of the management itself. The decision to establish a supervisory committee was confirmed by the third convention of the Federation of Labor at the end of 1927. The resolution stipulated that the committee would engage in setting the fund's budget, oversee the work of the fund's management (i.e., the Kupat Holim directorate), serve as an arbitrator in differences of opinion between the directorate and the branches, oversee outlay of funds, acquisitions, investments, and sales, approve contracts, and choose members of the Kupat Holim directorate. Furthermore, it was resolved that the committee would be comprised jointly of representatives of the insurees, the Federation of Labor, and Kupat Holim.

The first supervisory committee of Kupat Holim was appointed in 1928. Dr. Moshe Beilenson, a medical doctor and journalist, was appointed head of the committee. Other committee members were chosen from among longtime Federation activists and leaders in the Yishuv: Yosef Baratz from kibbutz Degania, a member of the Federation of Labor's inner circle and a member of the executive committee; Neta Goldberg-Harpaz, a member of the Agricultural directorate (the representative body of the cooperative agricultural sector); Dr. Avraham Katznelson, who had been a member of the secretariat for health matters of the National Committee; Pinchas Rashish, a member of the executive committee of the Federation; Yaakov Ori, a member of Hapoel Hatzair; and Golda Meirson-Meir, a member of the women laborers' council. One can assume that the standing of the personalities chosen to serve on the supervisory committee in practice determined the importance and degree of authority allotted the supervisory body within the organization itself and the stature and weight of the body in external affairs as a representative body of Kupat Holim vis-à-vis the Federation. Examination of the lineup and their stature within the Federation hierarchy reveals that none hailed from among the most prominent leaders of the Yishuv at the time, and most lacked any political clout. Only Dr. Moshe Beilenson, the chairperson of the supervisory committee, was a member of the editorial board of *Davar* and a personal friend of Berl Katznelson, a person of influence. The appointment of individuals who were not key figures reflects the status of Kupat Holim as an institution of secondary importance among an array of Federation of Labor institutions (for instance, of lesser importance than Solel Boneh). One may assume that the choice impacted on the degree of influence the committee wielded within the Federation of Labor and beyond.

In practice, the supervisory committee served as the supreme body within the Kupat Holim hierarchy, and its members were the ones who formulated policy and directed the management in the fund's operation. This mode of operation remained in effect until the establishment of the state of Israel in 1948.

THE KUPAT HOLIM BUDGET IN TIME OF CRISIS

The willingness of Kupat Holim to implement the conclusions of the inquiry committee and coverage of Kupat Holim's deficit by the Zionist directorate did not solve the health fund's operational difficulties from a fiscal standpoint, although these steps eased the crisis and forestalled bankruptcy. In 1927 the crisis in the economy reached new heights: Solel Boneh stood on the verge of bankruptcy, spreading demoralization within the Yishuv. The unemployment rate among salaried workers reached 35% (the unemployment rate for 1926), thousands left the country, and immigration came to a standstill. Kupat Holim was forced to treat thousands of unemployed who ceased to pay their dues but still enjoyed coverage. On the 24 August 1927 the Kupat Holim directorate announced in *Davar* that four thousand unemployed members of the fund who had not paid their dues continued to receive health services, that payment of the parallel tax had been suspended for firms such as Solel Boneh, and that an outbreak of malaria further exacerbated a trying situation. In a public proclamation, members of Kupat Holim turned to the executive committee of the Federation of Labor demanding

> that all members, every farm, kibbutz and institution, should help Kupat Holim to the best of its ability. Every member working in any kind of work is called upon to pay his dues promptly; every member, institution and farm that owes money to Kupat Holim is called upon to make all efforts and liquidate what is coming to the institution. Our members must remember: any delay of their payments to Kupat Holim endangers the existence of the institution and also deprives us of the ability to extend assistance to workers and those without work during these trying times.[34]

At the same time, the Kupat Holim directorate, for the first time, turned to the finance department of the Yishuv's health committee in order to prepare the health fund's 1927–1928 budget with the health committee's assistance and collaboration, as part of implementation of the inquiry committee's decisions. In a letter accompanying the health committee's comments on Kupat Holim's draft budget, Dr. Yehuda Rokach wrote in the name of presidium of the health committee:

> Regarding setting the budget for Kupat Holim in the year 1927–1928, the health committee perceives two goals: a) to adjust the fund's expenditures to the objective capabilities that constitute sources of revenue for the institution, the lack of employment among members of the fund, decline in revenue from work providers, the economic state of the Zionist directorate and other [factors]. b) To formulate a plan to fully liberate the fund within a number of years from the burden of debts that the institution carries—debts that were incurred over the last 4–5 years.[35]

According to the decision of the health committee and the conclusions of the inquiry committee, the Kupat Holim budget was cut by

20 percent. However, collaboration between the Yishuv's health committee and Kupat Holim over responsibility for the budget was not a matter of charity, but constituted official recognition of Kupat Holim's special stature and importance. From the beginning of the 1920s the fund had sought economic aid from the Zionist executive and the health committee. Obtaining such support was viewed as recognition of Kupat Holim's exclusive status as *the* body destined to address the health needs of the Yishuv as a whole. The Zionist directorate and the health committee, while supporting financial backing for Kupat Holim according to their abilities, viewed Hadassah and not Kupat Holim as the central party in health matters of the Yishuv. The inquiry committee's findings that lead to collaboration and sharing of financial responsibility were what changed to a large extent the attitude of the Yishuv's health committee and the Zionist executive towards Kupat Holim. In an appendix to Kupat Holim's budget, Dr. Rokach wrote:

> One should hope that this great settlement endeavor—the only one in the field of health in Eretz Israel—will succeed in encompassing in the near future all the tens of thousands of the working public.[36]

Indications of the change in the status of Kupat Holim in the eyes of Zionist institutions can be found in the words of Yitzhak Kenivsky-Kenev, a member of the Kupat Holim directorate who wrote in *Davar* on the 23 October 1923 under the heading "Kupat Holim for the Year 1927–1928":

> Zionism has recognized its indebtedness to Kupat Holim, not only because it has extended medical aid to new points of settlement, but because the working public bears the arduous burden of building the country and conquering new places [that are] dangerous to health, and it is transparent that the colonialist [settlement] institution must participate in outlay of medical assistance for the pioneering part of the Zionist movement.

PARALLEL INVESTIGATIVE COMMISSIONS OF THE HEALTH SYSTEM IN ERETZ ISRAEL

The Fifteenth Zionist Congress opened in Basel on the 30 August 1927. The deliberations focused on the economic depression in Eretz Israel, the decline in immigration, and election of a new Zionist executive under the leadership of Harry Sacher. The new leadership, elected under pressure from Dr. Chaim Weizmann, was neutral from a political and party standpoint. Its main goal was to seek solutions to the economic crisis, to curtail deficits that had been accrued in past years, and to revitalize the economic state of the Zionist movement and settlement in Eretz Israel. Part of the congress's deliberations dealt with Kupat Holim's difficulties and the findings of the inquiry commission. The commission's findings were accepted by the new leadership of the world Zionist movement, but not their conclusions. Most of the opposition focused on the recommendation that the Zionist leadership cover the fund's deficit. Hadassah delegates participated in the deliberations, calling for a thorough examination of health services in Eretz Israel and the establishment of a unified and coordinated health system. In September 1927, in light of the commission's conclusions and Hadassah's demand for revamping health on a national level, the Zionist Congress called upon the Zionist executive in Eretz Israel and the Yishuv's health committee to establish immediately two parallel inquiry commissions: an external body from abroad—a "commission of experts" (Dr. Rozenau and Dr. Velensky)—and a local commission comprised of members of the health committee. (The congress established a similar dual configuration to examine agricultural settlement, a field of endeavor that faced a severe crisis similar to Kupat Holim's in 1925–1927.)

The congress also demanded that representatives of the Zionist directorate in Eretz Israel (Harry Sacker, Henrietta Szold, and Colonel Kisch) prepare a comprehensive plan for overall organization of health services for the Yishuv, in collaboration with all relevant health bodies (Hadassah, Kupat Holim, municipalities, and local governing councils) and with Mandate officials who were responsible for health services in both a financial and practical level. The plan was to be based on the proposals of the two parallel investigative commissions. The target date for submission of the plan to the executive committee of the Zionist Federation was set for the summer of 1928. The Fifteenth Zionist Congress even called upon the Mandate government to legislate a compulsory health insurance law, similar to the one in Great Britain. The congress hoped that with the establishment of a Labor government in the U.K., passage of such legislation would be easier—a hope that did not materialize.

On 7 June 1926, the Zionist Congress' executive received the suggestions of the parallel investigative committees for organization of health services in Eretz Israel. The two proposals called for abolition of Kupat Holim's independent status and for it to be placed under the auspices of the Zionist directorate in Eretz Israel or under the wing of Hadassah; the two bodies—Kupat Holim and Hadassah—were to provide health services to the Yishuv. Kupat Holim would have representation on the health committee or on the executive committee of Hadassah but would be subordinated to them from a fiscal standpoint. According to the proposal of the health committee's commission, Kupat Holim would enjoy partial autonomy in the operational domain and would be entitled to provide medical services by itself, stipulating that the services should be limited "[t]o the extent that [they were] needed according to local conditions and special needs of members of the fund."[37]

That is, its operation should be concentrated primarily in the agricultural sector, a domain where Hadassah had no interest in being active. The "commission of experts" from abroad on the other hand, held that Kupat Holim should curtail its mission, stipulating that the health fund should "concentrate its operation only in the field of insurance. Its medical role [should be] transferred to the health department of the Zionist executive."[38]

That is, Kupat Holim should function solely as an insuring organization and cease providing medical services as it had done up until then. The experts' prognosis reflected the decisions of the Fifteenth Zionist Congress which sought, for reasons of economy, to deliver administration of all health matters in Eretz Israel into the hands of one body—Hadassah or the Zionist executive—subsequently curtailing the role of the Kupat Holim. In the closing deliberations on the two proposals, it was stipulated that the health system in Eretz Israel should be reorganized and the details of how to do so should be worked out in separate negotiations with Hadassah, Kupat Holim, and other parties in the health field operating in Eretz Israel.

In August 1928, Kupat Holim entered into negotiations with Hadassah and representatives of the Zionist executive concerning the 1928–1929 budget, as part of efforts to implement the recommendations of the parallel investigative committees and in keeping with new directives of the Zionist Congress. Negotiations were conducted in Berlin; Eliezer Perlson and Dr. Moshe Beilenson, head of the supervisory committee of Kupat Holim, took part. In a survey for internal consumption of the Kupat Holim directorate detailing negotiations, it was cited that Kupat Holim's fiscal demands had been accepted as is, but budgeting hinged on the health fund accepting the Congress' reorganization plan in accordance with the recommendations of the commission of experts and the health committee. Kupat Holim gave its consent for execution of the plan.

Why did Kupat Holim agree to a plan that threatened its independence? From internal correspondence within the Kupat Holim directorate between August 1928 and January 1929, it becomes evident that the heads of Kupat Holim questioned the ability of the Zionist executive to carry out, in practice, any comprehensive examination of health services in Eretz Israel. Their experience had taught them that affairs were dictated by realities in Eretz Israel, not plans designed by experts from abroad. From their viewpoint, obtaining a regular budget from the Congress, even through the auspices of Hadassah, was a far more important step than coping with a general plan whose details were still fuzzy. In a summary discussion with Henrietta Szold concerning this matter, Perlson and Beilenson noted that they had been given to understand that "this question would be raised for in-depth clarification in negotiations in Eretz Israel."[39] Thus, there was no reason not to agree in general principle. The Congress had not set forth, expect in general terms, how health matters should be handled, and the details were to be settled between Hadassah and Kupat Holim—that is, things were not set in stone. In addition, in the summer of 1928, with publication of the reorganization plan, Kupat Holim had received aid from Hadassah that allowed the building of the fund's Jezreel Valley Hospital (in place of the hospital in kibbutz Ein-Harod). Kupat Holim began to expand its operation into the hospitalization realm, which until then had been solely the province of Hadassah. It seemed that prevailing conditions were stronger than re-organizational principles set by the congress and designed to neutralize Kupat Holim and undermine its primary source of strength.

During the years 1928–1929 the reorganization program accompanied budgetary discussions between Kupat Holim and Hadassah over and over again. In the summer of 1929, it was again raised, at the

Sixteenth Zionist Congress in Zurich, but even this time, the delegates refrained from taking any practical action. Unlike the previous Zionist congress, this convention took place in a more relaxed atmosphere, due to improvements of the economic situation in Eretz Israel. The congress's resolutions were general in nature and did not make any changes in Zionist policy. Tranquility in the security realm after dissipation of the 1922 disturbances[40] also moved the question of relations with the Arabs to the sidelines, the delegates having presumed wrongly that opposition to Zionist endeavors had dulled. Most of the deliberations focused on economic issues and Dr. Chaim Weizmann's efforts to establish a "Jewish agency" that would mobilize capital from Jewish capitalists (Zionist and non-Zionist) that would spur renewed economic development of the Yishuv. A review sent by the Kupat Holim directorate to the supervisory committee on the fund's operation stated:

> Negotiations in the health committee of the Congress was tense and the positions of the two institutions, Kupat Holim and Hadassah, were contradictory on a number of questions. During this negotiation it became apparent to us that on one hand it is common in Hadassah circles in America to seriously oppose the reorganization scheme of the health committee regarding Hadassah, and on the other hand, to date, managerial circles in Hadassah believe that the medical work of Kupat Holim must be concentrated in the hands of Hadassah. We must cite that lobbying activity filled with evidence, facts and statistics in this matter, extending over 7–8 years, have not proven anything to Hadassah circles including madam Szold as well, although in the health committee there is a general belief (expect for I. Kleigler) that calls for Kupat Holim's independent medical [sic] institutionism.[41]

Thus, the health committee reiterated its stand from 1926 concerning the importance of Kupat Holim. The committee argued that Kupat Holim must be broadened and not targeted for members of the Federation of Labor alone. That is, it should be come a core institution of and for the entire Yishuv, parallel to Hadassah. In a letter to

David Kaminsky, the Kupat Holim delegate in the United States Perlson wrote that the reorganization scheme and the question of Kupat Holim's role in it had generated acrimonious debate within the Hadassah leadership in the United States.

Henrietta Szold, who supported reorganization (with minor changes), found herself in the opposition and lost her position of power in Hadassah leadership. Dr. Reuven Kleigler, a member of the Yishuv's health committee, and Rose Jacobs and Irma Lindheim from Hadassah leadership in the United States opposed the changes proposed by the Zionist Congress putting Hadassah in charge of Kupat Holim's budget. Jacobs and Lindheim even threatened to withdraw from the Zionist Federation of America and to join the "non-Zionists" in Eretz Israel if the reorganization plan were carried out. The two feared in particular the heavy financial burden placed on Hadassah's shoulders under the scheme due to the unlimited support in underwriting Kupat Holim that it entailed, and the unending energies that would have to be invested in obtaining the necessary budget from the Zionist Congress for this purpose. The differences of opinion between the Zionist Federation of America and Hadassah disrupted to some degree regular payments by Hadassah to the Kupat Holim budget, but indirectly eased the pressure on Kupat Holim from the Zionist executive and the Zionist Congress over actualization of the reorganization plan: It was no longer Kupat Holim's "fault" that the reorganization plan was not being implemented. It was Hadassah's fault.

In August 1929, renewed Arab violence aimed at foiling Zionist aspirations broke out in Jerusalem and rapidly spread throughout the country. Due to the scope of the 1929 disturbances and the large number of fatal casualties (133 Jewish inhabitants), health matters were pushed onto the sidelines in deliberations within the Zionist Congress. A short time later, in October 1929, the crash of the stock market on Wall Street signaled the beginning of the Great Depression. The Great Depression had a negative impact on Hadassah and led to a marked curtailment in the scope of its activities in Eretz Israel, undermining its stature compared to Kupat Holim. Under the new circumstances; the congress's scheme for a thorough reexamination and reform of health services in Eretz Israel sunk into oblivion, and was never realized.

The Role of Kupat Holim in the 1920s

In the mid-1920s, Kupat Holim began to publish its own house organ, *Briut Haoved* (Worker's Health). The first issue opened with an editorial signed by Dr. Avraham Mendelberg entitled "The Way of Kupat Holim," which addressed the question: What should be the roles for Kupat Holim? This was, indeed, one of the most fundamental questions facing the health fund.

There were two basic approaches held by members of the fund and its management. The first viewed Kupat Holim's future as providing comprehensive medical services and caring for the social welfare of the entire population. The other viewed Kupat Holim's role in a narrow sense—providing primary care services solely to laborers. Both approaches found expression in the press and in deliberations at Kupat Holim conventions during the 1920s.

The question of Kupat Holim's future role was not merely a theoretical issue. It had deep economic ramifications that impacted immediately on the way the fund functioned.

The role of Kupat Holim as set forth by Dr. Mendelberg was not planned or carried out within a formal framework. The matter became part of the agenda because the fund stood at a crossroads that forced it to choose between acting as a key player in realization of national goals (settlement, aliyah, and so forth) and only providing medical assistance to the working public.

In Mendelberg's opinion, Kupat Holim had a national duty to defend the worker and provide him with comprehensive social insurance, and its operation should not be limited to ambulatory services only. Kupat Holim had a core role to play in settlement activity: "To settle means to make healthy—became the first rule of all the great settling Peoples."[42]

In addition to a national role, Mendelberg stressed the duty of the fund to play a role in the advancement of local medicine and

> [t]o develop our operation and our medical institutions and to establish them on strong scientific foundations on one side, and on the other hand to delve into the special pathology of Eretz Israel, partake in clarification of the medical geography of Eretz Israel.[43]

As for the fiscal difficulties that were likely to arise as a result of the expansion of Kupat Holim in the future, Mendelberg said that this issue should be solved without impairing the other missions of the fund.

A similar opinion was presented by Yitzhak Kenivsky-Kenev, a member of the directorate. Kenev-Kenivsky said that Kupat Holim must assume all the responsibility for welfare services and social insurance of the Yishuv (that is serve as both a health fund and as a framework for social security). Moreover, Kupat Holim should, together with the Federation of Labor, assume the care for *all* social classes, not just laborers as set forth in the fund's founding ordinances. In Kenev-Kenivsky's opinion, it was possible to do so through cooperation among all the settlement institutions and employers (even through legislation). Kenev-Kenivsky argued that legislation would make it possible to require all members of the Federation to join Kupat Holim, and vice versa. When the number of members would increase, the fiscal deficit would diminish, and Kupat Holim would be transformed into the core body in the realm of health services in Eretz Israel. He opposed limiting the fund's operation to immediate medical care "dictated" by the prevailing economic circumstances of the fund—an approach supported by the minimalists. Fiscal problems should be solved by increasing the number of members and expanding the fund's operations, he believed.

Examination of the ordinances in the Kupat Holim formulated by the Second Federation of Labor council in 1922 and amended in 1924 reveals another outlook on the role of the fund. According to the ordinances, members were promised health services only, not sick leave and coverage of convalescence. The ordinances were worded in concise cut-and-dry language and there is no mention whatsoever of Kupat Holim's role in Zionist settlement activity, social legislation, preventive medicine, educational activities, or responsibility for the entire Yishuv—not even expansion of the scientific foundations of medicine in Eretz Israel as proposed by Mendelberg and Kenev-Kenivsky. The ordinances' approach is pragmatic and minimalistic, confines itself solely to medical assistance in keeping with available funds, and does not perceive Kupat Holim's role in a broader national perspective. In an article entitled "The Question of the Worker's Health" Dr. Shaipra, a physician at the Hadassah Hospital in Haifa, wrote:

> [It is said that] "one who seizes too much, is left holding nothing" and it would be better if Kupat Holim will strive to stand high within the domain of its core work, the job of medical assistance to its members.[44]

When Kupat Holim opened clinics in Tel Aviv, the minimalists expressed their opposition, arguing that Kupat Holim should have continued to utilize Hadassah clinics in the cities: "Why these new and superfluous expenditures? What does it give and what does it add to Kupat Holim?"[45]

In rebuttal, Perlson as head of Kupat Holim wrote that the fund, as part of its full responsibility to provide health services to members, had to open clinics in urban neighborhoods because Hadassah's clinics did not address the special health needs of the laborers. Disregard for these needs would be a shirking of responsibility on the part of Kupat Holim and breach of trust of the membership. As for Hadassah's proposal that Kupat Holim doctors in the city confine themselves with referring the sick to Hadassah's clinics, Perlson responded:

> Kupat Holim with objectives such as this, would not be able to continue to exist in the fashion of offices that accept dues and give chits to Hadassah only, without a strong and organic tie with arranging actual medical assistance....A Kupat Holim such as this will be a machine without a soul, bereft of the ability to fulfill its public role in solving the social-medical problems it faces.[46]

In Perlson's estimation, Kupat Holim had to aspire to independence and expansion, and not satisfy itself with the role of an intermediary or agent for providing health services. A curtailed and minimalist Kupat Holim would not function properly and would deny its own mission. Perlson struggled with this question often, despite the resoluteness in his public defense of the "maximalist" vision: He had to deal daily with fiscal problems in the framework of his work, and more than once was forced to curtail the scope of the fund's operations due to budgetary pressures, scaling Kupat Holim's operation to its financial abilities, postponing certain national missions to a later day when things would improve.

In December 1925, the Kupat Holim council was convened, in part in order to end the consternation that surrounded the fund's operation and the need to define Kupat Holim's role.

THE FIRST KUPAT HOLIM COUNCIL AND THE CONTROVERSY OVER KUPAT HOLIM'S ROLE

In December 1925, soon after the convention of the Sixth Federation of Labor council, the Kupat Holim council called its first convention. The directorate's announcement explained that

> [t]he inability to clarify our fundamental questions in all their scope in the Federation of Labor council makes it necessary for us to seek another avenue to engage our public in solving the question, so that [the public] can influence the institution directly and bear responsibility for its operation. Only a special council on Kupat Holim matters and insuring the workers, can focus on these problems to discuss the fund's direction and its manner of operation in the future.[47]

These "problems" also stood at the center of media reports on the council's deliberations. Dr. Avraham Katznelson, a member of the secretariat on health matters of the National Committee, wrote in *Hapoel Hatzair*:

> This council has not come to deal with organization of the daily work of the fund, rather its primary role was to bring about clarification of the basic questions of Kupat Holim, to examine its manner of operation and development, as well as to set forth the independent organizational framework of the institution.[48]

Eliyahu Monchik-Margalit, the founder and director of the "Hasneh" Insurance Company wrote in *Davar* on 13 December 1925:

> Among all the questions under clarification in the upcoming council of Kupat Holim…the question

> of curtailment of the parameters of Kupat Holim or its expansion will surely hold an important place, as well. The aspiration to expand the borders of Kupat Holim's operation and encompass within it matters of insurance and responsibility are evident.[49]

The debate in the council centered on differences between the minimalists and the maximalists. The minimalists demanded that Kupat Holim's operation be tailored to the fiscal means available to the fund, and that the services of the Hadassah Medical Unit be utilized as much as possible. The maximalists—"devotees of the inflationary mode," according to the *Davar* writer —argued that what was needed was sustained growth, and the work of the fund should be expanded without taking into account prevailing finances. In his survey of the proposals raised in the council, Monchik-Margalit noted in a positive tone a proposal that called on Kupat Holim to be part of a compensation fund that the Federation of Labor would establish that would address *all* welfare and social insurance matters. According to that proposal, Kupat Holim would turn over all its fiscal assets to the Federation of Labor, and the Federation for its part would oblige itself to budget Kupat Holim on the basis of a detailed contract. Thus, the financial burden for managing the fund would be transferred to the Federation and the health fund could focus its energies on providing health services. Monchik-Margalit held that the council should reorganize on the following basis:

> The parameters of Kupat Holim should not be broadened, and as for the matter of responsibility, [for this] a special institutions must be created in the Federation. Each institution would fulfill its own role for which it was created.[50]

Monchik-Margalit claimed that if Kupat Holim's mission was broadened, it would be detrimental to medical services and the financial standing of the fund. Yet, it is fair to assume that Monchik-Margalit's position in favor of integration of Kupat Holim within a social welfare system provided by the Federation to its members was partly influenced by the fact that a year prior (1924) Monchik-Margalit himself had been responsible for the foundation of Hasneh insurance, serving as its director.

In the keynote speech before the council entitled "According to Ability or According to Needs?" Eliezer Perlson stressed that budgetary difficulties stood at the heart of the matter. Perlson held that the solution was not choosing between needs and abilities, but a compromise between them:

> There is only one way—via totally matching the needs of the institutions and its objective abilities; increasing ability to the maximum and maximal reduction in needs in times of inability.[51]

Perlson did not publicly oppose the view championing a broad public role for Kupat Holim, but situated it within the framework of the health fund's fiscal abilities. His words generated opposition, particularly among the maximalists. In a discussion on a conceptional level that followed his keynote address, the majority of the members supported curtailment of Kupat Holim's role and harmony between scope of operations and budget, while the maximalists—who "rejected vehemently economic axioms requiring adjustment of ability to needs"—were left in the minority. Despite the polarization in positions among council members as to the future role of Kupat Holim, and despite that fact that the majority supported Perlson's position that needs must be tailored to abilities, the resolution taken was more in the spirit of the minority who supported expanding the Fund without taking into consideration budgetary difficulties.

The position of Reuven Shenkar, treasurer of the fund and a member of its directorate, is particularly interesting. Of all people, Shenkar, a person engaged in financial matters, held that the fund must develop and grow. In his estimate, if the role of the fund were expanded, Kupat Holim could become a going concern, while merely striving to maintain the status quo would lead to regression and only perpetuate the prevailing economic distress. In a summary article of the council's deliberations in the paper *Contras* Shenkar wrote:

> In two decisions the council marked a new period in the development of the institution....The council expressed its desire that Kupat Holim be transformed from an institution purely for arrangement of medical assistance...to an institution that embraces all questions touching on the working public's health in Eretz Israel...and the second

> thing decided [by the council was] the need particularly for collaboration of all social welfare activities in one large comprehensive institution.[52]

Shenkar went on to express his own personal opinion that the fund's economic difficulties made it imperative that Kupat Holim grow and expand and break out of the limited framework in which it had operated to date:

> On the basis of this mutual assistance and in the name of fulfillment of the pioneering role of the working public, Kupat Holim must first and foremost amplify its operation in places of agricultural settlement and in the Jewish agricultural villages and to aid the worker conquering [the land] with broad assistance without any additional payment above that of the worker in the city, and establish a series of various medical institutions in Eretz Israel, necessary institutions that do not yet exist and that will not be established by others[53]

Shenkar added that one must envision Kupat Holim as "an institution that in time must become a ministry of health & social insurance of the working society in Eretz Israel."

The decisions taken by the council were not anchored to any time schedule for realizing the fund's roles and mission. They dealt primarily with formulating Kupat Holim's direction in the future and finding a solution to its financial difficulties.

In a summary article on the debate in the council Dr. Avraham Katznelson wrote:

> These questions that engaged the council for two days, did not find their full resolution, and the core organizations of the Federation of Labor will have other opportunities to deal with them, but the very fact of clarification of questions in a special council of Kupat Holim members, that brought about a harsh war of opinions within the council, should be viewed as an important step forward toward a full solution of the problems with which the Kupat Holim directorate struggles in its war on behalf of consolidation of the institution.[54]

Scrutiny of the identities of the speakers in the Kupat Holim council reveals that rank-and-file members who partook in the council's deliberations as delegates of cooperative settlements or workers' councils constituted the majority who opposed expansion of Kupat Holim's role beyond care for sick workers. They sought no more than good accessible and inexpensive medical services. Among those who favored expansion of Kupat Holim's role as an institution with a core social role were Reuven Shenkar and Yitzhak Kenivsky-Kenev, founders of the fund and members of the Kupat Holim directorate from its beginnings. It seems that the controversy over the role of Kupat Holim was largely a split between the fund's functionaries and member-recipients of its services.

Increasing economic difficulties of Kupat Holim, the controversies with Hadassah over funding and domains of authority, the inquiry commission of Kupat Holim's functioning, and curtailment in its operation in the wake of the commission's findings were all contributing factors in placing the question of Kupat Holim's role on the public agenda. The issue became all the more acute in the wake the Federation of Labor's third convention that convened in July 1927 in the shadow of a growing economic depression in Eretz Israel.

KUPAT HOLIM AT THE THIRD FEDERATION OF LABOR CONVENTION

The Third Federation of Labor convention devoted little attention to Kupat Holim. During the convention, despite the expectations of the fund's directors, no serious discussion of the role of Kupat Holim and its future took place. Most of the convention energies focused on Solel Boneh's dire straits and the war on unemployment among workers. Discussion of Kupat Holim was limited to technicalities: amendments to the health fund's ordinances, adjustment of membership fees, and establishment of the supervisory committee. The supervisory committee was established in order to enhance supervision by representatives of the insurees over the work of the management and to separate the policymakers (the supervisory committee) and the executive (the Kupat Holim directorate). The convention, therefore, stipulated that the supervisory committee would constitute a board of directors for the Kupat Holim and be comprised of representatives of the insurees, the Federation, and the fund.

The only matter of principle discussed at the convention was implementation of the principle that all members of the Federation of Labor must be members of Kupat Holim. It was the Kupat Holim people who pressed for passage of this resolution, for members of the Federation who were better off financially often abstained from membership in the health fund, availing themselves of the services of Hadassah when in need of medical care. Kupat Holim argued that passage of the resolution was an expression of the principle of mutual aid to which all members of the Federation and the health fund were duty-bound. Of course, fiscal motivations were an underlying motivation behind this demand, and the realization that the membership base would be enhanced by the addition of members of means whose regular dues-paying would contribute to balancing the fund's deficits and expansion of services.

While the convention accepted Kupat Holim's demand for reciprocal membership, in practice nothing was done to implement the decision and in practice nothing changed much. The Federation refrained from compelling its members to be members of the health fund, fearing that many would choose to leave the Federation if faced with an ultimatum.

DISCUSSION OF KUPAT HOLIM'S ROLE, 1927-1928

Due to the Federation of Labor convention's failure to address the role of Kupat Holim and the Federation's evasion of a showdown with recalcitrant members over implementation of reciprocal membership, and due to growing dissatisfaction with services among Kupat Holim's membership, the media were filled with a wave of articles concerning Kupat Holim's debts/obligations and its role.

In a major piece published in *Hapoel Hatzair*, Yosef Baratz, a member of the executive committee of the Federation of Labor and the Kupat Holim directorate from kibbutz Degania, leveled sharp criticism at curtailment of the fund's operation and inclinations to tailor provision of needs to the fund's economic capabilities. Baratz attacked Kupat Holim for failure to stand firm in demanding that reciprocity in membership be carried out, arguing that the moral foundations of the fund were liable to be eroded by too much emphasis on fiscal matters: "Accounts and matters of the budget cannot always accompany saving souls, the fate of human beings." Kupat Holim, he argued, must put itself above daily accounting, to force the Federation to increase the number of its members in the fund and to return to and lay the foundations for the principle of mutual assistance:

> When Kupat Holim will become the institution as I have described it to you, then its members will multiply, its revenue will grow and it will be able to fulfill the important role placed upon it.[55]

Baratz's words constituted the opening shot in a renewed battle over the role of Kupat Holim.

A short time later, in June 1928, Kenivsky-Kenev wrote an article in *Davar* devoted to "Timely Roles for Kupat Holim." Kenivsky-Kenev argued that Kupat Holim must choose its path: "whether as an institution of mutual assistance to all members of the Federation of Labor or as an insuring institution as the health funds in Europe."[56]

In his opinion, Kupat Holim should work towards social legislation that would encompass the entire Yishuv, anchor Kupat Holim's position, and ensure compulsory health insurance and social insurance for all. To do so, the Mandate government must be mobilized to support and recognize the status of Kupat Holim as the leading public health organization in the Yishuv. Kenivsky-Kenev, like Baratz, argued that Kupat Holim's primary weakness was that not all members of the Federation of Labor were members of the health fund, and lack of implementation of the principle of reciprocal membership eroded the public stature and the economic capabilities of the fund. However, unlike Baratz, Kenivsky-Kenev did not ignore Kupat Holim's chronic budgetary problems and emphasized that the difficulties must be taken into account in planning the basket of services that the fund provided to its members.

An important juncture in the debate over the role of Kupat Holim was witnessed on the eve of the second Kupat Holim convention.

THE SECOND KUPAT HOLIM CONVENTION

In May 1929, the second Kupat Holim convention was scheduled to assemble. For the first time, convention delegates were elected by a general assembly of the membership and not appointed by an inner circle. Elections were proportional and conducted according to a combined list of local and national candidates, based on one delegate for every 150 members. Those settlements with less than fifty members were supposed to organize as a group and choose a delegate who would represent them at the convention. In addition to local elections, a national list was also drawn up, based on party and federation affiliation. Fifty-six settlements conducted local elections in which some 8,000 members participated (55% of the total Kupat Holim membership); 3,720 members participated in the national elections. All told, fifty-two delegates were chosen: thirty-four local representatives and eighteen national representatives. More than half (56% came from rural agricultural settlements and the remainder (44%) from the cities. Among the fifty-two delegates, there were only four women, and only one of them came from the cooperative settlement sector.[57]

The elections were not free of criticism, and during the tally, tens of ballots were left blank, testifying to a show of nonconfidence in the elections among some members. Members of the "Valley" Workers Group, lodged at the time in the village of Rishon le-Zion, protested publicly in writing in opposition to the use of party-federation affiliation as the basis for drawing up the national list in an institution such as Kupat Holim. The Valley Group argued that such an arrangement was discriminatory and detrimental to those members who participated in the local elections.

The fifty-two delegates were not the only participants in the convention. Delegate status was also granted to the three members of the Kupat Holim directorate, Eliezer Perlson, Yitzhak Kenivsky-Kenev, and Dr. Glicker from the Kupat Holim medical department, Dr. Chaim Yaski, director of Hadassah, Dr. Moshe Beilinson, chairperson of the supervisory committee, and six members of the supervisory committee. All in all, the convention was comprised of sixty-one voting delegates.

In an announcement to the press the supervisory committee stated:

> In that this convention will have a decisive value in determining the development and operation of Kupat Holim in the future, it is important that all members in their localities will prepare themselves for the convention and propose questions that they believe should be clarified at this convention.[58]

As was the case at the first Kupat Holim council held in 1925, lively discussion in the media preceded discourse at the convention, focusing on the expected ideological debate.

> In his article "Toward the Convention" Shlomo Lavie, a member of kibbutz Ein-Harod, criticized the conduct of Kupat Holim for curtailing services: "Concern for the fund devoured concern for the member…there was lack of action and lack of consideration of the means of the members here."[59]

Lavie questioned the way in which Eliezer Perlson had set priorities for Kupat Holim in the wake of the fund's financial crisis."The aspirations of the Kupat Holim directorate is the health of the fund…[I]t has nothing to do with the health of the worker." The fund, Lavie said, should have concerned itself with providing service for its members and not engaged in other matters. He even dared to suggest that Kupat Holim should not assume welfare functions such as care for the chronically ill and rehabilitation patients, and that other Federation bodies should take upon themselves these duties.

On the other hand, Dr. Yosef Meir, the fund's medical director argued in an article published in *Davar* entitled "Toward Kupat Holim's Convention" that Kupat Holim should expand, not only by enforcing membership in the fund on all members of the Federation of Labor, but also by providing services to others who were not members of the Federation, including individuals who were not members of the proletariat but wished to avail themselves of its services. This was a very daring proposal for its day from an ideological standpoint, not only in regard to Kupat Holim, but also for the entire Federation of Labor. Similar views were voiced previously by Kenivsky-Kenev and Shenkar, members of the Kupat Holim directorate, but their sentiments were worded with utmost care—relating to "all classes of the public." Dr. Meir was the first to say so openly.

In the three months that preceded the convention the Kupat Holim issue remained solidly in the headlines in the workers' newspapers, mainly in *Davar*. Readers who were members of the fund expressed their opinions in the "Members' Letters" section in *Davar*. Many wrote that there was a need to amend Kupat Holim's ordinances in light of the social and economic changes the country was undergoing (unemployment, the growth of the urban proletariat, and so forth). Others dealt with questions such as "mutual assistance or donations," "mutual assistance or a cooperative of consumers of medical assistance," and other issues.

In a comprehensive article entitled "The Problems of Kupat Holim" (published in *Davar* 6 May 1929), Dr. Katznelson took the Federation of Labor's council to task for refraining from conducting a serious discussion of questions facing the health fund. He presented the positions of those in favor and opposed to reform that would expand the role of Kupat Holim. The opponents argued that those against reform and broadening of the fund's roles sought to "backpedal" to times when the Federation and Kupat Holim were just beginning. Those in favor argued that the health fund could no longer remain a sectarian body:

> Kupat Holim can't be a party-based institution or a Federation institution. It is not a class institution in the normal sense of the word, but rather it is a national institution based on a certain state legislation....The upcoming convention should continue in this direction and recognize Kupat Holim as a general health fund for Hebrew laborers in Eretz Israel.

It was predictable that most articles written at this time would deal with the role of Kupat Holim and the question of "needs versus means" in light of the ongoing financial difficulties in which Kupat Holim found itself during the 1926–1928 depression. There seemed to be no solution in the foreseeable future, and signs of improvement began to appear only in 1929.

In light of the flood of coverage in the press concerning Kupat Holim on the eve of the organization's second convention, it was hard to image that the convention's participants could ignore the public mood. Many feared that deliberation would be to a large extent a repetition of discourse in the December 1925 Kupat Holim council and that the convention would close without any operative resolutions.

The second Kupat Holim convention that convened in May 1929 in Haifa was fundamentally different from the Kupat Holim council that met in 1925. The first gathering was overshadowed by the worst economic crisis in the history of the Yishuv and at an hour that the fund stood on the verge of total bankruptcy. At the time of the second gathering, clear signs of economic recovery were visible in all branches of the economy and the state of the fund had improved. The change for the better was reflected in the opening welcomes given in the name of Henrietta Szold who spoke in the name of the Zionist executive of the World Zionist Organization:

> The Zionist executive views Kupat Holim as the foundation for a mode of general social insurance in Eretz Israel, and it is one of the important factors in raising the level of health and hygienic culture of the worker in Eretz Israel.[60]

Such warm support from Henrietta Szold, who usually held up Hadassah as the leading health service organization in the country, was extremely significant. To a large extent this was a repeat of the words of the Yishuv's health committee in the inquiry commission report presented to the Zionist executive, and Szold's sentiments reinforced the "winds of change."

According to the agenda, the key speakers were to be Dr. Beilinson, chairperson of the supervisory committee, and the three members of the Kupat Holim directorate, Eliezer Perlson, Dr. Glicker, and Yitzhak Kenivsky-Kenev. The closing address of the opening plenum session was to be delivered by Yosef Baratz. After the speeches, a general discussion among the members was to take place. According to the list of speakers, the majority of whom were veteran managers in Kupat Holim, it is possible to guess the content of what would be said, for Perlson, Kenivsky-Kenev, and Glicker had already expressed their views more than once over the role of Kupat Holim—first in the council in 1925, later in the daily press and in the fund's house organs. Dr. Beilinson, however, had yet to publicly express his views on Kupat Holim, and his speech, scheduled to open deliberations, was met with tense expectation.

Dr. Beilinson spoke in a similar vein to Henrietta Szold's:

> And we have a dream, a dream that is also "imperialistic," for the nationalization of all of the health profession. All this work, for curative medicine, maintenance of health, must be built on popular public foundations. We are proud of our 15,000 dues-payers, however we are part of the overall Yishuv, a small handful compared to the

> huge Yishuv that will arise in this country. Kupat Holim must be an agent for nationalization of medicine, just as the workers' farms [cooperative settlements] must be the agent for agricultural settlement of the entire nation, and the workers' organization must be the agent for independent political life of the nation.[61]

Beilinson's words left no doubt as to his position vis-à-vis Kupat Holim's mission: Kupat Holim must be the core national body for health services in Eretz Israel. As part of its mission, it must treat all classes of the public and not just laborers, members of the Federation of Labor. Contrary to the Kupat Holim council of 1925 where the focus of discussion was the question "according to need or according to ability," Dr. Beilinson refrained from raising the question of fiscal capabilities in his delivery. On the contrary. He was adamant on this point:

> When we will improve Kupat Holim in its present scope we will not say this is enough for us. Our political aspirations are not limited to a parallel tax….There is a whole network of social legislation. Particularly [in regard to] the law for insurance for invalids [disability insurance] our work is not restricted to curative medicine. There is preventive work, protecting the worker against illness—social medical work, a domain that is perhaps the most important. However, it is possible to say: Due to daily cares, we have yet to begin it.[62]

Not only did Dr. Beilinson's speech at the opening session of the convention decisively clinch the question of Kupat Holim's mission; it flew against all media-generated expectations of a stormy debate on this issue. Instead of discussing the issue for which the convention had been convened—What was the role of Kupat Holim and how should it operate in the future?—the convention ended up discussing how best to actualize in practice the role of Kupat Holim as it had been set forth by Dr. Beilinson in his opening address: primarily, how to increase revenues in order to realize Beilinson's vision of tomorrow's Kupat Holim in practice.

Thus, Dr. Beilinson had a decisive impact on the course of the convention's deliberation. Even Perlson, scheduled to survey the fund's operation following Beilinson's speech, closed his own keynote address with a call "for the convention to open a new era in the development of Kupat Holim until it shall be a forceful and comprehensive institution for social welfare." Similar sentiments were voiced by Dr. Glicker and Kenivsky-Kenev.

Although the Yishuv had yet to extricate itself from the economic crisis, Kupat Holim under the leadership of Dr. Beilinson set forth to mobilize funding, not only to cover its deficit, but to establish new enterprises in the health field. Subsequently, a second floor was completed at the Arza convalescence facility near Jerusalem; a convalescence facility was established on the Carmel (primarily for mothers and children); construction of the [Jezreel] Valley Hospital near Afula was embarked upon; and new clinics were opened in the cities. Dr. Beilinson mentioned all these in his address before the convention when he added: "Now there is a bit of a respite. Now there is the possibility to bring various proposals for broadening assistance and its improvement."

Despite the "lofty" quality of his address regarding the role of Kupat Holim, Beilinson did not ignore the fund's troublesome financial straits. In detailing deployment of the fund's services throughout the country, Beilinson took pains to note that expansion of Kupat Holim must be carried out in keeping with available resources. The question now on the agenda, he said, should be how to realize Kupat Holim's mission, particularly how to obtain the financing to transform the fund into the type of organization he envisioned:

> Anyone who suggests improving the institution with an operational branch of this or that nature, must also bring a proposal for income along with the proposal for expenditures. [We should] forbid building an artificial conflict between the institution's coffers and the institution's operation, between the "health of the fund" and the "health of the laborer," and therefore the proposals of the supervisory committee should be formulated in such a way that against all expansion of assistance stands a [corresponding] growth in revenue.

In the same context, Beilinson argued that Kupat Holim must demand that the Mandate government legislate a compulsory social insurance law and participate actively in underwriting health services for the Yishuv by participating in Kupat Holim's budget.

> From this convention must go out a demand to the government to issue a law that will require the work-provider and the government itself to participate in the worker's social insurance.

Similar sentiments had been voiced earlier by Yitzhak Kenivsky-Kenev at the Health Fund International Organization in Vienna in September 1928 where he served as Kupat Holim's first delegate to the body.

Dr. Beilinson did not tell the audience that even prior to the convention, an informal request had been submitted to the Mandate government though the auspices and with the support of the Yishuv's health committee and the Zionist executive. It would have been improper to request that the convention take a stand on a move that had already been taken. Within days after the adjournment of the convention, however, the Mandate government rejected the request.

KUPAT HOLIM AND SOCIAL LEGISLATION INITIATIVES

The need for broad social legislation under the leadership of Kupat Holim was also the main topic of Yitzhak Kenivsky-Kenev's address before the convention.[63] In his survey of "A Health Fund Law," he reiterated the message presented by Beilinson regarding the role of Kupat Holim: "It is clear that we must not curtail the medical assistance to members. Just the opposite: It should be broadened and improved."

Kenivsky-Kenev emphasized Kupat Holim should operate on an autonomous footing:

> [Kupat Holim] must operate through independent work. Provision of assistance [must come] through institutions and personnel of the fund itself, for in this manner economy is ensured and suitable management of public medicine.

In practical terms, this meant that Kupat Holim should sever its ties to Hadassah's hospitalization services and establish its own independent hospitalization capabilities.

Dr. Glicker, Kupat Holim's acting medical director who was filling in for Dr. Meir, was of the same opinion. He called upon Kupat Holim to organize the Federation and all the Jewish settlements in the country to "go to war" with the Mandate government—through strikes, legal action, and so forth—on behalf of social legislation for which the British refused to take responsibility. Akin to other speakers who preceded him, Dr. Glicker viewed Kupat Holim as the leader in ensuring health services, an organization with a national mission. Glicker perceived the convention as a kind of "legislative body" whose role was to determine the means and the statutes by which Kupat Holim should operate in the future.

On May 13, following the opening addresses, general discussion was opened to the floor.[64] The air of optimism and the positions of the keynote speakers impacted on the positions adopted by the participants. If the keynote speakers spoke primarily on principles and general direction, the convention participants who took the floor focused on the "nitty-gritty" of Kupat Holim's roles. From the list of subjects that concerned those who spoke in the plenum session it seems that most of the members agreed with the new vision of Kupat Holim as a national rather than solely a sectarian institution—agreed, that is, that Kupat Holim, while responsible for the health of the worker, should also be charged, within the framework of its mission, with broadening its services to encompass other sectors in the Yishuv (Arab workers and persons who were not members of the Federation of Labor).

Stressing their common working-class background, a good number of participants raised the issue of opening Kupat Holim to Arab laborers—whether by establishing a separate health fund under Federation auspices in the Arab community, or whether by integrating Arab workers into the existing Kupat Holim system. Similar proposals had already been raised in years prior to the convention when Jewish laborers had worked shoulder-to-shoulder with Arab laborers in the railroad maintenance workshops in Haifa. At the time, the Arab workers received medical assistance in an informal unauthorized manner from Kupat Holim-appointed doctors. Others spoke of the need to initiate health education and preventive medicine; some called upon Kupat Holim to put special emphasis on the health of women and establish a national network that would engage in guidance and care for mothers, newborns, and children. Most of those who spoke demanded that the fund work toward enactment of social legislation and apply pressure on the Mandate government in this area. Many tended to blame the Mandate government for most of Kupat Holim's financial troubles, especially its refusal to pay the parallel tax. It is possible that this is the reason why no in-depth discussion was conducted concerning weaknesses in the performance of Kupat Holim itself and ways of improving its own management. The general tendency was to blame externals, a third party. The only reservation was voiced by Reuven Shenkar—and even here, his reservations had an optimistic tone:

> From the report [by Perlson] one can get the impression that the crisis period is behind us and from now on a new era of consolidation and quiet endeavor has arrived. This is a mistake. Anyone who looks will learn that heavy debts continue to burden the institution. Income from 1928 has dropped in comparison with 1927. There is no room to talk of reducing dues and increasing expenditures.

Nevertheless, Shenkar did not voice any opposition to the picture drawn by Dr. Beilinson vis-à-vis Kupat Holim's roles. Shenkar as well believed that Kupat Holim should open itself up and broaden its perspective until it became the primary body for health services in Eretz Israel.

On the afternoon of the May 14 the convention drew to a close. The main resolutions passed were as follows:

> 1. Demand for social legislation that would recognize Kupat Holim's exclusive status as "the only institution in the field of health insurance in Eretz Israel," as well as a demand that the Mandate government relinquish its estranged attitude toward Kupat Holim.
> 2. Demand that the government enact legislation that would require every employer to pay the parallel tax.
> 3. "Realization of the duty of all Federation members to be members in Kupat Holim."

Other resolutions dealt with expansion of community services of Kupat Holim, opening of consultation stations for mothers and children, supervising the health of schoolchildren, amplifying awareness of the benefit of physical exercise, and more. The convention's resolutions said nothing about limiting Kupat Holim's operations to its fiscal abilities or more comprehensive use of Hadassah institutions in lieu of broadening the functions of the fund. The overall tone of the convention's resolutions was purely positive and infused with unbridled optimism, dealing for the most part with expansion of Kupat Holim services in all health areas and social insurance.

THE SECOND CONVENTION'S RESOLUTIONS AND THE MISSIONS OF KUPAT HOLIM

It is hard to pinpoint the factors that brought about the change in perceptions of the roles of Kupat Holim that the heads and the members of Kupat Holim struggled with during the convention of 1924. It may have emanated from the personality of Dr. Beilinson who aspired to broaden the ranks of Kupat Holim by bringing in members who were not members of the Federation (such as small merchants and crafts persons), to transform it into a large organization operating in accordance with his own social outlook. And it may merely be that after four years of discussion, things crystallized into a concrete platform. It may also be that members of the convention, chosen from among regional councils and cooperative farming communities, sensed a heavy responsibility as public servants. And it may be that things coalesced as they did due to the fact that previous attempts to curtail operations in order to rehabilitate the organization had failed, and therefore participants in the fund came to the conclusion that this was not the way. All the factors together, even some alone, whatever their individual weight, were sufficient to bring about the change in approach and point a new way for Kupat Holim in the future.

Historian Zeev Tzachor believes that the 1926–1927 economic crisis and the failure of members of the non-Socialist Fourth Aliyah to rise to the occasion and play a significant role in addressing core needs of the Yishuv cast into stark relief the dominant role of the labor movement and to a large extent strengthened the Federation of Labor and its institutions, generating public consensus on the Federation's hegemony. Tzachor writes:

> The Federation of Labor is today [1928] the largest organized power in the Yishuv.... They are

> from this time [forward] a public authority of great importance vis-à-vis other bodies in the Yishuv, toward the Mandate regime and toward the Zionist movement.[65]

Tzachor believes that the rise in the Federation's power caused many members of the Fourth Aliyah to join, not due to ideological motivations, but rather to the social security it could offer them. It may be that the rise in the power of the Federation also impacted on the participants in Kupat Holim's second convention—that visions of growth and broadening services that would transform Kupat Holim into the primary body in the health field in the Yishuv drew inspiration and the courage "to dare" from the experience of the Federation.

Historian Anita Shapira stresses that 1929, the year of the second Kupat Holim convention,

> marked a turnabout year in this history of the Yishuv and the Zionist movement....[A] dynamic era that changed the priorities of the Zionist movement began....[T]he economic and financial problems were what stood in the center of the movement's world.[66]

Shapira says that all the activities of the Zionist movement now circled around Dr. Chaim Weizmann's initiatives to establish a Jewish agency, with the hopes that such a body would bring about new economic momentum in Eretz Israel and make the influx of Jewish capital (including non-Zionist investments) in the movement and the Yishuv possible. One may surmise that intensive involvement of the Zionist movement at the time in renewal of economic progress was felt in Eretz Israel and had a degree of influence on the course of deliberations during the second convention of Kupat Holim.

From an historical standpoint, two important questions occur. First, were the convention's resolutions regarding the roles of Kupat Holim operational (did the fund's leaders indeed strive to realize them)? Second, what was the Federation of Labor's response to the resolutions?

Examination of the summary report of the Kupat Holim directorate for the year 1929–1930 and of the subjects raised in the third convention of Kupat Holim (1933) reveals the following: In the summer of 1929, Kupat Holim and the Federation of Labor together established a fund for those suffering from chronic illnesses that operated adjacent to Kupat Holim; opened physiotherapy institutes, lung disease institutes (together with the League for a War on Tuberculoses), and dental clinics; expanded the number of beds in its convalescence facilities; initiated regular seasonal educational gatherings on health issues headed by a Kupat Holim doctor focusing on health maintenance; began comprehensive supervision of the health of working youth in the country; signed an agreement with the Dead Sea Works and factories in the Haifa and Tel Aviv area to provide on-site medical assistance—the first steps taken by Kupat Holim in the field of industrial medicine; established consultation stations for women and initiated negotions with Hadassah over the opening of mother and child stations to be operated in conjunction with Kupat Holim; and completed construction of the Valley Hospital in Afula-city, which opened in late April 1930, becoming the first independent Kupat Holim hospital in the country. In January 1930, the Federation of Labor and Kupat Holim submitted a proposal to the Mandate government for compulsory health insurance legislation designed to encompass all employees in the country, through Kupat Holim.

Thus, the second convention's resolutions regarding Kupat Holim's mission did not remain solely "on paper." An article published in 1933 under the heading "Toward the [Third] Kupat Holim Convention," reveals in retrospect an interesting situation:

> In the 3rd convention, the members must plot a plan for fortification of Kupat Holim and expansion of its activities: increasing the number of fund members…increasing Kupat Holim's revenue…continuing improvement of medical work…expansion of preventive work and care of mother and child…expansion of Kupat Holim's activity among laborers in the agricultural villages…[demanding that] the government…enact compulsory insurance…[and fulfill] our demands by the municipalities.[67]

The key words —"fortification," "growth," "expansion"—speak for themselves. There was no discussion of the role of the fund, no calls to curtail operations or limited operations to provision of health services to laborers only. After some ten years of weighing and discussing various paths, Kupat Holim had chosen to embark on a course of growth and expansion, with the goal of consolidating its hegemony as a core social institution, the primary health service provider in Eretz Israel. The ideological period in Kupat Holim's history drew to a close and was not destined to reappear until the establishment of the state of Israel when the question of the fund's status within the framework of the fledgling state arose.

THE POSITION OF THE FEDERATION OF LABOR VIS-À-VIS KUPAT HOLIM'S ROLE

Examination of the protocols of the Federation of Labor's executive committee and council gatherings reflect the Federation's attitude toward changes in Kupat Holim. During the 1920s the Federation of Labor did not conduct any comprehensive ideological discussion of Kupat Holim's roles. From this standpoint, Kupat Holim was not constrained by binding precedents, enjoying great latitude in the conduct of its first convention. Even in the wake of the second convention at which a new course for the fund was charted, the Federation of Labor did not conduct any deliberation on this matter, and limited itself to confirmation of the convention's resolutions.

On the surface, it looked like the Federation approved the course that Kupat Holim had chosen. But in practice, examination of Federation actions in the wake of Kupat Holim's decisions reveals a far more complex picture. Two aspects of Kupat Holim occupied the Federation: enforcing compulsory membership in Kupat Holim on all Federation members, and expansion of Kupat Holim to embrace persons who were not laborers or were not members of the Federation of Labor. Despite repeated requests from Kupat Holim that reciprocal membership be enforced and despite the Federation's own 1927 decision concerning duel membership, the executive committee postponed implementation for ten full years (until 1937). In the early 1930s, the decision remained a dead letter, and delayed the growth of Kupat Holim.

As for expansion of Kupat Holim services to the Yishuv as a whole—a step that was designed to transform Kupat Holim into a core element in health matters in the Yishuv—it seems that the Federation of Labor refrained from supporting the health fund, except in places where assistance served the Federation's own corporate interests. Kupat Holim could not operate independently to expand its membership rosters among Jews who were not laborers or among nonmembers of the Federation without the approval of the executive committee, which chose to deal with each case separately. Under such circumstances, it was hard for Kupat Holim to increase its numbers, its fiscal means were limited, and expansion of services to the Yishuv as a whole—as resolved at the second convention—was unfeasible.

Thus, while the Federation of Labor did not conduct any discussion of Kupat Holim's role and the decisions of the second convention, its conduct seems to have been guided by a well-defined outlook. The Federation supported the aspirations of Kupat Holim to grow and expand, but solely within the framework of the Federation and under its own close supervision—and only so much as expansion was not detrimental to the Federation or in conflict with its own corporate interests. Whenever a conflict of interests arose, the Federation chose to protect its own corporate interests, even at the price of undermining the growth of Kupat Holim.

Shabtai Tevet, author of a biographical study of David Ben-Gurion, argues that the behavior of the Federation in such cases reflects primarily Ben-Gurion's attitude toward Kupat Holim. According to Tevet, Ben-Gurion viewed Kupat Holim as a first-rate organizational tool in the hands of the Federation. He was the driving force behind "engineering" the fund to operate first and foremost for the benefit of the Federation, and only afterwards for its own benefit. Too large a health fund was liable to threaten the executive committee's hegemony over such a crucial social institution. Thus, Ben-Gurion and his colleagues sought to slow down actualization of the convention's decisions regarding Kupat Holim's broader mission. It seemed that the Federation's decision to avoid implementation of the duty of reciprocal membership was also motivated by similar calculations—reflecting a combination of ambivalence and vested interests, both personal and corporate, that permeated the attitudes and actions of the Federation of Labor vis-à-vis Kupat Holim.

The heads of Kupat Holim, in both the supervisory committee and the Kupat Holim directorate, largely acquiesced in the position of the Federation of Labor, and other than a handful of comments about Kupat Holim being pushed onto the sidelines and inadequate support on the part of the Federation in, for instance, pressing for payment of the parallel tax, there was no open opposition to the

Federation's position. Kupat Holim's operation in the 1930s was largely the outgrowth of this relationship. Moreover, most of those who fulfilled key positions in Kupat Holim and in the supervisory committee were executives, not politicians, and therefore sought to achieve what was possible under prevailing conditions, rather than embarking on a political struggle.

In conclusion, in the late 1920s one finds that Kupat Holim took important steps torward crystallizing its raison d'être and defining its roles. From this point forward the fund had to deal with difficulties emanating from realization of its resolutions on its own, while coordinating its actions with the Federation of Labor and its wishes. Under such conditions, core issues arose as to the development of Kupat Holim in the 1930s until a "joint dues framework" (1937) took form that made membership in the Federation and Kupat Holim reciprocal.

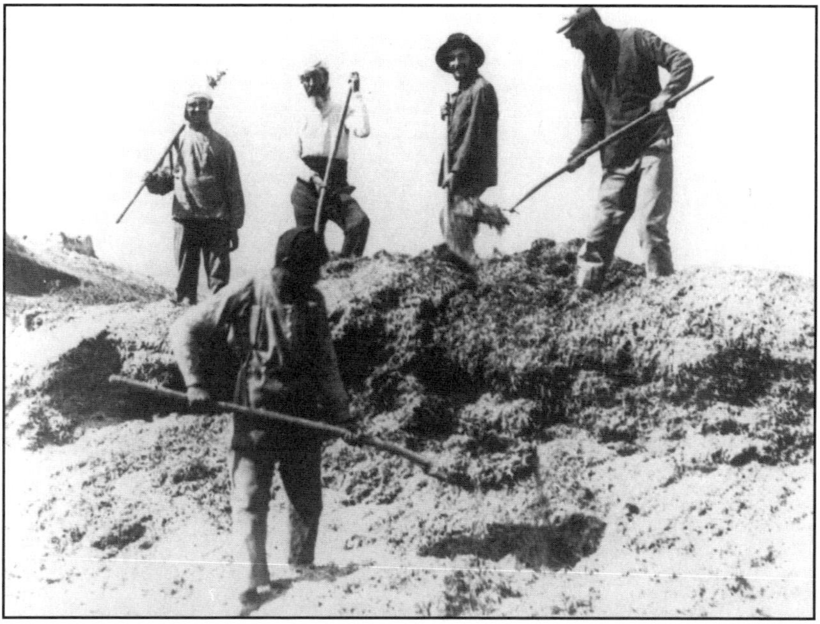

1. Workers from the Second Aliyah, 1905.

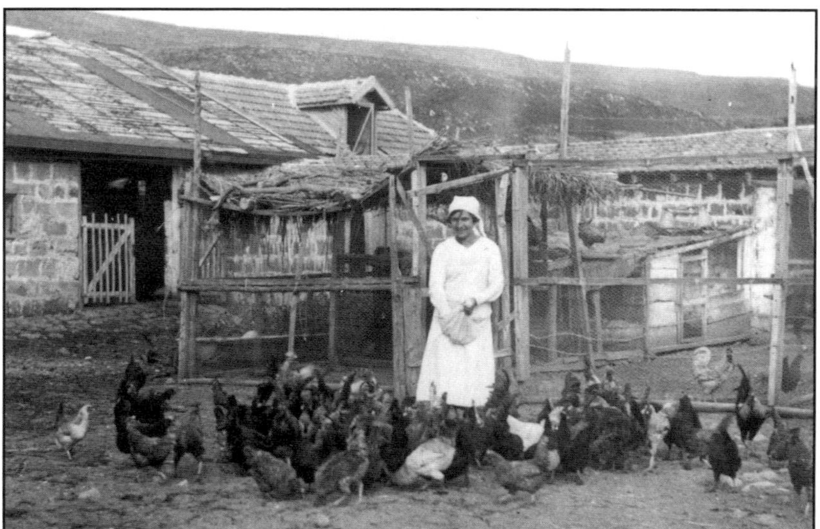

2. Kinneret, the Women Workers' Farm, 1907.

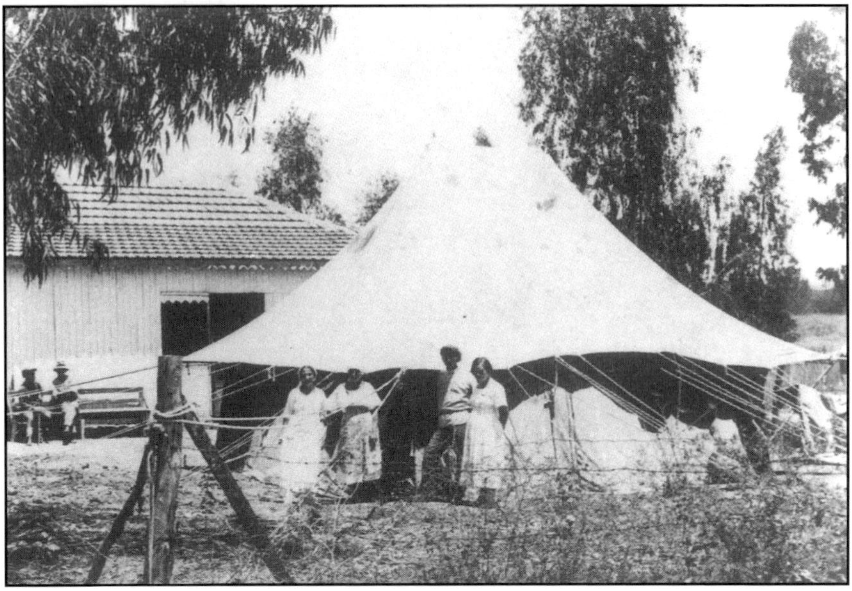

3. The tent: Kupat Holim's first clinic in Petach Tikva, 1912.

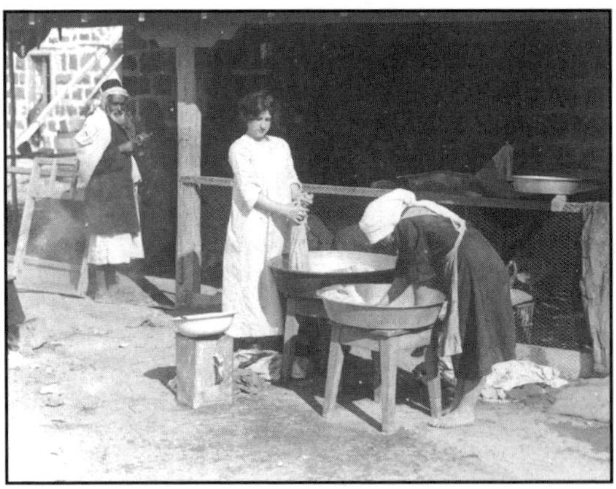

4. Living conditions at Kinneret, the Women Workers' Farm, 1907.

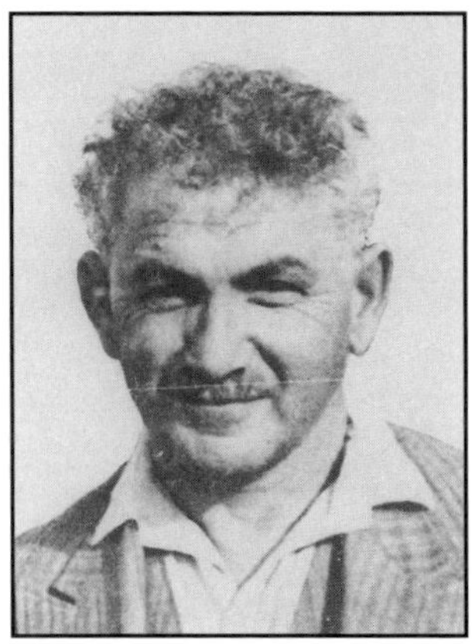

5. Berl Katznelson, labor leader and Kupat Holim founder.

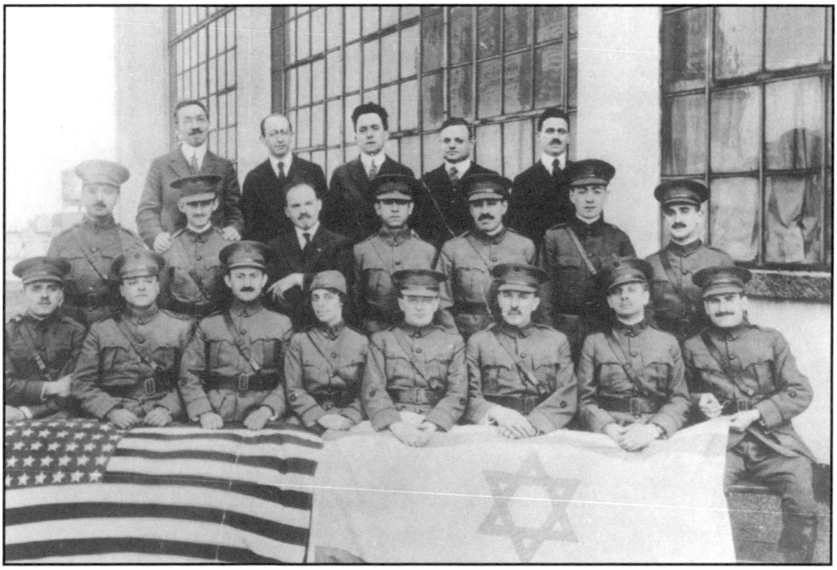

6. The American Zionist Medical Unit to Palestine, 1919.

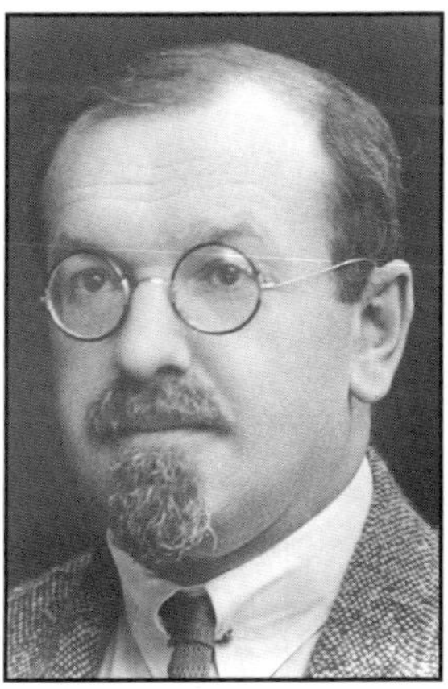

7. Dr. Isaac Max Rubinow, Director of the American Zionist Medical Unit and the first director of the Hadassah Medical Organization in Israel.

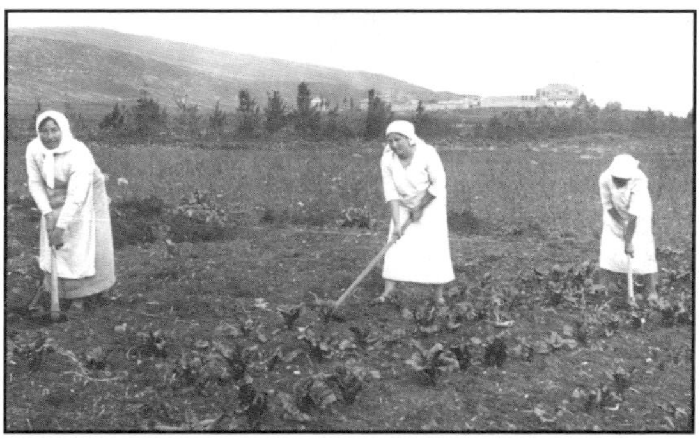

8. Women workers at the Kinneret Farm, 1913.

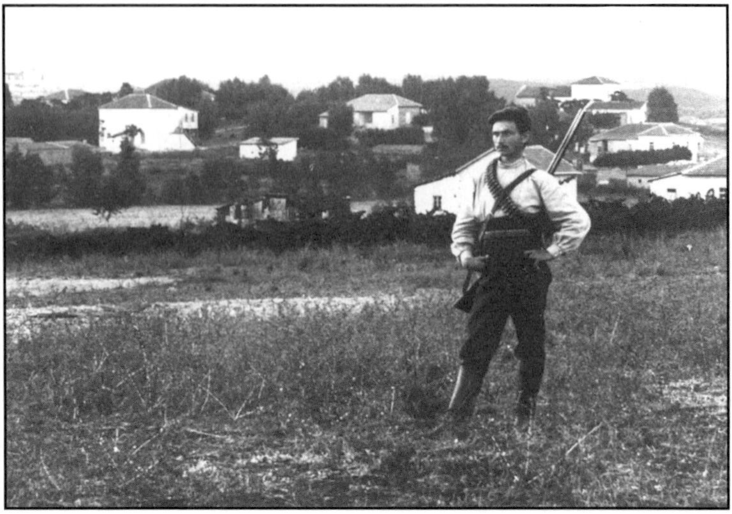

9. A Jewish watchman-worker guarding one of the villages, early 1920s. The watchmen worked in the fields during the day and guarded them by night.

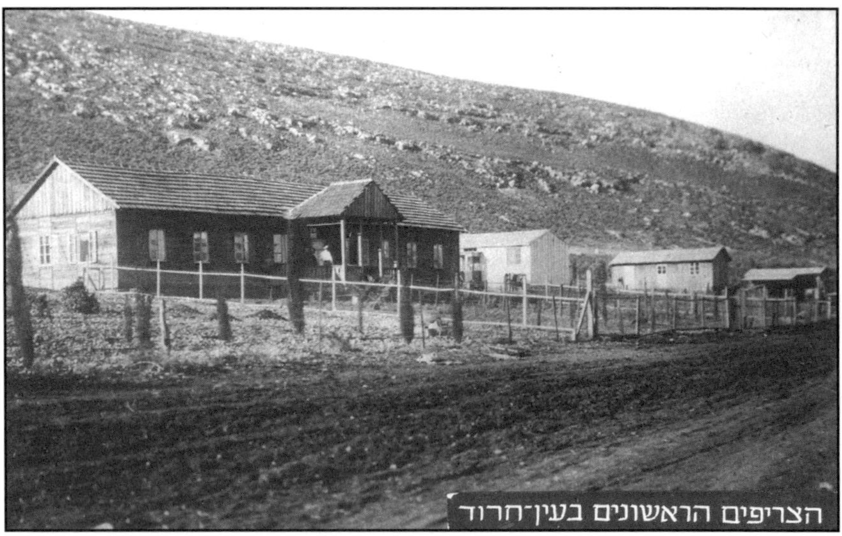

10. Kibbutz Ein-Harod in the Jezreel Valley, 1921.

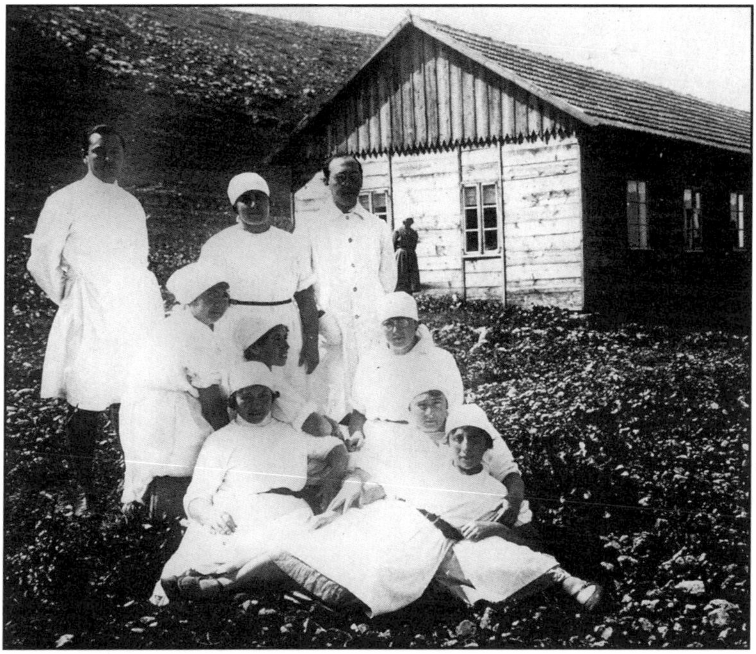

11. The Workers' Hospital in Ein-Harod, 1924.

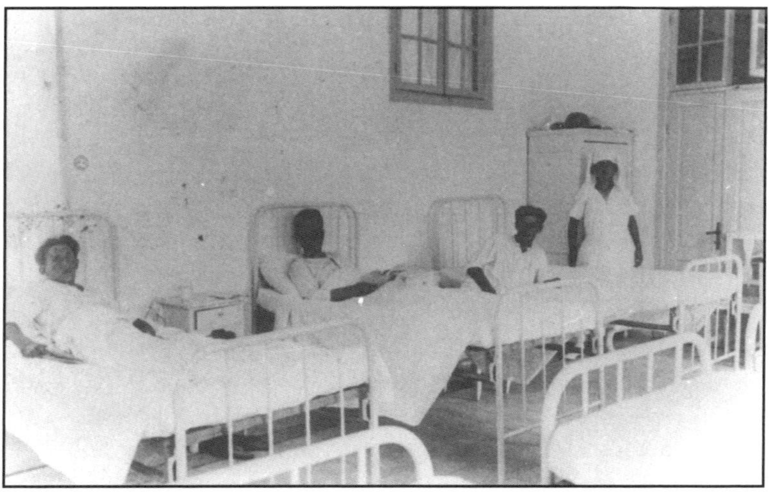

12. Workers' Sick Room in Kibbutz Ein-Harod, 1924.

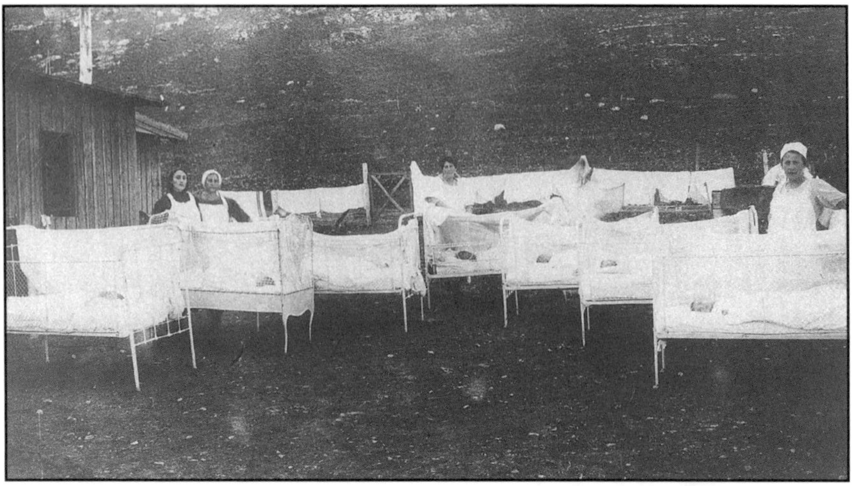

13. Nurses at The Workers' Hospital give children a sun bath, 1926.

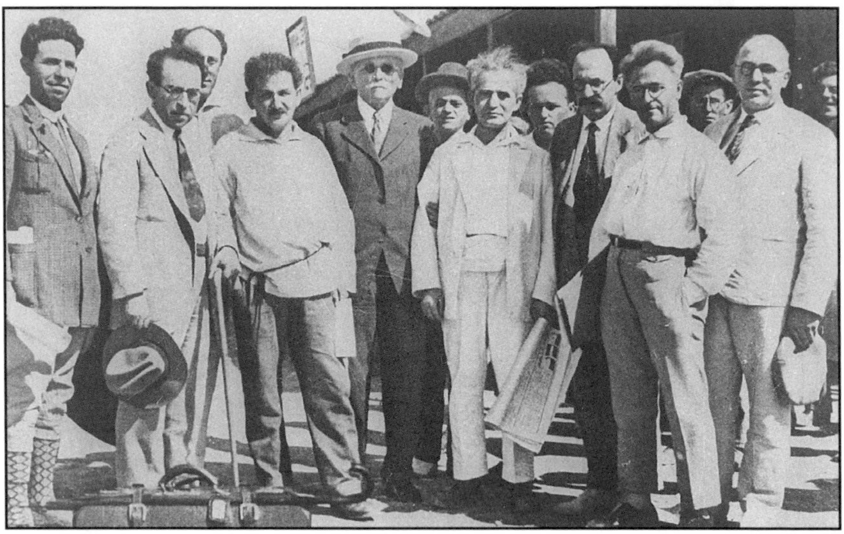

14. The opening ceremony of "Haemeck" (Emek) Hospital in the Jezreel Valley, 1930. British High Commissioner in Palestine Sir John Chancellor (center), Zionist labor leaders Berl Katznelson (left) and David Ben-Gurion holding the workers' newspaper *Davar* (right).

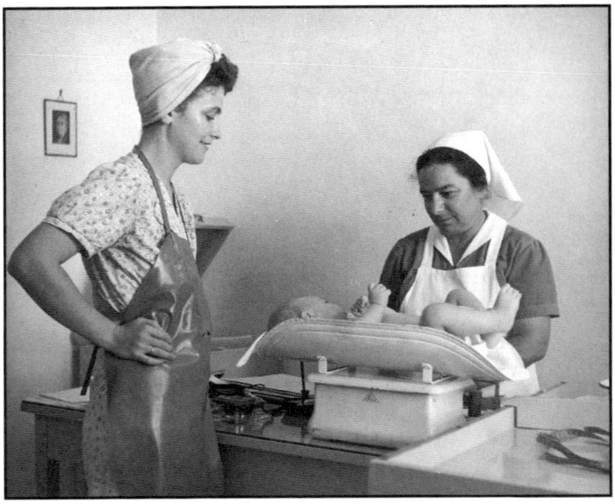

15. Tipat Halav ("A Drop of Milk") Maternal and Child Care Center, early 1930s.

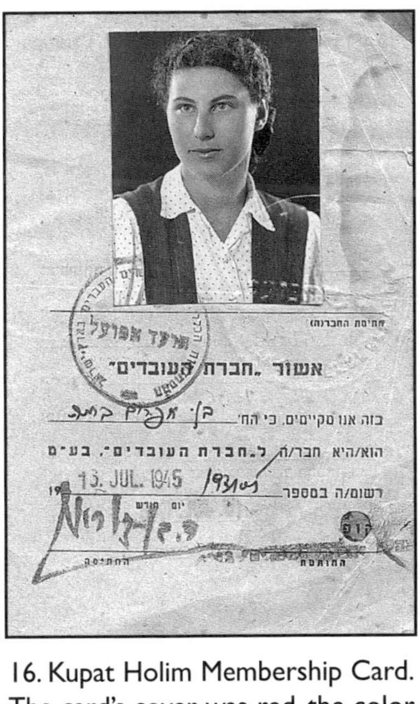

16. Kupat Holim Membership Card. The card's cover was red, the color of the International Workers' Movement, and signed by David Ben-Gurion, Secretary General of the Federation of Labor at the time.

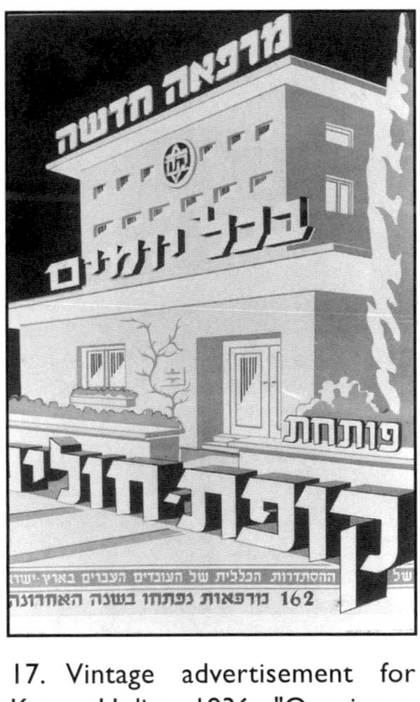
מרפאה חדשה
פותחת
קופת חולי
של ההסתדרות הכללית של העובדים העברים בארץ ישר
162 מרפאות נפתחו בשנה האחרונה

17. Vintage advertisement for Kupat Holim, 1936: "Opening a new clinic every two days, 162 clinics were opened this year."

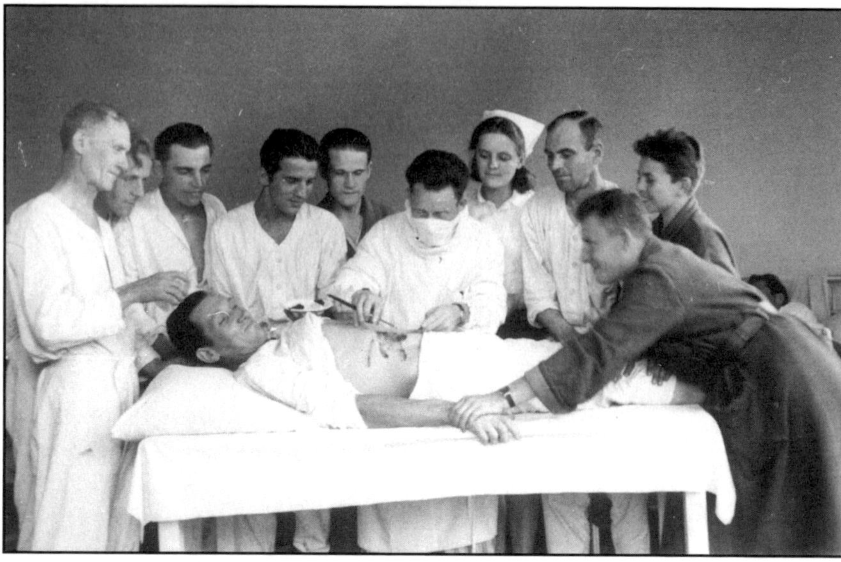

18. Bedside teaching at Beilinson Hospital, Kupat Holim's leading hospital near Tel Aviv, 1936.

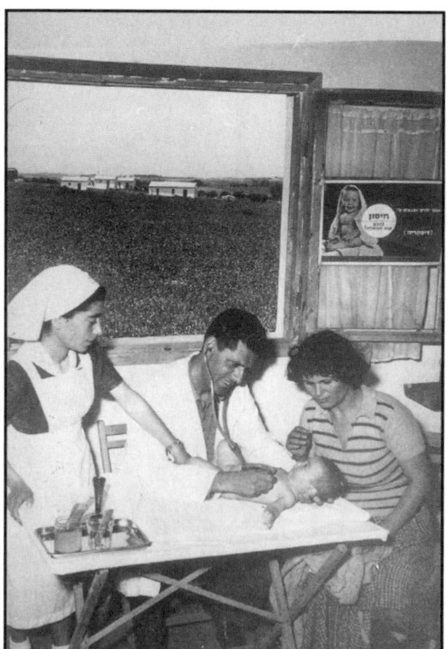

19. Kupat Holim's primary-care clinic in the Jezreel Valley, late 1930s.

7

Confrontation and Cooperation between Kupat Holim and Hadassah, 1920-1930

Hopes and First Struggles (1918–1922)

In August 1918, the American Zionist Medical Unit ("the Unit") began its operations in the health field in Eretz Israel. The medical mission headed by Dr. Rubinow "championed full socialization of medical services, and therefore began to establish a centralized medical service, based on a national network of hospitals and clinics all subordinate to the central management of the organization."[1]

The first attempts of workers' organization in Eretz Israel to establish a working relationship with the Unit, which they called simply "Hadassah" in their conversations and correspondence, began shortly after its arrival. In a letter to members in Rechovot, members of the Hapoel Hatzair detailed the reasons behind the decision to seek medical aid from a philanthropic organization:

> Difficulty in acclimatization that causes frequent illnesses does not allow us, unfortunately, to arrange medical assistance on the basis of self assistance only, and we must also utilize the aid of the entire nation through the Zionist Federation.[2]

The Unit was subordinate to the Zionist Federation in Eretz Israel, and was therefore viewed as "aid from the Jewish People" as a whole, thus making acceptance of aid kosher in their perspective, even a matter of a duty on the part of the givers:

> We can't consider the Hadassah group as [the same as] the American Red Cross, that runs philanthropic work in medicine in Eretz Israel....It emerges as an emissary of Zionism and as an organization of the Hebrew Yishuv.[3]

Expectations and hopes among the Yishuv ran high. At the outset of 1919, Yitzhak Izakovich from the Judea Workers Health Fund turned to the Unit's management, requesting an interview "to clarify the question of arrangement of medical aid in Eretz Israel henceforth."[4]

The degree of response on the part of the Unit to the health fund's request for assistance was described in a letter published in 1919 in *Contras*, the house organ of Achdut Haavodah:

> We conducted negotiations with it from the time of [the Unit's] arrival in Eretz Israel and in the end it became evident that the only thing that we will be able to do (if we suggest it)—is that [the Unit] will accept our sick people without pay. According to the prevailing situation we could not gain from this much utility....Afterwards there were several cases in which we turned [to them] about an automobile for the sick, that had to be transported from place to place and it was impossible to transport them by wagon. Not even in one case were we turned down, not in one case were we [met] by a positive response. There were various reasons for delay.[5]

A report by one the workers to the Jerusalem branch of Achdut Haavodah on 24 November 1919 emphasized:

> What did "Hadassah" or the Doctors' Association [The Hebrew Medical Federation] do to improve the hygienic conditions of workers? Even in the organized workers' groups, where conditions are easier overall, there isn't even minimal supply in a hygienic sense...and it is not at all surprising that the health situation among the workers is so unsound....Local sanitary conditions are entirely shabby, really a reversal to the cave dweller period.[6]

The workers were angry not only because the Medical Unit rejected their demands; they also objected to the Unit's interference in their political matters. Dr. Rubinow, director of the Unit, used his position and influence to demand (through the use of veiled threats) that the health funds, based on political affiliation, be amalgamated for reasons of economy—a move that *both* workers' parties opposed vehemently. While Rubinow sought only to reorganize health services in Eretz Israel according to American standards—on a professional and economical basis—his actions show his lack of understanding of the political culture in Eretz Israel among Unit staff and the role of health services, like other emerging institutions, as a power base and source of political clout in ideological struggles over the future of the Yishuv.

Relations were undermined when Rubinow fired three drivers, members of Achdut Haavodah, after they were accused of theft and fraud, ignoring Ben-Gurion's explanations after Rubinow issued an ultimatum that each office of the health fund must submit a monthly financial report to the Unit if it wished to receive financial assistance in underwriting medical assistance. A series of conflicts between the Unit and the workers' organizations cast a shadow on relationships between the sides, creating a growing gap between the Unit, which aspired to improve the efficiency of health services and the desire of the workers to receive medical assistance.

The workers' health funds were sorely disappointed with what they perceived as a desire to evade provision of substantial assistance as they had requested, and the treatment they received at the hands of Hadassah. Hadassah had a different perception of what constituted suitable assistance in improving the health of workers. According to Henrietta Szold, most work should concentrate on preventive medicine, thus one of the first steps was to establish sanitation groups in the cities whose job it was to supervise garbage collection, oversee conditions in food outlets, inspect meat in slaughterhouses, supervise hospitals, disinfect the belongings of new immigrants, and seek avenues to fight malaria. Economic assistance to the workers' health funds and transport of the sick in cars to hospitals was not part of the program.

In understanding Hadassah's position vis-à-vis the laborers' requests, one must know that while the workers perceived themselves as a Zionist vanguard entitled to special favor and a sector with special needs, numerically the workers' organizations had only several thousand members at the time, and membership in the health funds was limited to no more than 3,000 individuals out of 55,000 Jews living in the country. Hadassah provided assistance solely relative to their numbers. The large urban population was in no better shape than the workers. Thus, one can understand the considerations that guided the Unit's actions in "ignoring" the appeals of the workers to a certain degree and focusing most of their operation on the urban sector. Yet, the workers believed that as the spearhead of the Zionist movement they were entitled to special treatment, despite their small numbers. The American Zionist Medical Unit, isolated from the nuances of local society and unable to appreciate the achievements of the workers' organizations in transforming society, founded their medical operations solely on objective criteria of numerical weight and relative urgency solely in terms of health needs.

At the outset of 1920, with the establishment of British civil government, encampments of Jewish laborers were established in the Jezreel Valley and the Galilee; Hadassah sent doctors, nurses and sanitation personnel to oversee nutrition and hygiene in the encampments. The work of the health officers also served as a source of friction between the workers and Hadassah. Dr. Yosef Shapira, who was sent to the workers' encampment in Migdal on the Sea of Galilee, populated by five hundred laborers, reported that the workers refused to receive inoculations against typhus. They rejected his call to cease drinking water directly from the lake without purification, and claimed their living conditions carried no danger to their lives. The physician's claim that every worker in the camp was affected by malaria due to neglect of hygiene and sanitation fell on deaf ears, and when Shapira sought to purify drinking water by force, the workers organized a boycott. The nurse, Berta Landesman, also sent by Hadassah, sought to change the diet in the camp in Migdal in order to improve the health of the workers and raise their resistance to disease, but the workers also boycotted her efforts and refused to eat the food she prepared. It was only after numerous endeavors that she was able to win their trust and cooperation. One of the primary sources of mistrust was simply lack of a common language and culture; most of the Hadassah staff did not speak Hebrew and their contact with the laborers was conducted in Yiddish or through the auspices of a translator. Moreover, the foreignness of their "American ways" in the eyes of the Eastern European pioneers was further exacerbated by the medical staff's snobbery and patronizing attitude toward the pioneers.

In mid-1919, differences of opinion arose between the Unit and the Committee of Delegates, who viewed themselves as the supreme administrative authority in management of the Yishuv's affairs. According to Menachem Ussiskin, head of the Committee of Delegates, the Unit and its work should be subordinate to the Committee which had been appointed both by the Zionist Federation and the British as the official representative of the Yishuv. Dr. Rubinow and members of the Unit held that they were responsible solely to the American Zionist Federation. The Unit's personnel held that for the sake of order and efficiency in medical work, authority for administration and operations should be clearly delineated, particularly as to who was their direct superior. The Unit believed that the best formula was that they be answerable to the American Zionist Federation, and particularly its women's wing, Hadassah. Hadassah, after all, was the body behind organization of the American Zionist Medical Unit at the request of the World Zionist Federation, as well as being one of the partners underwriting the Unit's operation, together with the JOINT and the Palestine Restoration Fund.

Hadassah's demand for autonomy enjoyed the support of the American Zionist Federation, who viewed the labor movement in Eretz Israel in a negative light. The workers, on the other hand, viewed autonomy as an attempt to break ranks with Zionist control of the Unit's operation in Eretz Israel—a step that they feared would force the Yishuv to accommodate itself to Hadassah's wishes due to the need for its services. In 1919, the Hapoel Hatzair newspaper charged:

> The Hadassah Medical Group has liberated itself from the onus of outside interference and demands and it dwells in its [own] abode and speaks the tongue of its [own] people [i.e., English]....This event is undoubtedly symptomatic for us...dismantling the burden of Zionist discipline....As our ill fate would have it...to be destined [to the authority] of dwellers in [sic] cloud scrapers [i.e., skyscrapers] who together, from the president in Washington to some doctor of Hadassah in Eretz Israel, are joined in the shared belief that money buys everything—opinion and authoritative power to rule....Signs of this tendency to lord over us together with the politics of East Broadway are being done more and more outwardly and in secret... preaching morality with which the conceited authorities with rules of good manners...guide these dwellers of a wild and uncultured land.[7]

The acid tone adopted by Hapoel Hatzair vis-à-vis Hadassah is indicative of the open hostility harbored by the working public toward Hadassah and the decline in Hadassah's status by 1919. Hadassah, it was charged, acted solely in its own self-interest, not in the better interests of the Zionist movement. It was accused of being a snobbish organization that viewed the Yishuv as an inferior element that did not know what was good for itself and had to be taught how to behave, while totally ignoring the achievements of the Yishuv to date. Hapoel Hatzair even suggested boycotting Hadassah in response to its condescending manner and its aspirations to operate as a separate body, beyond the institutional framework of the Yishuv.

Hapoel Hatzair's rabid attack on Hadassah was not left unanswered. Zeev Jabotinsky wrote in the independent newspaper *Haaretz* on 14 December 1919: "The way [the Zionist idea] is sacred, but creative endeavor [i.e., the work of Hadassah] is more sacred," therefore "we must welcome the work of Hadassah in all its facets."

Moshe Smilansky a worker and a writer responded on 19 December 1919: "We cannot fight Hadassah....We don't have the capability to bring this [sacrificial] offering."

For a full year, the labor press continued to attack Hadassah and accuse it of misdoings. Hadassah, it was said, opposed the Zionist idea, made light of the achievements of the Yishuv, and sought to impose a foreign culture upon the Yishuv via the power of the purse. The attacks only worsened after the physical clash between Dr. David de Sola-Pool, manager of assistance of the Committee of Delegates, and Avraham Hartzfeld over levels of monetary assistance to the health funds. Hartzfeld's party newspaper *Contras* wrote, following the incident:

> The clerk [Dr. de Sola-Pool) warden for America's money...could not bear the vehement demands of comrade Hartzfeld and raised a hand against him. The scandal left a harsh impression throughout the entire country among various circles, also in Jerusalem, and also in Jaffa well-attended protest meetings were held.[8]

The workers succeeded in dragging the Zionist Federation, the delegates committee, and Hadassah into the commotion over de Sola-Pool's affront to Hartzfeld.

Roots of the Conflict

What were the primary objections of the workers' parties and their health funds to the manner in which Hadassah conducted its operations in Eretz Israel? Examination of Hadassah's correspondence with the health funds' offices in the years 1919–1920 reveal some of the core factors in the conflict.[9] The main controversy was the demand of each of the sides to determine by itself what to do with the monies earmarked for medical assistance.

Hadassah, which controlled the funding, refused to hand over money without receiving a detailed report and without supervising the ways in which the funds would be utilized. The health funds considered the demand an affront and sought to decide by themselves where to use funding without submitting a detailed account to Hadassah. The funds considered the demand for an account as an expression of lack of confidence, even contempt of their abilities to run their own affairs. Dr. Rubinow wrote to the Hapoel Hatzair health fund:

> What a strange notion about the relation between the AZMU [American Zionist Medical Group] and your federation.You can't tell AZMU what it must do, and you can't expend money on AZMU's account without our approval….This is not my idea of supervision your federation.

In another letter Rubinow wrote:

> I request that you let me know the amount of your debts at the beginning of the month...what was this amount at the end of that month, what was its scope at the end of the year? I must know if your debts are becoming smaller and going down or whether they are continuing to grow….If I won't be shown that you are trying to make amendments in your health fund's ways, according to the letter that I sent you, I won't be able to recommend to the committee, support in the future.

In a letter addressed to Achdut Haavodah in Jaffa, Rubinow wrote: "I want to notify [you] in writing of the conditions that I believe are necessary for proper inspection of your expenditures."

Rubinow went on to request a detailed list of all members and branches, and that the list be sent to Hadassah, adding that only Hadassah would determine which doctors would be authorized to provide treatment to the workers, to authorize travel for examination in Jerusalem, and to refer patients for hospitalization. Moreover, Hadassah demanded that allocation of medications be carried out solely through pharmacists associated with Hadassah or from Hadassah's own medical supply depot. Hadassah refused to pay for medical expenditures that were not in accordance with these directives. The supervision that Dr. Rubinow and Hadassah imposed was not, however, solely in the financial and medical domain. Members of Hadassah even checked the medical files of patients to approve or reject referrals of laborers for medical assistance. The case of Yaakov Dagani, a laborer and member of Hapoel Hatzair, is a case in point. Rubinow wrote Yaakov Aphter, treasurer of the Hapoel Hatzair health fund: "I cannot depend on your testimony. After Mr. Degani will be checked by a committee of doctors in Jerusalem I will let you know what needs to be done to help him."

Elsewhere Rubinow wrote in regard to the worker Yaakov Degani: "[S]urely we will not come to the aid of a person…only because he limps a bit." And in a later correspondence, Rubinow wrote in response to an appeal by Hapoel Hatzair of Hadassah's decision not to treat Degani: "If Yaakov Degani has slight pain and pricking sensations this doesn't mean one needs to give him support for all the days of his life."

In an article *Contras*, members of Achdut Haavodah protested the "rude tone" of Dr. Rubinow's letters to health fund officials. They said that Dr. Rubinow employed the claim that health fund officials were wasting money and making unacceptable demands, while his true purposes were merely to curtail funding transferred by Hadassah to the health fund. The Achdut Haavodah paper sarcastically accused Rubinow of poor judgment:

> Had we reduced the number of the average account by one day [i.e., referring to the number of sick days] then you could have saved 25 Egyptian pounds. What's in your method of sending people home (by train) when they can walk (by foot)?…We of course were not able to carry out Dr. Rubinow's cutbacks in practice because the sick were not willing to be sick one day less. And we could not send

> the sick who came to Jerusalem—the medical center—home to kibbutz Kfar Giladi for instance, a distance of some hundreds of kilometers by foot, not only because such walking home on foot could send a patient that had just risen from his sick bed back to bed, but also out of reasons of economy—for we would have needed to give the sick person on foot provisions for the road for a week.

The Achdut Haavodah Health Fund presented the most extreme examples in its responses to Dr. Rubinow's demands, but even when dealing with regular patients, Hadassah's demands were far reaching and hard to implement, both in terms of curtailment of sick days and demands that the sick be sent home on foot. The demands made in regard to treatment of Yaakov Degani were not out of the ordinary. The supervision that Dr. Rubinow sought to impose on the health funds was extremely rigid and caused difficulties in the operation of the fund.

The funding for medical assistance transferred to the health funds was not solely Hadassah's monies. It also included funding from a host of other organizations—the Zionist Federation, the Foundation Fund, the JOINT and other Jewish bodies—who funneled money through Hadassah for use in addressing health needs in Eretz Israel. From this standpoint, claimed the health funds, Hadassah was merely a pass-through organization for monies it received from others, beyond its own operating budget. The workers' organization argued that these funds belonged to the Yishuv as a whole, and they objected to the centralization imposed by Hadassah. Donald Miller wrote in his work on Hadassah that these clashes over finances and power plays were part of a larger clash for hegemony between members of Hadassah and the Committee of Delegates, and in the early 1920s between Hadassah and the Yishuv's health committee.[10] The historian Doron Netherland, on the other hand, views the conflicts over centralization as emanating primarily from Hadassah's management culture—the centralized administration that characterized the work of Hadassah in Eretz Israel, whether the outgrowth of a model of business administration or a reflection of the personality of its chief executive, Dr. Rubinow.[11]

A summary report regarding Kupat Holim's tie with Hadassah, published in 1923 by the Federation of Labor, noted:

> Up until 1922, relations between Hadassah and Kupat Holim were not orderly and organized. There was no reciprocal agreement based on an abiding coherent foundation [or] a framework for collaborative work. The results of this situation were immediately apparent. Due to the absence of a unified work plan in the same places and the same groups in which the two institutions opened their operations, things came to a collision. This was caused to a large extent by the fact that Hadassah as a strong medical federation whose budget was large and ensured, did not consider it necessary to take into account an institution of mutual assistance of laborers that had yet to crystallize and develop. On one hand, these relations resulted in expenditure of energy and resources in vain, and on the other hand the workers' groups were forced to bear a double burden of expenditures....If the budget that to date was received and expended by Hadassah would be delivered directly to our authority, this would impact significantly on the authority of Kupat Holim, on growth of its members and its overall fiscal strength. It will bring the institution closer to its goal—organization of proper and rational medical assistance based on mutual assistance, totally in keeping with the needs of the Yishuv and aliyah."[12]

It appears that the Federation of Labor was accusing Hadassah of hindering the work of Kupat Holim by an over-strict supervision of the Unit in medical matters and by Hadassah's desire to set the agenda for expenditures. All that the Federation of Labor requested was receipt of financial assistance from Hadassah, without preconditions.

Hadassah of course viewed things from an entirely different perspective. In a report on the relationship between Hadassah and Kupat Holim Henrietta Szold noted:

> Hadassah can hold to its credit that it was one of the parties that brought Kupat Holim to its present level....It was then in the difficult days of 1920–1921 when roads were paved [only] in the [Jezreel] Valley and the north of the country....Two health funds existed, a special fund for every workers' federation that received part of the work. Each federation demanded ambulatory services of a hospital from Hadassah....Hadassah could not agree to this demand. And thus the merger of the two health funds took

> place, not only due to internal necessity, but also due to the explicit demand of Hadassah. From the day of the merger, education of the worker and the work-provider in insurance in case of illness began. Kupat Holim is rightly proud of the degree of public participation it ensured through expenditure on medical treatment, but one should not forget that the presence of Hadassah made it possible for Kupat Holim to rapidly develop a comprehensive social system, for Hadassah liberated them from the exigency of caring for hospitalization of its members.[13]

Similar sentiments were voiced in the summary report of two decades of work in Eretz Israel, published by Hadassah in 1939. In the introduction to the volume and in the report dealing with the early 1920s, Kupat Holim was not mentioned at all as a significant factor in the health domain, and Hadassah preferred to take full credit for medical treatment provided Jewish pioneers in labor encampments during these years.

Hadassah chose to crown itself for achievements of others, even claiming to be the "moving force" behind unification of the Eretz Israel labor movement's two health funds. Such an attitude shows the inability of Hadassah's personnel to grasp the political culture in Eretz Israel at the time. The two health funds did not unite, and would not have united, under pressure from Hadassah; they would have done so only in keeping with the decisions of their own party and own political leaders. Generally, health matters were of little consequence in deciding political matters. When party ideology was weighed against medical assistance, ideology usually won out and health considerations were pushed to the sidelines. This was the nature of labor parties at the time and also reflected considerations that fueled the health funds which were part and parcel of the political system and subordinate to the directives of the party.

The basic contrasts between Henrietta Szold's report and the articles against Hadassah published in the Eretz Israel press reflect the differences in the way Hadassah and Kupat Holim viewed one another. Kupat Holim regarded Hadassah solely as a source of funding, while Hadassah viewed Kupat Holim as an unorganized body unable to operate effectively without both monetary *and* organizational assistance. The differences burdened and overshadowed attempts to work in collaboration, and served as an ongoing source of conflict between Hadassah and Kupat Holim throughout the Mandate period.

First Agreements Between Hadassah and Kupat Holim

In 1920, British military rule, imposed with the conquest of Eretz Israel in the latter stages of the First World War, was rescinded and a civilian administration was organized under the British Mandate. The change in the regime called for a change in the deployment and organization of the American Medical Unit. In the years 1918–1920, the Unit had operated as a temporary rescue organization that engaged primarily in immediate medical assistance and burning needs. The advent of the British Mandate required that the Unit assist in the establishment of a health system that would provide ongoing medical care on a permanent basis to the Yishuv. Such a mission could not be carried out by an ad hoc organization; moreover, Hadassah sought to transform the Unit into a permanent, autonomous institution. After a year of deliberations, the Twelfth Zionist Congress, convening in Carlsbad in September 1921, resolved to transform the Unit into an independent medical federation that would operate in Eretz Israel as an autonomous body, though subordinate to its parent organization, Hadassah in America. At the same time, the congress resolved to establish a health committee that would take upon itself management, organization, and coordination of all health activities in the Yishuv.

It was clear to Kupat Holim, which began to operate on an organized footing under the leadership of Eliezer Perlson in early 1922, that in order to take the high road, Kupat Holim must establish a working relationship with the Hadassah Medical Federation.

In November 1922, after prolonged negotiations, the first working contract was signed between the two organizations. David Ben-Gurion and Eliezer Perlson were the signatories for the health fund. Henrietta Szold, Shoshana Yaakobi, and Irma Lindheim signed in the name of Hadassah.

The opening clauses of the contract stipulated that Hadassah would supply Kupat Holim with medications and assist it in equipping itself and in hospitalization of workers in Hadassah's institutions. Kupat Holim would bear half the expenditures. Opening of clinics and mobilization of additional employees by Kupat Holim would hinge on agreement between the two sides and be in keeping with Hadassah's budgetary capabilities. Furthermore, it was stipulated that

> all work at laborers' points [of settlement] would be done in accordance with a reciprocal agreement. Actualization of the resolutions would be carried out by Hadassah....Hadassah negates the right to arrange special contracts between itself and individual groups of workers.[14]

The contract served the interests of both organizations. Kupat Holim sought to return to a framework of mutual assistance in lieu of philanthropic assistance, and even protect itself from organization of groups of laborers outside its own framework; Hadassah remained the administrator of the operation of the medical system and continued to hold the right to make decisions in medical matters. Assistance to Kupat Holim had no negative impact on Hadassah's regular budget, for Hadassah's commitment did not go beyond the existing budget.

The agreement with Hadassah strengthened Kupat Holim greatly: The health fund was recognized as the exclusive body entitled to operate among the working public, free of any competition; the entire working public was "handed over" to Kupat Holim en bloc. A laborer who sought medical assistance through his place of work at a modest price had to join Kupat Holim, and had no other reasonable alternative. The contract with Hadassah enabled Kupat Holim, for the first time, to increase its membership rolls and its revenues by a significant margin, and expand the framework of its operation. In the first year following the signing of the contract, Kupat Holim established fifteen mobile sick rooms (tents) with a total of two hundred beds, and the number of Kupat Holim members grew by 60 percent—from 4,000 to 6,000 members.[15]

But, the contract was not long-lived. In July 1923, Hadassah sought to open negotiations for a new contract, due to the large outlay (more than expected) incurred in the wake of the Hadassah–Kupat Holim accord. Now Hadassah demanded that Kupat Holim bear the full burden of expenditures for medications and additional expenditures of food, lodging, and travel by patients, not half the cost as stipulated in the original contract. Kupat Holim opposed this and announced to Hadassah that it could not operate under the new conditions, and if Hadassah did not lower its demands, the health fund would turn to the Zionist Congress (that stood to convene in Carlsbad in September 1923) and demand that the fund's budget allocated by the Zionist Congress be funneled directly to

Kupat Holim. The Yishuv's health committee supported Kupat Holim's position on this matter. Hadassah announced it could not change its demands prior to the convening of the congress, which stood to approve Hadassah's own budget; if the congress did increase its budget, Hadassah could compromise with Kupat Holim on the conditions laid down in the new contract. Until a new contract could be signed, Hadassah promised to provide Kupat Holim with one-time intermediate funding of 6,000 Egyptian pounds. Kupat Holim agreed to wait and shelved its appeal to the congress, but demanded it receive representation on the Hadassah management. A voice in the management would enable Kupat Holim to present its case in matters concerning the health fund; under the current framework, all members of the management resided abroad and important decisions that concerned the health fund were made in New York.

In retrospect, Kupat Holim's shelving of its appeal was a great mistake. Hadassah's budget was not increased by the congress and Kupat Holim missed the opportunity to obtain a separate independent budget for itself. On the new Hadassah management only one place out of five was allocated to Kupat Holim, and the fund refused to fill the chair since such representation would lack any real significance. A short time afterwards, Kupat Holim was forced to sign a new contract with Hadassah under far worse terms. One of the clauses in the contract stipulated that "transfers from various places that will be carried out in light of this accord and dismissals will be set according to the needs of Hadassah (and the sites interested in such)."

Furthermore the contract also dictated that general administration of health services in the Yishuv would be in the hands of Hadassah, and Kupat Holim would be required to submit to Hadassah detailed monthly reports on expenditures and to submit to the following operating regime:

> Hadassah management will have the right to visit all the local medical stations of Kupat Holim and give orders to the station management and to demand all reports necessary. As well, [Hadassah] has the right to withhold providing medicines from those stations that will not fulfill the demands they receive or curtail the scope of medicines.

As for payment for hospitalization and medications, the contract required Kupat Holim to pay 50 percent of all medical expenditures and all expenditures on food, lodging, and beds in sick rooms for medical staff and hospitalized workers. The only area where Kupat Holim enjoyed total independence was in convalescence facilities, for Hadassah had neither interest nor fiscal obligation to assist in such matters.

The new contract put Kupat Holim in an impossible position. On one hand it had to ensure that ongoing medical aid dependent on Hadassah would not be stopped; on the other hand, the terms of the new contract doubled its expenditures and led to a huge deficit. When Kupat Holim asked Hadassah to ease the terms of the contract, Hadassah agreed, on condition that the health fund would waive part of the subsidization it received on medications.

Power Struggles between Kupat Holim and Hadassah

Already in mid-1922 Hadassah management moved to greatly curtail its medical assistance to workers in order to balance its budget, which had been impaired by losses incurred in supply of medication to Kupat Holim at reduced prices, and to cover other fiscal problems stemming from a drop in the organization's revenues in the United States. Consequently, Hadassah closed its hospital in Tiberias, curtailed the number of hospital beds in Safed, closed the surgical ward in Jaffa, curtailed maintenance bills on patients, decreased supply of medications (primarily quinine), and reduced the length of hospital stays for malaria patients to a maximum of seven days (insufficient time for full recovery). Those most affected by the cutbacks were the working public in the Galilee and the Jezreel Valley, for closure of the hospital in Tiberias forced the laborers to turn to Hadassah's hospital in Haifa, a facility that was almost always full. Kupat Holim's request that Hadassah establish a special hospital for malaria cases, whose operation would be low-cost compared to regular hospitalization costs, was rejected. Thus Kupat Holim was forced to take upon itself roles from which Hadassah withdrew, resulting in an increase in medical expenditures beyond what had been budgeted.

Fierce criticism was voiced in the press over curtailment of Hadassah's operation, a move that was worst felt among the laborers. Members of the Yishuv's health committee also condemned the cutbacks and claimed that Hadassah should not save expenditures at the expense of Kupat Holim. But Kupat Holim had misgivings about an open battle with Hadassah, despite the support of the health committee, primarily because it did not have enough personnel and medical institutions of its own to operate alternative health services. In retrospect, it became evident that Hadassah's moves indeed impaired the health of the workers. Due to economic pressure applied by Hadassah on Kupat Holim, and the health fund's inability to take steps to remedy or at least mitigate the situation, Kupat Holim found itself in deep economic trouble. In the end, Kupat Holim came to the conclusion that it could not depend on Hadassah nor count on Hadassah's medical assistance over time. The conclusion was that Kupat Holim must embark on establishment of health facilities of its own, if it wished to free itself from dependence on the benevolence or good will of others.

Why did Hadassah lock Kupat Holim into such a harsh contract? The official explanation was of course budgetary problems in the organization's operation in Eretz Israel that forced Hadassah to curtail its assistance to Kupat Holim. For the same reason, Hadassah signed a contract in mid-1923 with the JOINT for joint financing of the operation of four Hadassah hospitals in Eretz Israel. The agreement brought about appointment of two members of the JOINT to the Hadassah management in New York (out of a four-member executive). There is substance to the suspicion that the admission of the JOINT, a non-Zionist Jewish aid organization, to Hadassah management, and its involvement in financing Hadassah's operations, ultimately impacted in Hadassah's work in Eretz Israel. In the wake of the agreement, all Hadassah activities in Eretz Israel came to be managed from New York, and the local Hadassah management had little influence on its decisions. Moreover, Kupat Holim did not receive more than one representative on Hadassah's local management. It seems that the Hadassah management sought to hide its own internal difficulties from the eyes of the heads of Kupat Holim, using fiscal difficulties as a ploy.

Reuven Shenkar, chief executive for financial matters in Kupat Holim, viewed Hadassah's moves as stemming not from financial difficulties but rather from Hadassah's opposition in principle to Kupat Holim's intention to establish its own health institutions. Hadassah sought to keep Kupat Holim under its wing, so it could serve as a broker or agent between the fund and the insurees. Shenkar claims that most of the controversies between Hadassah and Kupat Holim in the years 1922–1924 focused on this issue.

One can find support for Shenkar's claims in an episode in the summer of 1923, when the questions were raised about an independent Kupat Holim clinic in Jerusalem and the transfer of the Labor Battalion's hospital in kibbutz Ein-Harod to Kupat Holim. According to Perlson, Hadassah opposed these initiatives and viewed them as an invasion of a privileged Hadassah domain (medical aid in the cities and operation of hospitals). In a July 1923 letter to the heads of the Federation of Labor and Kupat Holim, Henrietta Szold wrote in the name of the Hadassah executive committee in Eretz Israel that the Kupat Holim initiative to open new service centers without coordinating such steps with Hadassah and without its approval was unacceptable and therefore would not be covered by the health budget. Kupat Holim was called to order—that is, told to listen to Hadassah from now on.

Further substantiation for the supposition that budgetary problems alone did not stand at the foundations of Hadassah's behavior can be found in a report written by Professor Rosental, a physician and a Zionist leader from the U.S. who visited Eretz Israel in 1922. Rosental noted: "Had it not been for the latter [Kupat Holim], Hadassah would have been forced to outlay on medical assistance to laborers…sums several times the amount now." The professor recommended that Hadassah spread its institutions around the country, and rely on local institutions of Kupat Holim, stressing that "There is no doubt that the independent operation of the workers eases and lowers costs of Hadassah's work."[16]

One may safely assume that the controversy between Hadassah and Kupat Holim derived not only from the intention of Kupat Holim to break ties with Hadassah in the future, but also from rivalry over control: which organization would control medical services in Eretz Israel? The vision of the two organizations was fundamentally different. Hadassah was a philanthropic body aspiring to establish a nation-wide health system on a broad centralized base. Kupat Holim was a voluntary organization that rejected any non-collective professional mold and believed it was its duty to establish an equalitarian nation-wide health system on the basis of mutual aid.

Another issue, besides the disagreement over the terms of the second contract, was monetary aid to Kupat Holim from the health committee of the Zionist executive. The funding was obtained after much effort on the part of Kupat Holim, in which Reuven Shenkar was particularly instrumental. At the close of 1925, with the agreement of Henrietta Szold, Dr.Yosef Burger, a Zionist activist from Kovna, approved a yearly budget to Kupat Holim, and one-time coverage of the health fund's deficit. But despite Henrietta Szold's agreement, the Hadassah management in Eretz Israel disapproved of the additional funding. They viewed it as assistance to the workers in organizing independent medical assistance (which they opposed on principle) and invasion by Kupat Holim of a domain that was the prerogative of Hadassah (the financial sphere). The issue of a separate budget for Kupat Holim was not new. Already in September 1921, prior to the twelfth Zionist congress in Carlsbad, Dr. Rubinow wrote to the Zionist executive: "Kupat Holim should not engage in arrangement of medical assistance while this is the role of Hadassah, and anyway no special budget is needed for Kupat Holim."[17] The heads of Kupat Holim knew that they could receive a separate budget that would free the health fund of its dependence on Hadassah, but in the early years of Kupat Holim, they were apprehensive over a fight with Hadassah, for the health fund was still very dependent on Hadassah's medical faculties that had no substitute. For the same reasons, Kupat Holim did not carry through the decision of the Yishuv's health committee of October 1922 that clarified: "Kupat Holim has the full right to receive its budget directly and not through Hadassah."

Only after Hadassah's cutbacks led to a sustained impairment in medical services to workers did Kupat Holim actualize its right to receive a separate budget from the Zionist executive. This was, in essence, the first step taken by the fund on the road to independence.

The power struggles between Hadassah and Kupat Holim and impairment of health services for laborers were not limited to a handful of officials in both camps, but were discussed in detail in the press.

A Federation of Labor report concerning the attitude for Hadassah towards Kupat Holim was published in the Federation of Labor's organ, *Pinkas*, in 1923:

> In light of the above, the question arises as to the role and manner of operation of Hadassah. It is clear that in its present state this Federation [i.e., the Hadassah Medical Federation] cannot realize its plans—to provide for the medical needs of the Hebrew Yishuv in accordance with its development and needs. The Hadassah management is

> distanced from interests of the inhabitants. There is not one delegate on the [Hadassah] management from the Yishuv or the part of it most interested in medical assistance, and from here [emanates] the same inappropriateness between work modes and its forms, and the needs of the Yishuv. This is also the reason that cutbacks made by Hadassah are in total opposition to our interests and are being made not in accordance with real needs.

In a long article in *Hapoel Hatzair* 15 March 1922, under the heading "As to the Way of Kupat Holim," the worker Avraham Kosovsky, a Kupat Holim activist, called upon Kupat Holim to sever its ties with Hadassah and organize its work on a different footing, separate from Hadassah:

> We amused ourselves with the hope that Hadassah would provide workers with all the medical assistance in the country. However this hope is dissipating, and realities prove to us that one should not depend on philanthropists. The time has come to begin creating elementary medical institutions suitable to conditions in the country, the state of medical assistance in general and all this within the boundaries of our capabilities.

Henrietta Szold challenged Kosovsky's call in the press, trying to prove through statistics that cutbacks in Hadassah had not impaired medical services for laborers, but Kosovsky replied that despite the objective difficulties facing Hadassah, it should first cut back administrative manpower and not the health services themselves. (Kosovsky cited as an example the closure of the hospital in Tiberias, which Henrietta Szold did not deny.) Kosovsky added that Hadassah should not claim its innocence and pretend that curtailments had merely been forced upon it and that the best interests of the workers had always been one of Hadassah's concerns, for everyone knew how Hadassah had operated in Zionist institutions—working against a separate budget for Kupat Holim, then imposing harsh terms on Kupat Holim in a joint contract.

The Management Crisis in Hadassah

From the outset of Hadassah's work in Eretz Israel in 1920, Henrietta Szold was forced to deal with management problems within the organization in Eretz Israel, and frequent turnover of its directors. Hadassah was unable to find a permanent replacement for Dr. Rubinow after the director left his post in 1922, following Rubinow's "battle of wills" with local leadership of the Yishuv,[18] Szold was forced to take over management of the organization for the time being. Toward the end of that year, Szold asked Rabbi Judah Leib Magnes to substitute for her, so Szold could return to the United States. A year later in November 1923, Dr. Shimon Meshulam Tannenbaum from the Beth David Hospital in New York was appointed director. In October 1924, Dr. Tennenbaum left due to adjustment problems, and again Henrietta Szold was forced to appoint a temporary director—Dr. Alexander Selkind—but within several months Dr. Selkind returned to New York due to illness, and again Hadassah was left without a permanent director of its affairs in Eretz Israel. At the beginning of 1926, after four years of temporary leadership, finally Hadassah found a permanent (and, so it seemed, a suitable) director: Dr. Efriam Blueston from Mount Sinai Hospital in New York. Dr. Blueston committed himself to serve at least three years as director.

Dr. Blueston had a promising record. He was the son of a Zionist family and a physician and surgeon with experience as a military doctor in the First World War who despite his age (35) was considered a very able administrator. Yet, Dr. Blueston was a technocrat—cold, determined, and not given to compromise with ease. With his arrival, he had very clear ideas how he thought Hadassah should be managed although he knew little about the status of the Yishuv or Kupat Holim's work, the state of health of the laborers, or the workings of Hadassah on the local level. He viewed his mission as an economic one, and was very apprehensive in regard to Kupat Holim officials whom he assumed sought to take advantage of Hadassah's philanthropic assistance without any attempt on their part to streamline their operation. Not surprisingly, troubles soon developed.

A short time after his arrival, news appeared in the Yishuv that the new director's salary was $10,000—ten times of the wages of the average workers—and immediately the new director found himself under attack in the media by a united front comprised of heads of the Federation of Labor, Kupat Holim physicians, and newspaper editors. Dr. Blueston did not anticipate such an attack and requested that Henrietta Szold annul his contract so he could return to New York, but Hadassah management stood behind him and convinced him to stay. In July 1926, Henrietta Szold reported to Hadassah management that Dr. Blueston's work was based purely on professional calculations; Dr. Blueston refused to take into account "Zionist considerations"—particularly when they stood in contradiction with his professional opinion. Thus, he was opposed to Hadassah's part in the operation of hospitals in Tel Aviv and Haifa, rejected decision-making procedures in medical matters, argued that the Yishuv's health committee was a "serious threat to the independence of Hadassah," and indirectly set himself in opposition to any tie between health work in Eretz Israel and the Zionist Federation.

The "Certificate of Poverty" Episode and the 1927 Accord

The primary "casualty" of Dr. Blueston's work was Kupat Holim. His first step as director was to abolish the linkage between Kupat Holim and hospitalization of its members in Hadassah hospitals set forth in the 1922 accord. From January 1927 forward, all discounts given to Kupat Holim by Hadassah were cancelled, and the hospitals were given orders to change the admission procedure for Kupat Holim members. The hospitals were

> not to receive members of the Health Fund [for hospitalization] on the strength of Health Fund documents as was customary until now, but rather as patients are received from the rest of the Yishuv (by documents from the Community Committee or other institutions vouching for poverty, and so forth.[19]

Dr. Blueston held that "there is no place in Eretz Israel for a class-based institution for laborers." Unemployed laborers in need of hospitalization were now forced to turn to all sorts of institutions and request a "certificate of poverty" in order to be hospitalized in a

Hadassah hospital. It is hard to imagine how demeaning this requirement was for the working public. In a sweep of his hand, Dr. Blueston had abrogated the very essence of Kupat Holim's existence as an institution of mutual assistance.

Attempts to negotiate with Dr. Blueston were of no avail, and even the intervention of Colonel Kisch, director of the Zionist executive, failed to move him. For Kupat Holim, Blueston's move was paramount to a "declaration of war," and the health fund mobilized all its forces to do battle not only against the decision, but the director behind its adoption. In the main cities, mass protests were organized against Hadassah, particularly its director. The protesters called upon Hadassah to recall Dr. Blueston to the United States, change Hadassah's work modes in Eretz Israel, and allow members of the Yishuv to participate in management of Hadassah affairs in Eretz Israel. In meetings there were calls to denounce the "anti-settlement" activities of Hadassah and calls to boycott the organization.

Dr. Blueston's response was swift. In a letter to Eliezer Perlson, director of Kupat Holim, he wrote:

> We deny most emphatically that Hadassah has any intentions to subjugate the organized working public or engage it in a war, at all. The most incisive proof is the fact that we are providing our services to members of the organized working public under the same terms that we offer to all classes of the Yishuv [i.e., via requirement of a Certificate of Poverty]....The war that Your Honor speaks of is the fruit of your imagination and the fruit of Kupat Holim's actions, and not of Hadassah's.[20]

In America where Dr. Blueston was raised and educated, a Certificate of Poverty was an acceptable "means test" that enabled the lower classes to receive free hospitalization, and was not viewed as a requirement that demeaned the holder. Consequently, he could not understand what the protest among the laborers and Kupat Holim was all about. He could not even fathom what a Certificate of Poverty signified in the eyes of unemployed Zionist pioneers, who felt such a requirement stripped them of their dignity, for membership in Kupat Holim had always ensured medical care to unemployed members of the Federation as an entitlement, not a matter of charity or compassion.

Due to the acrimonious dispute with Hadassah and the difficulties entailed in finding hospitalization for its members, Kupat Holim decided to send those in need of hospital care in the Haifa area to the German mission hospital in the city. The repercussions of the dispute reached the Zionist executive and Dr. Blueston's reputation was damaged by the controversy. Henrietta Szold and the Hadassah management in New York also felt that Dr. Blueston's decisions directed against Kupat Holim and his attempts to rid himself of the authority of the health committee representative of the Zionist executive in Eretz Israel were erroneous decisions, for they failed to take into account "the good of the Yishuv" and Zionist interests. Henrietta Szold held that Zionist considerations *should* be the foundation of Hadassah's work in Eretz Israel.

In April 1927 a special session of the Zionist executive was called to deal with the dispute. Participating in the gathering were Henrietta Szold, Shoshana Yaakobi, and Irma Lindheim as delegates of Hadassah, and David Ben-Gurion, Eliezer Perlson, Yitzhak Kenivsky-Kenev, and Reuven Shenkar as representative of Kupat Holim and the Federation of Labor. In two prolonged sessions it was agreed to renew collaboration between Kupat Holim and Hadassah as stipulated in the new contract, and update pay schedules for hospitalization of Kupat Holim members in Hadassah hospitals. Dr. Blueston was not invited to be party to the deliberations at the Zionist executive, while Eliezer Perlson, director of Kupat Holim did participate in formulation of the new agreement—a clear demonstration of non-confidence in Bluestone's leadership that also underscored Henrietta Szold's displeasure with his management style and the negative public image he had acquired. Consequently, in February 1928, Bluestone submitted his resignation, but agreed to stay another few months until a replacement could be found.

In the April 1927 agreement, not all issues were resolved, and disagreements between Hadassah and Kupat Holim continued. Hadassah continued to demand that unemployed members of the health fund present Certificates of Poverty if they sought free hospitalization (in which case, Kupat Holim was not billed for their care) and that Certificates of Poverty be issued by community institutions, holding that Kupat Holim's confirmation of the individuals economic state was not sufficient. Hadassah suspected that Kupat Holim was issuing Certificates of Poverty on behalf of health fund members in need of hospitalization in order to dodge payment of the fund's part in the cost of hospital care. Hadassah claimed that they had uncovered, among the "free patients," members of Kupat Holim who had paid dues (and therefore were apparently not indigent), and rejected the health fund's explanations that such cases were the outcome of innocent mistakes and were not deliberate acts. Kupat Holim argued that its officials were in a better position to know the economic state of their members than any community institution, and therefore their confirmations of inability to pay were far more reliable and should be honored. Dr. Blueston charged that Kupat Holim sent Hadassah only its free patients, while those who would be required to pay were referred to other hospitals whose hospitalization tariffs were lower. Blueston was referring to hospitalization of health fund members in the German hospital in Haifa between January and May of 1927. While the daily costs of hospitalization in the German hospital were indeed lower, the practice was initiated by the fund as part of Kupat Holim's dispute with Hadassah, not as an economy move.

Only after protracted negotiations did Hadassah agree to rescind its demand, abolish the demeaning concept of Certificates of Poverty, and renew recognizing of permits issued by Kupat Holim to its members referred for hospitalization. In one of the last letters written to Eliezer Perlson, Dr. Blueston wrote:

> Hadassah Medical Federation does not want, just like Kupat Holim, to employ expressions that could hurt the feelings of the patient. We attach herein a copy of the circular to our branches in which we request they cancel the name "Certification of Poverty."[21]

In September 1928, Dr. Blueston returned to New York and in his stead Dr. Chaim Yaski was appointed director of Hadassah operations in Eretz Israel. In a long eighteen-page report summing up Hadassah's activities in Eretz Israel, submitted at a press conference held under the auspices of the World Zionist Movement's Fund, Bluestone mentioned Kupat Holim only parenthetically in the section "Relationships between Hadassah and Other Health Institutions in Eretz Israel." In a brief paragraph—no more than nine lines—Dr. Blueston spoke of the treatment provided sick laborers by Hadassah. The dispute with Kupat Holim was not mentioned at all.

The appointment of Dr. Chaim Yaski, a Zionist pioneer in his own right who had received his medical training in Odessa, met the approval of the Yishuv, after over a decade marked by tension and discontent. Unlike the directors who preceded him—all of them individuals schooled in the American system that were perceived as outsiders by the Yishuv—Dr. Yaski was born in Eastern Europe, had a clear Zionist perspective, and could understand the complexities of local society and the demands of the Yishuv in health matters. Yaski served as Hadassah director for twenty years, until his untimely death in 1948 during Israel's War of Independence. He was one of seventy-eight medical personnel and escorts killed in the convoy of doctors and nurses on their way to the Hadassah Hospital complex on Mount Scopus, attacked by Palestinian Arab insurgents in mid-April 1948.

Under the leadership of Dr. Yaski, Kupat Holim and Hadassah again assumed a collaborative relationship. While disagreements did not cease, controversy was dealt with in a businesslike manner, mostly focusing on matters such as funding, financing of medications, calculation of hospitalization time, coverage of new immigrants, and so forth. It was clear to Kupat Holim that they could find a ready ear in Hadassah management, even if in the framework of his post, Dr. Yaski had to work primarily for the good of Hadassah.

Despite the vast improvement in relations between the two bodies, the heads of Kupat Holim and the Federation of Labor never forgot the harsh clash with Dr. Blueston, particularly the impotence they felt when Hadassah closed the doors of its hospitals to Kupat Holim members, and the health fund's weakness and almost total dependence on Hadassah for hospitalized care. The lesson learned was that Kupat Holim must expand independent ambulatory institutions and establish a large hospital that would operate under their own auspices. The decision to establish an independent Kupat Holim hospital had begun to take shape earlier, but became all the more urgent during the crisis with Hadassah. With the conclusion of the dispute, the decision was taken: To establish a central hospital of its own in the Jezreel Valley.

8

The Emek (Jezreel Valley) Hospital

In April 1930, the new Emek (Jezreel Valley) Hospital was opened on the slopes of Mount Moreh near Afula city. The inauguration ceremonies were attended by the heads of Kupat Holim, representatives of Zionist institutions in Eretz Israel and from abroad, a crowd of residents of the Valley, and the laborers who worked on construction of the hospital. None of the participants in festivities imagined that the opening of the hospital would mark an important turn in the development of Kupat Holim for years to come, and was destined to impact on the structure and role of Kupat Holim and the face of the health system of the state of Israel to this day.

Hospitalization Services in the Valley

The Emek Hospital had its beginnings in the hospital established by the Labor Battalion at kibbutz Ein-Harod. The hospital consisted of one wooden hut with twenty-two beds that was established at the advent of Jewish settlement in the Jezreel Valley in the early 1920s, a facility that served primarily as a treatment center for the numerous malaria cases plaguing the Valley. The director of the Ein-Harod hospital, Dr. Ben-Zion Hershovitz, was assisted in his work by members of kibbutz Ein-Harod, although most lacked any professional training in nursing or medicine. In 1924, in the wake of the political crisis between the Labor Battalion and the Federation of Labor (see chapter 5) the hospital was turned over to Kupat Holim. The number of beds was increased to thirty-two, a special hut was added for maternity cases under the direction of Dr. Hugo Cohen, a gynecologist who had emigrated from Germany, and in April 1926 work was begun on the establishment of a pediatrics department under the direction of Dr. Gerta Unger. Despite expansion of the hospital, in the mid-1920s it became evident that there was a need to replace the wooden structures with stone buildings in order to meet hygienic standards becoming of a modern hospital, as well as to provide room for the much-needed labs, an x-ray institute, and so forth.

In December 1925, amid discourse in the press in preparation for the convention of the Kupat Holim council, Yitzhak Kenivsky-Kenev wrote of the need to establish a building for the hospital in the Valley. Kenivsky-Kenev was one of the first to envision Kupat Holim as a core body in health services in Eretz Israel and to argue that Kupat Holim should break away from Hadassah and operate the health fund as an independent body. He was one of the first to call for "building anew" the hospital in the Valley to serve members of Kupat Holim in the vicinity. Kenivsky-Kenev noted that the constellation of Hadassah institutions in Haifa were not in a position to hospitalize members of the health fund from the Valley and provide them with suitable medical treatment:

> In the Valley today there are 700-800 children, and in the hospital in Haifa only 8 beds have been earmarked for children….It is clear that the Valley cannot enjoy [the services] of this department at all….Only a permanent building will save this important institution and allow putting it on proper footing….Without sophisticated medicine there is no hope for development of our public medicine….Only in suitable buildings can we realize our aspirations to establish a sophisticated hospital in the Valley with auxiliary institutions, such as a sophisticated laboratory, x-ray cabinet for diagnostics and so forth.[1]

Kenivsky-Kenev's public call to build a modern hospital in the Valley won the support of Dr. Ben-Zion Hershovitz, director of the Ein-Harod hospital. Three weeks after publication of Kenivsky-Kenev's article, Dr. Hershovitz published an apocalyptic article in *Davar* in which he described the dire state of the Ein-Harod hospital, warning of a pending crisis if nothing was done to rectify the situation. Dr. Hershovitz also argued that only establishment of a new modern hospital could save the health and well-being of Valley residents, members of Kupat Holim.

Kenivsky-Kanev's and Hershovitz's idea quickly struck a cord among members of the Kupat Holim directorate and Valley residents. In order to increase the number of supporters for the idea, Dr. Hershovitz set out to convince the heads of Kupat Holim and the Federation of Labor to adopt the idea. At the same time, veteran settlements in the Jezreel Valley—kibbutz Beit Alpha and kibbutz Ein-Harod, and the farms Kfar Yechezkel and Nahalal—applied pressure on the powers-that-be in the labor movement to establish a new hospital in the Valley and even committed them to play a significant role in realizing the vision. It was not difficult for Dr. Hershovitz to convince all those involve of the need to construct the hospital, for the health situation in the Valley was particularly troublesome. Yet, it was clear to all that even if the endeavor were approved (by the Mandate government, the Zionist executive, and the Federation of Labor) Kupat Holim could not bear the cost alone, and would have to mobilize a great deal of assistance in order to bring such a project to fruition.

However, Kupat Holim's appeal to the Zionist executive in this matter was met by total rejection, due to two factors: the difficult financial state of the Zionist executive, and objection on principle to Kupat Holim's entering the hospitalization domain where Hadassah enjoyed exclusivity. Of course, Hadassah also opposed the idea for the same reasons. Yet, having been stonewalled on all fronts did not dampen the determination of Kupat Holim's leadership. Eliezer Perlson, director of Kupat Holim, knew that in order to succeed, he needed to convince Henrietta Szold, influential with both the Zionist executive and the Hadassah management, of the logic of his cause. Perlson, Dr. Hershovitz, and Moshe Soroka (at the time coordinator of Kupat Holim operations in the Valley) wrote letters to Henrietta Szold describing the dire health situation in the Valley and arguing that if a new hospital would be built in the vicinity, it would greatly ease the pressure on Hadassah's hospital in Haifa. The letters had a positive impact on Henrietta Szold's position, and in retrospect was an excellent tactic in taking their cause forward.

Organization and Mobilization of Donors

At the outset of 1926, the idea of constructing a hospital in the Valley had already won over many supporters, yet timing was also in Kupat Holim's favor. Hadassah's Eretz Israel operation was struggling with its own management problems and lacked a permanent director. Thus, it was natural for the heads of Kupat Holim to turn directly to Henrietta Szold in an appeal for support, without offending anyone. It would seem that the management problems faced by Hadassah and its difficulties in providing Kupat Holim with an alternative for meeting the shortage of hospitalization facilities for Valley residents played a significant role in Szold's ultimate stand. She announced her support of the proposal. Moreover, Kupat Holim was fortunate to have gained her support prior to appointment of Dr. Blueston as director of Hadassah operations in Eretz Israel. Although Dr. Blueston himself opposed the idea, he was forced to accept the decision as a *fait accompli*. Henrietta Szold was won over by Perlson's and Soroka's arguments that one-time support for construction of a Kupat Holim hospital in the Jezreel Valley would free Hadassah entirely of the duty to care for members of the fund in the north. Perlson and Soroka promised that if Hadassah provided Kupat Holim with a one-time sum for construction of the hospital, the health fund would waive ongoing financial assistance from Hadassah's budget to cover part of the cost of hospitalizing members of Kupat Holim in the Valley, as Hadassah was bound to do under the terms of the contract between the two parties.

Henrietta Szold's support removed any objections within the Zionist executive and the Mandate government. Hadassah, the JOINT, and the Hebrew Doctors Association of America pledged a sum of 5,000 Eretz Israel pounds (approximately $25,000), and the Zionist movement's Foundation Fund committed itself to give the health fund an additional 3,000 Eretz Israel pounds (approximately $15,000) that had been donated by the Jewish community of Shanghai in China.[2] The Shanghai community's donation had not been earmarked from the start for the Emek Hospital, but had been given to the Foundation Fund for various objectives. At the beginning, the Foundation Fund planned to apply the money to expansion of the Hadassah hospital in Tiberias, but since this plan was not on the current agenda, the Zionist executive recommended that the Foundation Fund channel the sum toward establishment of a hospital in the

Valley, and the management of the Foundation Fund accepted the recommendation unanimously. In its recommendation, the Zionist executive wrote:

> The need for a hospital is urgent in that the state of the huts in Ein-Harod is very bad and until the building will be finished, [it] will become even worse.…The demand for beds in Haifa is so great that the hospital there is almost out of the question for the people of the Valley.[3]

The unanimity of opinion regarding use of the donation reflects the Zionist leadership's recognition of the need for a hospital in the Valley even apart from Henrietta Szold's support for the plan.

Now that the main sum had been ensured for construction of the hospital, the settlements in the Valley also mobilized to contribute their part—committing themselves to donate work days for realization of the project. The "Zion" Community group in Afula promised to lay the infrastructure to connect the hospital to the water system and the power grid. And the Mandate government undertook to pave a road that would link the hospital with Afula city.

On 3 August 1926, in the presence of Eliezer Perlson from Kupat Holim, Henrietta Szold from the Zionist executive, and Dr. Natan Rotnoff from the JOINT, a memorandum was signed in London between Kupat Holim and the Zionist executive for the construction of a Kupat Holim hospital in the Jezreel Valley. In the framework of the agreement, Kupat Holim committed itself to complete construction within three years, share decisions on the hospital plans and its exact location with Hadassah's management in Eretz Israel and the Zionist executive, and collaborate with the medical department (later the Faculty of Medicine) that was scheduled to be opened at the Hebrew University in Jerusalem. The fund also promised to provide medical care to *all* residents of the Valley, even those who were not members of Kupat Holim, when the hospital commenced operation. Moreover, it agreed to turn ownership of the hospital over to the Zionist executive if Kupat Holim could not live up to its commitment to operate the hospital on its own resources. This condition was hard to bear, for it carried no time limit, and stated: "If at some time, [Kupat Holim] will not have the strength to maintain this hospital, then it will deliver it to the Zionist executive."[4]

The wording sought to protect the financial investment of the Zionist executive in the hospital in the event of bankruptcy and to forestall transfer of its ownership to another body or sale of the asset to another party. From an economic standpoint, this condition was an indirect threat to Kupat Holim, underscoring that it had better manage its financial affairs wisely, and it allowed strict supervision of the hospital by the Zionist executive and Hadassah.

In its summary, the memorandum stipulated that a final contract would be signed in Jerusalem

> by assignees of the two sides. The power-of-attorney of the abovementioned committee [the Zionist executive, JOINT and Foundation Fund] in Eretz Israel shall be the Hadassah Medical Federation.

Despite the harshness of the terms of the agreement from Kupat Holim's standpoint, Perlson accepted all the conditions in the name of Kupat Holim. All knew that Kupat Holim had no choice. If it did not agree to the terms, Kupat Holim would not be able to obtain the money needed to build the hospital at all. The real Achilles' heel from Kupat Holim's perspective, however, was Hadassah's role in the plan. With the establishment of the hospital in the Valley, Kupat Holim hoped to liberate itself from its dependence on Hadassah, but again, found itself dependent on Hadassah to the same degree with realization of the plan. Hadassah had been appointed as a trustee for the Zionist institutions, given power-of-attorney to supervise planning of the hospital and its construction. The choice reflects Hadassah's own experience in operating hospitals, while Kupat Holim personnel lacked any previous experience in such matters. The individual appointed by Hadassah to supervise execution of the plan was Hadassah's new director in Eretz Israel, Dr. Blueston.

Bureaucratic Difficulties

The decision process that set in motion establishment of a hospital in the Valley and mobilization of backing to initiate the project was very rapid—nine months from the date Kenivsky-Kanev published his article. This objective was accomplished without any unnecessary delays, but implementing the decision encountered a host of difficulties. The first delay was caused by Dr. Blueston. In his opinion Kupat Holim should not have been allowed to establish its own hospital at all:

> May it be added that we supported with all force and support also now the building of a hospital in the Valley that will be open to all inhabitants without party distinction, and that will be administered by the only agency that was created to maintain the Emek Hospital in the country, that is the Hadassah Medical Federation.[5]

Blueston refused to cooperate in drawing up an abiding contact with Kupat Holim and thus to fulfill Hadassah's part as set forth in the London memorandum. But a short time after, he resigned from his post and Dr. Magnes—who had served as acting director of Hadassah in Eretz Israel— was appointed director in his stead. However, Magnes also delayed drawing up a final contract. He responded to numerous appeals from Kupat Holim officials at the outset of 1927 with the excuse that he had not received clear directives from America, and therefore could not consummate signing the final contract. From the contents of a letter from Harry Sacker, head of the Zionist Appeal in Great Britain, to Eliezer Perlson,[6] it seems that Magnes had deliberately adopted a "holding tactic," for like Blueston, Dr. Magnes was also opposed to establishment of a Kupat Holim-run hospital in the Valley. He felt it was wrong to turn over monies, which were donated in America for Hadassah, to Kupat Holim for establishment of a hospital, when the money was been earmarked originally to establish a university hospital in Jerusalem under Hadassah's auspices in the future.

In February 1927, Henrietta Szold came to Eretz Israel to facilitate the signing of the contract for establishment of the Emek Hospital, and arbitrate in the dispute that had broken out between Kupat Holim and Hadassah over the Certificate of Poverty issue (see chapter 7). While the two issues under dispute were not tied, the tension created by Blueston's opposition to the Emek Hospital made Szold's efforts to settle the Certificate of Poverty issue all the more difficult. Szold sought to finalize the terms of the contract with Kupat

Holim and solve the problems that had arisen on her own accord, but despite her presence, drawing up the contract was delayed—at first, until the Zionist Congress in Basle in August 1927 (a six-month postponement), then to the beginning of 1928.

All these delays did not prevent holding a cornerstone-laying ceremony for the Emek Hospital in August 1927, with all the relevant parties present. The event was festive and impressive and took place in the presence of most of the inhabitants of the Valley. Most of the attendees did not know that the final contract had yet to be signed, and a cornerstone-laying was somewhat of a gamble, based solely on declarations of intentions, not a binding agreement of any kind.

The opposition of the heads of Hadassah in Eretz Israel was not the only stumbling block on the road to establishment of the hospital. A short time after the decision was made and the memorandum signed in London, the settlements in the Jezreel Valley began to apply pressure regarding the location of the hospital—each settlement lobbying for the hospital to be built close to its own geographic location. In March 1927, when it became known that the special committee appointed by the Yishuv's health committee to determine the site of the hospital had chosen Afula city, the group of settlements dubbed the "Norris Bloc" (i.e., the eastern sector of the Jezreel Valley: kibbutzim Ein-Harod, Tel-Yosef, Beit Alfa, Heftziba, and KfarYechezkel farm) issued an ultimatum to the executive committee of the Federation of Labor and the Kupat Holim directorate demanding that the hospital be located near them. They argued that most of the residents of the Jezreel Valley resided in the eastern sector of the valley, and the distance from the hospital would be detrimental to them and particularly to the health of the children who needed its services, and that Kupat Holim would ultimately have to establish another smaller hospital in the vicinity if the site remained unchanged. Moreover, building the hospital in the eastern sector of the Valley would ease high unemployment and lower costs of hospital maintenance and operation that could be handled by members of the agricultural settlements in the vicinity (such as was the case with the hospital in Ein-Harod). They claimed that the Afula city decision was solely Dr. Blueston's and that the work of the committee had been restricted from the start to the Afula city area, while other sites in the Valley had not even been considered, as had been agreed upon at the outset. A memorandum sent by the kibbutzim Heftziba, Tel-Yosef, Geva, and Beit Alpha to the executive committee of the Federation of Labor in May 1927 sought to convince the special committee of the logic of their position, adding that the climate was better in their area, and that it was only fair that the hospital be built close to those who would need it most—that is the agricultural communities—while the residents of Afula city could avail themselves of health services in Haifa. But the pressure of the rural settlements was to no avail. The special committee opted to establish the hospital near Afula and made transfer of funds for construction contingent on fulfillment of their decision.

In a letter to the east Jezreel Valley farming communities, Eliezer Perlson revealed Kupat Holim's sentiments and the forces at play:

> While we want to build the hospital in the Norris Bloc [i.e., the eastern Valley], indeed you know of the terms that concern building the hospital don't leave any hope of receiving even a farthing of the 8,000 Egyptian pounds that we stand to receive for the building, if we won't build it in accordance with the decision of the committee of experts elected by the health committee. We stress that any delay or postponement for new clarifications truly endanger the very building of the hospital by us.[7]

Perlson and Reuven Shenkar, the Kupat Holim treasurer, supported the agricultural farms' demand, and would have preferred to build the hospital adjacent to the old hospital in Ein-Harod, but since they could not sway the decisions of the committee, they accepted its decision as the least worse possibility, as long as the primary objective—a Kupat Holim hospital in the Valley—would not be impaired.

The Jezreel Valley farms were not the only party that wanted the hospital built near them. A short time after it became know that the site of the proposed hospital was outside the municipal boundaries of Afula city, local residents turned to the Yishuv's health committee and the Zionist executive demanding that the hospital be built within city limits—with the intention that ultimately the hospital would become a municipal hospital, as had been the case in Tel Aviv. Behind the economic rationale were also political motivations. On the eve of the cornerstone-laying ceremony, the "Committee for Afula" together with the Afula branch of the "National Civil Association" demanded that the Zionist executive change directions:

> [W]ait with the building of the central hospital in the Valley until after the 15th Congress to demand from the Congress that the above-mentioned hospital be a general hospital not of Kupat Holim.[8]

Consequently the two groups asked the Zionist executive to cancel the planned cornerstone-laying ceremony.

The declaration of the "Committee for Afula" angered the farm community committee that had been working to change the site of the hospital, generating an abrupt change of tune. Aware of the inherent danger should a review be undertaken, the farm settlements decided to drop *their* call to move the proposed hospital site to the eastern sector of the Valley, mobilizing to stand firm behind the health committee's decision to build the hospital on the site chosen—under the proviso that the hospital would, indeed, be administrated by Kupat Holim as planned. In a letter to the Zionist executive in September 1927, a month after the laying of the cornerstone, representatives of the Jezreel Valley and Jordan Valley farming communities wrote:

> This hospital has to service all the inhabitants of the Valley 90% of whom are members of Kupat Holim. Its affiliation and administration must be turned over to Kupat Holim in keeping with our desires…and we will oppose vehemently any attempt to take it out of the hands of Kupat Holim.[9]

The Valley farming communities feared that because of the opposition by Hadassah directors in Eretz Israel and by the Afula residents' committee, the plans would be canceled at a juncture when the final contract had yet to be signed. Despite pressure, the Zionist executive held fast to the original plan to establish the hospital outside city limits adjacent to Afula, and did not even discuss the Afula residents' petition to make it a municipal hospital.

If the heads of Kupat Holim hoped that all the barriers, internal and external had been removed, they were sorely disappointed. At the outset of 1928, a new stumbling block appeared on the road to signing the contract. The member of the Zionist executive charged with drawing up the text of the contract, Harry Sacker, demanded that the hospital be approved and registered legally by the Mandate government before its construction, but the government awaited the final signing of the contract and asked to examine the plans first. Kupat Holim was caught in a blind alley—and with fiscal problems to boot—for the delay in signing the contract meant that the sums earmarked for beginning construction had also been held up. The first installment had been received and work on the foundations had commenced, but without a signed contract work could not continue. The urgency was amplified by deterioration in conditions in the huts that housed the Ein-Harod hospital and difficulties in admitting all those in need of hospitalization. Perlson's repeated appeals to Henrietta Szold and other parties to the plans were of no help. Only the contribution of workdays by the Valley settlers and donation of money by members of Kupat Holim keep construction going. In a report sent to the supervisory committee of Kupat Holim, Perlson wrote that the money earmarked for the Emek Hospital had been transferred to the country, but was being held by Hadassah and it was impossible to get the funding without a signed contract.

Only at the end of 1928, after two years of delays, while work on construction continued throughout, was the contract finally signed and the building permits obtained. Also in 1928, the prolonged arbitration between Hadassah and Kupat Holim over the Certificate of Poverty was finally resolved, ultimately leading to the resignation of Dr. Blueston as Hadassah director in Eretz Israel and the appointment of Dr. Yaski in his place—both changes that seemed to facilitate consummation of the contract between the Zionist executive and Kupat Holim. Only now was it possible to finally go forward with all speed towards completion of the Emek Hospital as planned.

The Building Plan: A Hospital "Made in Eretz Israel"

At the end of October 1928, preparation of the building plans began. The architect was Alexander Berwald from the architecture department of the Technion (Israel Institute of Technology), who was assisted by engineer Noyman. The hospital building committee that supervised the work was comprised of three members: Dr. Glicker from the medical department of Kupat Holim, Dr. Hershovitz, director of the Ein Harod hospital, and Dr. Rosental, the representative of the health committee. On-site inspection was handled by Moshe Soroka, the administrative assistant of Dr. Hershovitz and chief Kupat Holim administrator in the Jezreel Valley.

The planned hospital was to include four two-story pavilions with approximately fifty to sixty beds. Three of the wards were to house the main departments—internal medicine, pediatrics, and maternity—and the fourth, the administration and maintenance wing. It was decided to build two building first and use them for each of the four departments, and only later to add the buildings for pediatrics and maternity. Two factors were at work in the decision to opt for separate buildings and not one multi-story structure: the desire to accommodate the design to the rural population that the hospital would serve, and the construction workers' unfamiliarity with the building techniques that a multistory structure would require.

Dr. Hershovitz and Moshe Soroka were the moving force behind crystallization of the plans. The two were well acquainted with the health needs of the Valley's population, the lay of the land, and the climate and work methods employed by the hospital staff. In the design, environmental elements were taken into account such as dust, heat, and misquotes, and care was taken to find solutions to the large number of visitors expected at pediatric and maternity wards. Soroka, who oversaw construction, insisted on choosing the best of materials and was unwilling to compromise on quality, ensuring that maintenance of the hospital would be economical and simple. All those involved in the project knew that Kupat Holim was being put to the test in carrying out this project, and their performance would determine the future of Kupat Holim in the hospitalization domain.

In mid-1929 construction was at full-steam and the primary apprehension was that the work could not be completed by October, as stipulated in the contract. Delay carried the danger that the Zionist executive could choose to apply the clause in the contract that allowed it to take over the hospital, if Kupat Holim failed to fulfill its commitments. In the meantime, worries were complicated all the more by the condition of the maternity ward in Ein-Harod, which had begun to sink, thus making completion of the new hospital all the more pressing.

In August, when the 1929 Arab disturbances[10] broke out, work on the hospital came to a halt and was not renewed until the end of the year. Due to the unforeseen circumstances, the Zionist executive chose not to activate the "takeover" clause in the contact and allowed Kupat Holim to continue construction. In April 1930, after a several-month delay beyond the stipulated completion date, construction of the Emek Hospital was finished. Kupat Holim now faced the challenge of underwriting orderly operation of the hospital, as set forth in the contract.

The first burning question was equipping the hospital. In November 1929, Kupat Holim asked the secretariat for health affairs of the Yishuv's health committee to support a request for annual financial assistance from the Mandate government in order to equip the hospital. As a matter of course, the Mandate government supported municipal hospitals that treated Arab patients and employees of governmental concerns, as well as medical facilities involved in prevention and treatment of tuberculosis— domains that were the responsibility of the Mandate government. The Hadassah Hospital in Tel Aviv (later the municipal hospital) also received a yearly stipend of 2,000 Eretz Israel pounds.

In October 1929, in a letter from the Yishuv's health committee to the Zionist executive, Dr. Katznelson-Nissan, a member of the health committee supported the health fund's request, recommending that the executive intercede with the British Mandate government on behalf of Kupat Holim and the Emek Hospital. In his letter, Dr. Katznelson-Nissan said:

> The government health department's delegates who examined the site on various occasion expressed their satisfaction with the location as well as the building plan and its execution....Maintenance of the hospital costs approximately 5,000 Eretz Israel pounds per year. Seventy-five percent of the expenditure comes from payments of settlers [who are] members of Kupat Holim. The rest is budgeted by the Foundation Fund....There is no basis for placing the burden of maintenance of the Emek Hospital, that serves a certain rural area, solely on the young for the most part un-established farms and on the Foundation Fund, in that the government health department participates with decent sums up to 50% of the general expenditures for maintenance of hospitals in municipal

> areas Jaffa, Gaza, Nablus, Beersheva and Acre, and to a smaller degree also in maintenance of the hospital in Tel Aviv (with 2,000 Eretz Israel pounds a year)....Kupat Holim has taken upon itself right now all the expenditures of the building. It must now seek means to furnish the hospital. Kupat Holim has therefore the right from all standpoints to petition the government for suitable participation in the expenditures for maintenance of the hospital that serves not only as a general hospital, but also as a hospital for infectious diseases for all the Hebrew vicinity (as it is known, there is not in the entire north, the upper and lower Galilee, the Valley and the Samaria even one government hospital other than the small hospital in Haifa with 26 beds). I am honored to suggest Your Honor, that the Zionist executive will turn to the government with a petition to budget already for the coming year a suitable sum as participation in the Emek Hospital's expenditures and it is clear that Kupat Holim will agree to ongoing supervision by the government over the hospital management and in-house arrangements.[11]

A similar position was presented by the Zionist Executive in a memorandum from the Jewish Agency for Eretz Israel to the Mandate government's health department, and in many other letters. However, the British government stood behind its refusal to approve any support for the Emek Hospital. In a letter of 17 January 1930, the government secretary wrote:

> Much to its sorrow, the government will not be able to budget support today for this hospital, and the reasons are the difficult financial state of the government and the fact that the hospital will serve only a small section of the Valley residents.[12]

The Mandate government continued its refusal of support up to the end of British rule in mid-1948, and Kupat Holim was forced to find other sources of funding to augment the hospital's budget.

The positive note of Dr. Katznelson-Nissan's letter of recommendation, describing the Emek Hospital as successful and efficient, and capable of providing high standard health services, is noteworthy. Similar descriptions can be found in a host of other correspondence, and reflects the positive attitude within the Yishuv's health committee, the Zionist executive, and the Jewish Agency toward the hospital. During negotiations over the terms of the contract, the Zionist executive were extremely tough and raised doubts about the prospects of the entire project, while now, after Kupat Holim successfully completed construction of the hospital, and under far-from-ideal circumstances, the accomplishment was viewed as proof of the fund's executive abilities, and all doubts and apprehensions dissipated.

On 30 April 1930, the Emek Hospital was inaugurated at an impressive ceremony attended by many of the residents of the Valley, delegates from the Mandate government, Henrietta Szold, Dr. Chaim Yaski, and many guests from abroad. With completion of construction, after the project was consummated despite difficult budgeting problems and disruptions during the 1929 Arab uprising, the Emek Hospital was crowned a symbol of success, in the eyes not only of the inhabitants of the Valley and Kupat Holim, but also of the entire Yishuv—which dubbed the hospital, even in official documents "Kupat Holim's hospital" (rather than merely the Emek Hospital). The role of Henrietta Szold and the Zionist executive and the fact that the hospital had been financed largely thanks to capital from abroad were forgotten.

The First Two Years: Crisis and Operating Problems

After the opening of the Emek hospital, Kupat Holim immediately found itself embroiled in a new financial crisis. The Mandate government had turned down requests for assistance in equipping the hospital, and the health fund was prevented by the terms of the contract from requesting financial assistance from the Zionist executive and Hadassah to pay running costs. The hospital's functioning stood in question. The hospital had yet to be connected to the power grid or the water system; paving of the road from the hospital to Afula had yet to be completed; and there was not even a budget to transfer patients and the scanty equipment in the Ein-Harod huts to the new hospital. In the end, the patients were transferred by wagon, and only after a year, with the completion of the road and a modest improvement in Kupat Holim's financial state, did the health fund succeed in procuring an automobile for the hospital to transport patients and supplies. The question of living quarters for the staff had yet to be resolved. In Ein-Harod, they had resided adjacent to the hospital and were on-call around-the-clock. In the meantime, it was decided that the doctors and nurses would be required to live in the hospital compound and be on-call after hours, if need arose. They were forbidden from living outside the hospital complex. In the original plans, a building had been allocated for staff housing and the Mandate government had promised assistance in its construction, but work on the building had yet to begin.

The impact of the Emek Hospital was soon registered in the marked improvement in medicine in the entire area. Prior to the opening of the hospital, women in labor and sick children were sent to Haifa and Jerusalem: now they could be hospitalized them locally. Not only residents of the Valley availed themselves of the hospital's services, but all residents of the north, and at times even inhabitants of Samaria. In the summer of 1931, 45 percent of those hospitalized came from Samaria, the Galilee, and even from Haifa.[xiii] The importance of the hospital as a vital element grew in 1931 when the internal medicine department in the Hadassah hospital in Haifa was closed. The Yishuv's health committee even proposed that a surgical department be opened at the Emek hospital. Members of the committee praised the decisive role of the hospital in quickly stemming a typhus epidemic that broke out in the Valley in the summer of 1931. Due to the epidemic, occupancy in the hospital rose sharply and a hut was constructed in the compound (a gift from the Mandate government) to house the typhus patients.

Historian Idit Zartal noted the favored stature the new hospital quickly won for itself within the medical community:

> [The hospital] brought with it medical progress in concepts of the time….The pinnacle of aspirations for young doctors and new immigrants was the Afula hospital, where pioneering work was done in the treatment and study of diseases of the period.[14]

The hospital's laboratory conducted blood analysis to determine blood types and managed a central filing system to register blood types and medical histories of patients. It hosted monthly in-service training and one-day conferences for doctors in the Galilee and the Valley and brought in lecturers on special clinical questions. A special relationship developed between the hospital and all the Valley settlements. The doctors would go out on periodic visits (once every week or two) in settlements in the vicinity in order to inspect sanitation, and teach first aid and preventive medicine. The hospital's medications storehouse served as Kupat Holim's central storehouse for the area, and the hospital operated as a center for the war on malaria and headquarters for all Kupat Holim operations in the north of the country.

Despite its success from a professional standpoint—medical and organizational—operation of the hospital was a serious drain on the health fund's fiscal reservoirs. Kupat Holim was unable to keep up payments of staff salaries, postponed payment to suppliers for months, and failed to reimburse the railway for transport of the sick by train. In October 1931 Kupat Holim even ceased transfer of all funds to the Emek Hospital, and for five full months the hospital continued to operate with a budget and on an empty kitty. In March 1932, Dr. Ben-Zion Hershovitz wrote the Kupat Holim directorate that the hospital stood to close its doors if steps were not taken to cover its debts. Hershovitz wrote:

> There is no room to think that with some one-time sum the situation will be rectified. I will not be able to be responsible in any way for management of the institution if we will not be ensured a budget every month with the necessary amount.[15]

Kupat Holim had no solution. The treasury was empty, and there was nowhere to borrow money. In a letter to the management of the Jewish Agency, in the wake of Dr. Hershovitz's letter, Eliezer Perlson placed direct responsibility for the pending closure of the hospital at the doorstep of the Jewish Agency:

> Already five and a half months have passed without even one farthing being received for our budget from the Agency for 1931–32…and we believe it is our duty to inform you that if by the 25th of March, we will not receive from you payment of the budget for two months we will no longer be able to maintain the hospital in the Valley and it

> will close….The hospital has no right or ability to continue and go into great debt linked to maintaining the hospital without receipt of the minimal budget from the Agency.[16]

A month later, Perlson wrote a letter to the British High Commissioner describing the difficult circumstances of the hospital in the Valley and claiming that the hospital was entitled to receive a yearly budget like all other hospitals in the country. In his appeal to the government for assistance, Perlson argued:

> [The hospital] fulfills such an important role in the war on infectious diseases and provides its services to a whole rural area….Delegates of the government expressed on various opportunities their positive attitude toward completion of construction of the hospital in the Valley with the aid of a special budget from the government, and we hereby request that Your Majesty with agree to expedite realization of this matter.[17]

On 6 June 1932, following numerous appeals regarding Kupat Holim, the British high commissioner visited the Jezreel Valley in order to evaluate the situation first-hand. The commissioner was accompanied by Dr. Chaim Arlosoroff, a member of the Jewish Agency executive. In a letter "For Your Confidential Information" to the Kupat Holim directorate in the wake of the visit, Arlosoroff recommended that the directorate try to apply personal pressure on the high commissioner in order to obtain immediate financial assistance for the hospital. He said that he had brought the hospital's distress to the attention of the commissioner during their visit to the Valley. "It seems that the matter made a serious impression on the Commissioner. He noted the matter and promised to deal with it urgently."[18]

A confidential memorandum sent by Dr. Katznelson-Nissan to members of the National Committee a short time after the commissioner's visit presented a far less optimistic picture. Katznelson-Nissan related that he had met with Colonel Herron, head of the Mandate government's health department, and the director had spoken at length about the distressed health status of Arab residents of Eretz Israel, and had even said that the expenditures on health of Jewish institutions were much higher than those of governmental institutions, and therefore it was fitting that assistance be given to the Arabs or to hospitals of the mission whose financial state was also difficult. Dr. Katznelson stressed that as long as Colonel Herron was director of the health department, one could not expect that Kupat Holim and other Jewish health institutions would enjoy any assistance whatsoever. He suggested that the true motivations of the director were less patent:

> This man uses all sorts of excuses in order to prevent assistance of the government to Jewish endeavors, and his ambition is in fact not to raise the level of medical assistance among the Arabs, rather to lower as much as possible medical standards among the Jews and to force them to utilize the medical service of the government, to the extent that is exists.[19]

At the beginning of July, it became clear that Dr. Katznelson-Nissan's evaluation of the situation was correct: The Mandate government refused to provide any financial assistance whatsoever, and the Emek Hospital was closed. Warnings by Dr. Kreiger on behalf of the doctors' professional organization, that closure of the hospital in the summer—a season in which epidemics were most prevalent— constituted a clear health peril, had no effect. Kupat Holim was faced with a *fait accompli.* "Unfortunately" there were no major epidemics during the summer of 1932, and warnings that closure of the hospital would have a dire effect on health—a situation that might have spurred steps to mobilize funding to reopening the hospital—did not materialize.

The closure of the hospital also had political overtones. At the beginning of August 1932, Dr. Beilenson, head of Kupat Holim's supervisory committee, wrote a personal letter (hand-written and without any copies) to Dr. Arlosoroff dealing with some of the political aspects of the closure of the Emek Hospital. Dr. Beilenson agreed with Dr. Katznelson-Nissan that the Mandate government would not support the Emek Hospital, and even argued that its closure served the interests of the government. He held that Colonel Herron's refusal to assist the hospital was a move designed to maneuver Kupat Holim into an untenable position that would lead to closure of the hospital. The British government sought to take advantage of the situation in order to expand its own governmental health services and draw to them parties within the working public, with the aim of eroding their support of Jewish institutions whose autonomous stature had political implications. "Do we need our own hospital? Perhaps really it would be better to use the government's service and save the money we put out up until now to maintain the hospital?"[20]

Beilenson viewed closure of the Emek Hospital as a "political-Yishuv-labor danger" that was liable to undermine the status and clout of Kupat Holim and the Yishuv as a whole. Dr. Beilenson noted that the Emek Hospital was not just

> a hospitalization site but also a property testifying greatly to our power, our prestige, our talent for action....We must be swift in opening the hospital; it is clear that we do not want and cannot be misled by sudden commencement of our political activity, we don't want and we can't put you [Dr. Arlosoroff] in the position as if you have fought a false war, a staged war, therefore it is imperative that you study the question and find together a formula that will allow "a retreat backwards in the order of things," for instance: a donation that fell from the heavens, a "gentleman's agreement" with the government, that it take us into account if we open immediately and "liberate" it from the worry placed on it to prepare a new budget. There is no need to explain to you how extensive the damage will be for us from this precedent (lack of credibility [in the eyes of] the government regarding our each and every demand, lack of faith in our ability to bear our burden when it arises, and so forth) if we will not find an honorable out.[21]

Dr. Beilenson spoke of the political ramifications of closure of the hospital but did not mention the financial distress that had led to the closure at all in his letter to Arlosoroff. The impression is that he believed closure of the hospital was not an inevitable reality and was designed to pressure the Mandate government to budget financial aid. His comments on "an honorable retreat" are not tied to any financial settlement. Examination of the financial reports of Kupat Holim and the Emek Hospital from the corresponding period strengthen the authenticity of Dr. Hershovitz's and Eliezer Perlson's claims regarding the dire state of Kupat Holim's finances.

On the other hand, the general state of Kupat Holim from a financial standpoint—beyond the hospital—was in better shape. The genuine obstacle, it seems, was the demand of the Zionist executive that the hospital's budget not be integrated within the general budget of Kupat Holim and that there could be no transfer of monies between budgets. The heads of the Zionist executive meant to protect the hospital's budget from exploitation by Kupat Holim, and no one imagined that under certain circumstances the tables would be turned—that the hospital would find itself in financial trouble and in need of Kupat Holim's financial backing. Dr. Beilenson grasped the situation in a broader context and therefore was less worried about the financial situation, as long as a solution were found that would not impair the political prestige of Kupat Holim and the Yishuv's leadership. Loss of political prestige was liable to project negatively in other areas, such as the Yishuv's demand that the Mandate government grant the Yishuv autonomy in civil matters.

End of the Crisis and Reopening of the Emek Hospital

In October 1932, two months after the crisis, Hadassah announced it was prepared to assist in covering the Emek Hospital budget in lieu of the Jewish Agency's appropriation to Kupat Holim. An "honorable exit" from the crisis had been found, and it was possible to reopen the hospital, although the number of beds in the internal medicine department had to be curtailed. A month later Hadassah reneged on its promise, but the hospital had already begun to operate again, with the assistance of the general budget of Kupat Holim and the Jewish Agency allocations. The ups and downs in the hospital's fortunes impacted on its administration, but without the danger of closure of the facility. Despite the difficulties, the Zionist executive, ignoring the terms of the contract, did not request to transfer the hospital to its ownership, but rather mobilized to find a way out of the crisis and help the hospital in its distress. Kupat Holim came out of the crisis strengthened. The political importance of the Emek Hospital was proven beyond any doubt. Its professional work and contribution to the health of Jezreel Valley residents was highly praised, and these accomplishments served as a basis for Kupat Holim's demands for funding from other institutions, and primarily the Mandate government. Within Zionist national institutions there was unanimity as to the vital role of the hospital, and all agreed that a united effort should be made to resolve the crisis.

At the outset of 1934, the first apartment building for staff—who until then had lived in wooden huts—was completed. The Mandate government stood behind its original promise to assist in building quarters for staff (although refusing to participate in operating costs), and even undertook to build a second apartment building. Kupat Holim financed furnishing and equipment from its budget. It seemed that after prolonged crisis, work at the hospital had finally gotten onto the right footing. One could say that in retrospect, the Emek Hospital emerged from the crisis strengthened. Even in periods in the future when Kupat Holim found itself in financial trouble, the fate of the hospital was never questioned again.

The degree to which Kupat Holim itself emerged from the crisis strengthened and confident of its abilities to succeed in the hospitalization domain can be seen in mid-1933—less than a year after the closure and reopening of the Emek Hospital, when the Kupat Holim directorate proposed to build another hospital under health fund auspices for the agricultural villages in Judea near Petach Tikva. The new hospital (it later became known as Beilenson Hospital, and today is the Yitzhak Rabin Medical Center) was envisioned to be larger, more sophisticated and complex than the Emek Hospital. In a November 1934 letter, when plans were already well underway, Reuven Shenkar wrote:

> Only now have we the proof how important the role of the Emek Hospital was. Only thanks to it, hospitalization in the north of the country is more organized....We don't see a solution to this question [i.e., a shortage of hospital beds] without establishing a hospital in Judea similar to the Kupat Holim hospital in the Valley.[22]

Thus, the Emek Hospital was a turning point in the history of Kupat Holim in hospitalization care. It proved the ability of the health fund to establish a modern hospital, and run it on a professional basis, despite serious budgeting problems. The good name that the hospital won for itself was a contributing factor in the growth in membership that Kupat Holim witnessed in the 1930s and afterward. As membership grew so did the status of Kupat Holim and its importance within the Federation of Labor, and in the Yishuv as a whole.

Kupat Holim's entrance into the realm of hospitalization services changed the nature of the organization from a health fund for workers, designed first and foremost to provide primarily medical services to the working class in Eretz Israel on the basis of mutual assistance, to a powerful multifaceted organization. In light of the protracted and heated controversy that surrounded the question of the role of Kupat Holim in the years 1925–1929, the fact that its decision to enter the hospitalization realm took place without any thorough pubic debate appears quite remarkable. It seems that no one thought about or envisioned the ramifications such a step would have on the shape of Kupat Holim in the future. The establishment of the Emek Hospital was spurred by lack of hospital beds and the needs of the hour, yet was destined to contribute decisively to the development and growth of Kupat Holim as it was transformed into a key party in hospitalization services in Eretz Israel, ultimately to "inherit" the primacy of Hadassah in this area.

9

Kupat Holim and the British Mandate Government

In January 1930, Kupat Holim and the Federation of Labor presented a detailed proposal to the Mandate government for legislation of a compulsory health insurance law. The proposal was accompanied by a memorandum with a draft proposal formulated by a special joint committee of the two organizations. Members of the committee were the jurists Israel Barshira (Bashrovker), Chaim Eretzisraeli-Gavrieli from the Federation of Labor, and Yitzhak Kenivsky-Kenev from Kupat Holim. The proposal called for the government, the employers, and the workers to pay progressive compulsory health insurance, based on salary. The insurance would be managed by the high commissioner who would appoint a governmental committee to manage the insurance. Collection of dues and provision of health services would be placed in the hands of independent health funds that would be established by the insurees. The basket of services would encompass medical assistance, sick leave, disability pensions, and a maternity grant.

The same year Kupat Holim had a membership of 18,000 that together with their families provided coverage for 34,000 inhabitants—approximately 20 percent of the Jewish population in Eretz Israel.[1] Despite the marked increase in membership, the fund still found itself incurring a constant deficit. Had the Mandate government accepted the proposed legislation for compulsory health insurance, such a move would have enhanced the fiscal wellbeing of Kupat Holim significantly, and allowed it to expand and realize plans formulated at the second Kupat Holim convention in 1929. The heads of

Kupat Holim hoped that the rise to power of a Labor government in Britain and improvement in the economic situation of the Yishuv would motivate the government to approve the proposal.

The British high commissioner, Sir John Robert Chancellor, responded to the proposal with reservations. He also rejected the Federation of Labor's call for establishment of a joint committee between the Federation and the government to discuss the issue, and claimed that the proposal was not practical for fiscal reasons. Only under pressure from the International Labor Office and the Mandate's commission did Chancellor appoint a committee in October 1931 to discuss the proposed legislation. The International Labor Office based its demand on the authority of Great Britain to legislate a compulsory health insurance law within the framework of the League of Nations, and its obligation to enact this decision in all its colonies. The timing of the proposal was bad from a host of standpoints. It was Chancellor's last year at his post, and in the same year the Mandate government awaited the findings of the Shaw Commission concerning the 1929 Arab disturbances that had decimated the Jewish community in Hebron, and levels of tension between Jews and Arabs ran high. The Shaw Commission's report leveled fierce criticism at the Federation and its actions in the immigration and labor domain. This was followed by publication of John Hope-Simpson's report recommending that the status of Arabs not be jeopardized by Jewish immigration and that the status quo be maintained in demographic ratios between the two communities, under the guise that immigration of Jews could not be sustained economically. Next came implementation of the Passfield White Paper and the Ramsay MacDonald[2] letter that sought to institute an "even-handed policy" toward Arabs and Jews, back-pedaling on pro-Zionist sentiments enshrined in the Balfour Declaration, thus an anti-Zionist policy ultimately embodied in the 1939 White Paper that would severely limit Jewish immigration to Eretz Israel. All these anti-Zionist steps generated high tension between the Mandate government and the Yishuv. Under such conditions there was little chance that British authorities would give the Federation of Labor and Kupat Holim proposal for a compulsory health insurance law an objective review.

This was not the first time that the Mandate government had distanced itself from Kupat Holim initiatives, such as suggestions concerning services in industrial medicine, demand that employers' parallel tax be made legally binding, and attempts to broaden services for laborers in the cities. Almost from its founding, the Mandate government ignored Kupat Holim, while viewing Hadassah's work favorably.

The Legal Status of Kupat Holim and the British Mandate

Already at the outset of 1924, the chief secretary of the British Mandate government refused to recognize documentation of illness issued by Kupat Holim doctors to railroad workers who were also government employees. Only after numerous efforts did the government recognized the authority of the doctors, under condition that Mandate authorities oversee their work. At the same time the Mandate government caused difficulties when Kupat Holim demanded official recognition of the government as a non-profit public institution in the health domain, and asked to be registered legally as an autonomous association. Due to the delay, Kupat Holim was forced to pay higher taxes than other medical institutions and societies, such as hospitals and the Mission's clinics. In 1925, the fund gained its only dispensation—duty-free status from customs. In 1927, Kupat Holim again requested status as a non-profit public institution, and again was turned down on the excuse that without a binding charter, it was impossible to register it as such. Therefore in 1928 Kupat Holim turned to David Ben-Gurion, the general secretary of the Federation of Labor, and requested his assistance in formulating a binding charter and his personal assistance in completing the process of registering Kupat Holim as an association. Despite these efforts, the health fund's requests remained unanswered, except for one dispensation—exemption from payment of stamp taxes on receipts. The request for official licensing was not accepted.

The Mandate government delayed licensing Kupat Holim under various pretenses and until the end of the 1930s ignored entirely the difficulties this caused the health fund. Kupat Holim leaders blamed Colonel Herron, head of the Mandate health department who gave preference to Arab health services and government hospitals and patently ignored Kupat Holim and its operations. Herron held that the Yishuv and its institutions (that is Hadassah) knew how to care for themselves based on their own financial resources, and therefore it was the duty of the government to balance the situation and nurture health services for the underprivileged Arab sector of the population. He even sought to expand utilization of government hospitals and health services among the Jews, and consequently refrained from any action that would give Kupat Holim a relative advantage. This was the reason that all Kupat Holim requests to obtain additional exemptions from taxes as a public institution were stymied.

It should be noted that the Mandate government also discouraged any local initiatives in the Arab sector, and in place of encouraging the establishment of independent Arab health services, took upon itself full responsibility—financially and in practice—for providing health services to the Arab population.

Attempts to Legislate Heath Insurance in the 1920s

From the outset of its operation, Kupat Holim struggled with financial problems. Most of the members of the fund were laborers, members of cooperative settlements, and new immigrants from the Third Aliyah. Despite Federation of Labor declarations that membership in Kupat Holim was obligatory, the scope of Kupat Holim membership at the outset of 1921 was 30 percent lower than the scope of membership in the Federation of Labor, for most of the laborers could not bear the economic burden of paying membership dues to both the Federation and Kupat Holim. The Federation refrained from enforcing dual membership requirements, fearing that such a step would impact negatively on its own membership rosters, while the workers preferred membership in the Federation, which could protect their rights as workers and provide sources of employment that were irreplaceable, while Kupat Holim had a substitute—the modestly-priced services of Hadassah. Under such conditions, Kupat Holim could not realize its full potential in terms of revenues.

At the beginning of the 1920s, the number of members in Kupat Holim grew at a rapid rate. In 1922 the rosters registered 5,700 members (approximately 10,000 insurees including dependents). In 1924 that number had grown to 6,600 (approximately 15,000 including dependents). By 1926 membership was 15,000 (29,000 including dependents).[3] In 1924–1925 membership dues covered only 47 percent of the health fund's expenditures and the deficit—ongoing and accrued—devoured 50 percent of all expenditures.[4] The economic crisis at the start of the Fourth Aliyah exacerbated the situation and at the beginning of 1925 Kupat Holim stood on the verge of bankruptcy. In December 1925, Eliezer Perlson convened an emergency meeting of the Kupat Holim council to discuss the health fund's fiscal distress and seek a solution to its functional problems. At the close of two days of deliberations the council moved to make all efforts to increase Kupat Holim's revenue and to curtail expenditures, but no binding framework was formulated. Participants in the gathering called for implementation of the obligation of reciprocal membership and appeals to the Mandate government to legislate a compulsory health insurance law that would operate under the auspices of health funds. Among the "movers and shakers" behind the demand for compulsory health insurance were Reuven Shenkar and Yitzhak Kenivsky-Kenev. Kenivsky-Kenev even noted that "without an obligatory law Kupat Holim will not be able to solve its fundamental questions, to meet the needs of the workers and ensure their sustenance in times of illness."[5] Such legislation would have increased the number of Kupat Holim members and improved its financial situation. The heads of the health fund hoped that through such a law, they would also obtain governmental participation in underwriting health services, as was the case in Great Britain.

The proposal was based on the British law from 1911, whereby public associations were charged with collecting levies and providing services, employers were required to pay the equivalence of a parallel tax, and the government underwrote expenditures on administration and coverage for those unable to pay.[6] Unlike the law in Germany that required the establishment of health funds as the party responsible for providing health services and collecting payments, the British law satisfied itself with providing monetary compensation to the insuree, leaving the recipient responsible for obtaining health services needed by the individual. The doctors in Germany were required by law to sign agreements with one of the health funds in order to treat the sick, while in Great Britain the doctors remained totally independent and were not required to establish a tie with any particular health organization. Unlike the German system, which limited doctors to those associated with health funds, the British system entitled the patient to choose his or her own doctor. From this standpoint, the situation in Eretz Israel was closer to the German system than the

British one, but Kupat Holim was fighting for a principle, and the question of organization was secondary in its view. In an article published in the Kupat Holim organ *Briut Haoved*, Kenivsky-Kenev provided an overview of health insurance in Europe as an example of the system that should be established in Eretz Israel. He surveyed the ideological and economic base of health insurance in Europe and said that any labor organization that did not seek to enact compulsory health insurance for members was guilty of transgressing its own principles and subverting its own raison d'être. In closing, Kenivsky-Kenev said that without compulsory health insurance Kupat Holim could not prevail and fulfill its role for any length of time, because "[an element of] chance would always prevail in its condition."[7]

According to Federation ordinances Kupat Holim was obliged to receive the approval of the executive committee for every legislative initiative. Consequently, the Kupat Holim proposal for a health insurance law was transferred to the executive committee of the Federation of Labor prior to being submitted to the Mandate government. More than three years passed until the executive committee approved the proposal. Archival documentation within the Federation does not provide an adequate explanation to the delay. And examination of the deliberations of the executive committee during this period reveals that the subject was not raised *at all* on the agenda.

One can attempt to explain the Federation's position in a number of ways. The years 1925–1927 were years of economic hardship in the Yishuv. The Federation of Labor's institutions stood in danger of bankruptcy; agricultural settlements, Solel Boneh, and Kupat Holim were under scrutiny of investigative commissions; and the health insurance proposal may have been postponed while the Federation dealt with more burning questions. It may be that the Federation feared that a health insurance law would require membership in Kupat Holim by large groups in the population, primarily members of the Federation of Labor—a step that was liable to indirectly impact on the Federation's own budget. It is also possible that this was the reason the Federation had not enforced the reciprocal membership clause. Kupat Holim, on the other hand, hoped that through the law it would be able to gain what it had been unable to obtain from the Federation—enforcement of the obligation of membership in the health fund for all members of the Federation and other groups. Letters sent by the executive committee to Kupat Holim during this period reveal that the executive committee feared Kupat Holim would gain too much economic power should the Mandate government legislate a compulsory health insurance law. Concentration of power in the hands of Kupat Holim was liable to weaken the organizational control of the Federation of Labor over Kupat Holim. According to historian Shabtai Tevet, this fear accompanied the workings of the executive committee throughout this entire period.[8]

In mid-1927, the International Labor Office of the League of Nations passed a resolution calling for enactment of a compulsory health insurance law by all member nations. The resolution stated that such a law should also be enacted in protectorates—colonies and mandate states. The decision rekindled discussion concerning enactment of such a law in Eretz Israel as well.

In November 1928, more than three years after Kupat Holim submitted its proposal for a health insurance law for Federation approval, Kenivsky-Kenev wrote the executive committee and demanded that deliberations over the proposal be renewed. In his letter he noted the damage that threatened the health of laborers if the issue was neglected:

> This question of the obligation to insure workers against cases of illness is not only timely for us, without it Kupat Holim will not be able to develop, and the main thing is that without obligatory insurance the Eretz Israel laborer will not be able to reach the point that he will be secure in his existence in times of his illness.[9]

Kenivsky-Kenev emphasized two things in his letter: first, that the future development of Kupat Holim was tied directly to legislation of a health insurance law; second, that it was important to ensure the maintenance of the workers in times of illness with paid sick leave. He did not go into detail on ways to provide medical assistance or on its scope, but focused on the principle of sustaining laborers in times of illness, holding that "the Federation must take the necessary steps to obtain legislation for an obligatory Kupat Holim."[10]

In order to advance approval of the proposal in the executive committee, Kenivsky-Kenev suggested that a joint committee be formed between representatives of the executive committee and Kupat Holim to discuss and formulate proposed legislation to the Mandate government. According to his suggestion, the committee would be comprised of David Ben-Gurion, Dr. Moshe Zmora (head of the Yishuv's bar association), Walter Proise (an economist and member of the executive committee), and a member of the Kupat Holim management. Appointment of Ben-Gurion to the committee was designed to assure that the matter would be dealt with without delay in the Federation's institutions. Dr. Zmora was championed due to his professional standing and his good ties with the Mandate government. Walter Proise's presence was important in terms of both technical and financial value; as Kenivsky-Kenev noted, "He has the ability to obtain concrete assistance from the International Association of Health Funds and the International Labor Office in Geneva."[11]

Proise had indicated that the international labor and health organizations had pledged to help them convince the Mandate government to approve the initiative. Indeed, a short time after Kenivsky-Kenev sent his letter, a joint committee was established to examine Kupat Holim's proposal for a compulsory health insurance law. Ben-Gurion, Zmora, and Proise did not participate in the committee as Kenivsky-Kenev had requested, but rather the jurist Israel Barshira (Bashrovker), Chaim Eretzisraeli (Gavrieli)—the Federation of Labor's bookkeeper—and Yitzhak Kenivsky-Kenev himself. The appointment of Eretzisraeli, an individual lacking any clout or political stature, as the representative of the Federation on the committee suggests the degree of importance that Ben-Gurion and his colleagues in the Federation assigned the legislative initiative.

The media also dealt with the proposed legislation. In an article entitled "The Roles of the Day for Kupat Holim" the demand for legislation of a compulsory health insurance was cited among the three key demands that the Yishuv should place before the Mandate government (the others being a law that would put the parallel tax on a legal footing and government participation in Kupat Holim's budget).[12]

An article in *Davar* entitled "Kupat Holim and the Question of Governmental Insurance against Illness" described the state of health insurance in European countries and Kupat Holim's failure to bring about legislation of similar insurance in Eretz Israel. The article contained a detailed analysis of the pros and cons of health insurance legislation in the countries of Europe, the cost of services, the basket of services covered, and the size of the membership. The scope of information and degree of detail in the article reflects heightened awareness within the labor movement in Eretz Israel over questions of social security in general and health insurance in particular. In his summary, Kanievsky-Kanev wrote that a health insurance law should be one of the key issues on the agenda of the upcoming Kupat Holim convention (in May 1929), and stressed that

> There should be vigorous demands of the government legislation of a law of compulsory insurance against illness of workers, with participation in outlay on insurance of the workers, [on the part of] the employees and the government. One should not be so credulous to believe that the government will lend an ear immediately to this just demand, but the arguments on behalf of issuance of a law such as this are so just and so strong that there is no room for doubts....The Federation as a whole must open a bold war to realize this in the near future.[13]

On 12 May 1929, the second Kupat Holim convention opened in Haifa. In his opening remarks, Dr. Moshe Beilenson, chairperson of the Kupat Holim supervisory committee, said:

> From this convention must go out a demand to the government to issue a law requiring the work provider and the government itself to participate in social insurance of the worker[14]

Dr. Glicker, the medical director of Kupat Holim, even called for an open war against the Mandate government over the question of a health insurance law:

> We have but one path: A war with the government. We must single out the enlightened Mandate government in public, to repeat over and over our "j'accuse" until it brings about a radical change in the attitude of the government to the health of the inhabitants.[15]

Other participants in the convention voiced similar sentiments. The demand for legislation of a compulsory health insurance law was by this juncture a part of the overall outlook that had become widespread within the leadership of Kupat Holim. They now felt that the health fund must go beyond the narrow framework that had characterized its operation to date, work among the working public and members of the Federation of Labor, and strive toward becoming a key national health organization in the Yishuv. In the closing discussions of the convention, the participants were called upon to take immediate steps to advance legislation, and no objections were voiced.

The importance that the convention participants assigned health insurance legislation is registered in the place of the issue at the top of the agenda—the first clause in the resolutions:

> The convention calls upon the government in Eretz Israel for a fundamental change in its passive posture toward the problems of social insurance in event of illness....The government must: A. Work out in consultation with the institutions interested in compulsory insurance in event of illness and invalidism [i.e., disability] and publish it very soon....The convention demands that the Federation institutions begin to act with vigor to realize the demands cited above.[16]

Discussion of compulsory health insurance at the Kupat Holim convention raised several unanswered question, among them: Why did the majority of participants claim that it was only the Mandate government that was delaying legislation? Why was the Federation of Labor's foot-dragging not addressed? Even during the convention the proposed law had yet to receive the blessings of the executive committee and had not even been submitted to the Mandate government, which under such conditions could hardly be expected to express its stand vis-à-vis a proposal that it had yet to receive. Nothing was said about the protracted delay in addressing the proposal within the Federation that had stymied submission of the proposal for over three years. One may assume that the heads of Kupat Holim did not want to publicly finger the Federation of Labor as a guilty party, judging that such a step was liable to hurt chances that the law would receive the approval of the Federation. Consequently, all criticism was focused on the Mandate government. The resolutions of the convention regarding health insurance legislation were widely covered in the media, but here as well, not a word was said about the position of the Federation of Labor and the "holding-action" it had adopted—apparently due to similar expectations that an attack on the Federation would only undermine prospects of progress.

Despite all, even the Kupat Holim convention and its resolutions did not hasten approval of the proposal in the executive committee. On 24 June 1929, Kenivsky-Kenev wrote the secretary of the executive committee that due to protracted delay, an opportunity had been lost to raise the subject in the gathering of the Mandate's convention that was to convene on July 1. On June 14, three months after the close of the second Kupat Holim convention and nine months after establishment of the joint Federation-Kupat Holim committee to examine the proposed law, the Kupat Holim directorate told Dr. Zmora that the Federation's council had finally approved the proposal. The letter requested that Dr. Zmora word the proposed legislation in legal parlance, translate it into English, and submit the draft to the Mandate government in the name of Kupat Holim and the Federation of Labor. The Kupat Holim directorate even informed Dr. Zmora that the International Association of Health Funds backed the legislative initiative and stressed that the organization was willing to apply its influence on the Mandate government if it were requested to do so. With the letter, Dr. Zmora also received the evaluation of the International Labor Organization stating that the prospects that the Mandate government would agree to legislate such a law were extremely low, for the British government had not enacted social legislation in any of its colonies (in defiance of the resolutions of the international body passed in 1927). Nevertheless, the heads of the International Labor Organization were prepared to do all that was in their power to assist Kupat Holim advance legislation.

The Draft Proposal for Compulsory Health Insurance

On 20 January 1930, after four years of delays and "holding-actions," the Kupat Holim proposal for a compulsory health insurance law was submitted to the Mandate government in its Hebrew and English versions. The preamble to the draft legislation stated:

> It is inconceivable from both a social and health viewpoint that such an important matter should be left to chance and insecurity of income, and it is the government's duty to ensure the existence of the fund through a law that will

> require work providers, workers, and the government of the country to participate in issuing an arrangement for medical and financial aid to workers in times of illness. This law should induce the creation of similar health funds such as the one existing, also for Arab laborers. Laws such as these for social insurance in event of illness have existed for decades in various countries.[17]

The primary clauses in the draft legislation were as follows:

- All salaried employees in the economy would be required to join one of the health funds.
- Independent workers (farmers, crafts persons, and so forth) could join the health funds, but would not be required to do so.
- Collection would be carried out by the health funds that would be established for this purpose. The health funds would be non-profit organizations.
- A governmental health network would be established to supervise enactment of the law, oversee the operations of the health funds, and review their expenditures.
- Payment of insurance premiums would be shared equally between the employers (the parallel tax), the insurees, and the government. Each side would undertake to cover a third of the cost of the health insurance. Payments by insurees would be graduated by income.
- The basket of services would include medical assistance in keeping with the standards set by Kupat Holim: clinics, hospitalization, convalescence, medications, and assistance with medical equipment.
- Medical care would be provided to members and their families immediately after joining the fund.
- Sick leave would be arranged in a manner similar to insurance abroad. A sick employee would be entitled to sick leave from the fourth day of his illness and a maximum of twenty-six weeks a year. Eligibility for sick leave would be limited solely to those who had paid health insurance in the three month period prior to the illness.
- Disability annuities would be paid to a person in accordance with his last salary. Eligibility for disability was limited to those who had paid insurance for a year preceding the disability.

- Maternity grants would be granted to women with a minimum of ten months membership in the fund. The grant would be divided into twelve weekly payments, six prior to delivery and six after delivery.[18]

The British high commissioner did not delay his response for long. In mid-February 1930, a month after receipt of the draft legislation proposal, Chancellor sent his reply to the executive committee of the Federation of Labor:

> His Majesty believes that due to economic reasons, the proposal cannot be accepted at this time.…H.M. is unable to state, at what time it would be able to examine the program of compulsory health insurance for the workers in Palestine (Eretz Israel).[19]

The negative response of the British high commission to the proposal presented by Kupat Holim and the Federation of Labor sparked immediate response. Henrietta Szold, a member of the health committee of the National Committee, wrote her opinion to colonel Kisch, a member of the Zionist executive in Eretz Israel:

> The unsuccessful negotiation in this case proves again that negotiation with the government on individual issues and in a decentralized fashion cannot bring about the desired outcomes. It seems to me that it would be desirable that the above material be [in the hands of] the Zionist executive in London.[20]

As to the reasons for the failure of the negotiations, Szold suggested that efforts should have been coordinated for a concerted effort by all parties, citing a memorandum on "health matters and the government" that had been sent to London at the same time that the Zionist leadership in Eretz Israel was demanding passage of a health insurance law by the powers-that-be in Eretz Israel.[21] It may be that the initiatives of the Zionist executive, the Federation of Labor, and Kupat Holim regarding health insurance would have been crowned with more success, argued Szold, if all the parties had made a coordinated effort, rather than splitting their forces. Both Kupat Holim and the Zionist executive in Eretz Israel accepted Henrietta Szold's recommendations that further efforts to bring about legislation of health insurance be transferred to the Zionist executive in London—the seat of decision-making.

In December 1930, the Jewish Agency executive convened to discuss a proposal that all health projects in the Yishuv enjoying the Agency's support be transferred to Knesset Israel. Clause D of the proposal stated that in accordance with a demand from Kupat Holim, Knesset Israel would act to "investigate expansion of modes of social insurance in the event of illness."[22]

Dr. Katznelson-Nissan, a member of the secretariat for health matters of the National Committee, was charged with investigating the technical side of levying a health tax as required. The committee even voiced the opinion that "no less than a third of the revenues of Knesset Israel after deduction of operation costs of the management should be devoted to health needs."[23]

In a confidential memorandum, Katznelson-Nissan discussed the factors leading to the estrangement of the Mandate government from Kupat Holim and the health institutions of the Yishuv. The author suggested that the primary reason was that the government had not been made a partner from the start in underwriting health services and their organization. He quoted the words of Dr. Kleiger from the Kupat Holim management, who had said that "the only demand we have of the government is—Don't interfere."[24]

Katznelson-Nissan argued that this attitude was what had distanced the British from any involvement in health matters of the Yishuv, so that when they were subsequently asked for assistance, they ignored the needs of the Yishuv. Similar sentiments were expressed by Henrietta Szold and the Hadassah Medical Federation. Dr. Katznelson-Nissan concluded:

> Under such conditions, the government did not see for itself any role in the health field of the Yishuv, and if we add to this that at the head of the government's medical service stood from the start a man who is not at all eager for a constructive role in building the country [i.e., Colonel Herron], it is easy to understand how we got to such, that the government has withdrawn from all responsibly regarding provision of medical needs of the Yishuv.[25]

In summing up his memorandum, Dr. Katznelson-Nissan expressed the hope that legislative initiatives of Kupat Holim and the change in the position of the Zionist movement and Kupat Holim regarding the role of the Mandate government in health matters would slowly bring about an improvement in the situation, and in the future the Mandate government would participate in taking responsibility for the health of the Yishuv.

On 12 February 1931, the representative assembly of Knesset Israel ratified the resolution to transfer health facilities to the authority of Knesset Israel. From this point forward, the health projects became public bodies subject to inspection and coordination of the National Committee and subordinate to its legal decisions (such as the decision to allow enforcement of the parallel tax and so forth). On Katznelson-Nissan's recommendation, the assembly issued a call for the Mandate government to legislate a compulsory health insurance law covering sick leave and disability pensions. Along with the wording of the demand, the representative assembly also leveled harsh criticism at the Mandate government's health policy, which, they claimed, ignored the health needs of the Yishuv and was responsible for the increase in disease. The chronicles of the representative assembly were published in the newspapers on the same day the MacDonald letter to Dr. Chaim Weizmann was released (12 February 1931). This was the document in which the British prime minister sought to reassure the Jews that his government intended to stand behind the Mandate and had no intention of freezing existing conditions by cutting off immigration and absorption—meaning that politics (that is, Arab pressure) would not determine immigration policies. The pro-Zionist tone of the letter rekindled hopes within the Yishuv and Kupat Holim of a possible change of heart by the Mandate government on the issue of health legislation.

Attempts to Forward Health Insurance Legislation in the 1930s

On 10 February 1931, two days prior to publication of the resolution of the representative assembly and the MacDonald letter, Kupat Holim turned to Dov Hos, head of the Poalei Zion Alliance in London, considered to have good connections within the ruling Labor Party of Great Britain. In a long and detailed letter accompanied by a volume of material on Kupat Holim's operation in Eretz

Israel, Kenivsky-Kenev requested that Dov Hos do what he could on behalf of health insurance legislation, a parallel tax, and participation of the Mandate government in budgeting Kupat Holim. In approaching Hos, Kupat Holim sought to circumvent the opposition of Colonel Herron, head of the British health department. Kenivsky-Kenev described Kupat Holim's difficult financial straits that year, which had led to the closure of the health fund's only hospital, the Emek Hospital:

> We wish to note that if there are things that it is possible to gain from a workers' government [i.e., the Labor government] the issue of labor legislation being one of them, and if up until now we have not gained anything from the Labor government in this profession [in the health care field], in the near future we must take more energetic actions in this direction.[26]

On 21 May 1931, Dov Hos submitted a memorandum on the health situation in Eretz Israel to a group of socialist doctors in the British Parliament. Hos did not stress in his memorandum, as he was requested to do by Kupat Holim, that the draft legislation proposal included the Arab sector (in order to convince the British that the move was not solely for the benefit of the Jews), and he did not stress the importance of the law in light of the health conditions prevailing in the country. Moreover, Hos omitted Kupat Holim's request that the Mandate government participate in its budget, separate from the proposed legislation. In a response letter sent to Hos in June 1931, Kenivsky-Kenev expressed his disappointment with what he viewed as the slovenly manner in which Hos had handled things. He asked Hos to again act on behalf of the health fund, this time to concentrate on advancing the cause of health insurance legislation, and only as a secondary option working to secure participation of the government in funding Kupat Holim and putting the parallel tax on a legal footing: "The main thing is to work more forcefully and swiftly, because if this [Labor] government will fall, from whom will we demand laws protecting the worker?"[27]

From other documents we learn of Dov Hos's failure to advance legislation of health insurance via London. In September 1931, Kenivsky-Kenev wrote Dr. Chaim Arlosoroff, head of the political department of the Jewish Agency: "Our comrade in London did not achieve anything in the field of labor legislation."[28]

Kenivsky-Kenev requested Arlosoroff's intervention in advancing things in the health field. He described the lack of response of the Colonial Office in London to Kupat Holim's requests, its disregard for appeals from the International Labor Office and the International of Health Fund, and the failure of deliberations concerning draft legislation conducted in the in the Mandate's Commission (to a large extent due to the delay in approval of the draft by the Federation of Labor). Kupat Holim's proposal that the Mandate government establish a "commission to investigate the question" was also rejected. Consequently, Kenivsky-Kenev suggested to Arlosoroff that he draft a proposal for a health insurance law and raise it indirectly in the commission that was to be established by the Mandate government at the time, in order to prepare legislation that would protect working youth:

> If a commission of this nature will be established, it will be possible to demand revisions in a number of existing laws and also to realize other legislation, including a law for health insurance for workers (an obligatory Kupat Holim).[29]

Kupat Holim did not turn only to Dr. Arlosoroff, it also requested that Henrietta Szold use her influence on the Mandate government in order to integrate the question of health insurance among the subjects on the commission's agenda. One can surmise that the disappointment following Dov Hos's failure to advance legislation via London was the reason Kupat Holim abandoned the direct approach and began to seek other ways to realize its aims. The heads of the health fund hoped that if the draft legislation proposal could enjoy a hearing in the commission, the Mandate government would recognize its importance and perhaps take steps to put it into practice.

In November 1931, a short time after the multi-pronged action on the part of Dr. Chaim Arlosoroff and Henrietta Szold, Dr. Katznelson-Nissan told the Kupat Holim directorate that the chief secretary of the Mandate government had approved discussion of a health insurance law in the governmental commission for labor legislation that was about to be established, and that among its members would be Dr. Moshe Zmora and Dov Hos. In a letter to Henrietta Szold, Colonel Herron wrote that the Mandate government was not prepared in the near future to pass health insurance legislation, despite willingness to discuss the issue within the commission. Despite the pessimistic forecast of Herron, Dr. Katznelson-Nissan held that success was possible and hinged on how the issue was presented before the commission and the commission's final recommendations after the hearings. Consequently, Katznelson-Nissan suggested that Kupat Holim and the Federation of Labor's health committee form an internal committee that would advise the two representatives on the government commission. Kupat Holim was optimistic. For the first time in two years there was an official governmental body willing to discuss this important issue.

In December 1931 the government commission for labor legislation began its deliberations. The commission was comprised of seven officials—directors of government department, and two observers each from the Jewish and Arab communities. Most of the participants knew very little about the operations of Kupat Holim, and the discussion of health insurance was complex. During the course of deliberation, the commission invited a representative of Kupat Holim (Kenivsky-Kenev) to present the issue of health insurance and provide an overview of Kupat Holim's operation. Consequently, a detailed report on the health fund was submitted to each member of the commission. Most of the members (six out of seven government officials), however, opposed the Kupat Holim program, reasoning that "it was premature to realize compulsory insurance in the country" although the participants were impressed with the important role played by Kupat Holim in the health field. The minority opinion (five members—two Jews, two Arabs and one Englishman) was that the Mandate government should be called upon to legislate immediately a health insurance law through the auspices of Kupat Holim and with governmental funding, and for this purpose other health funds should be established as well. The proponents also recommended that Kupat Holim enjoy regular financial support. The commission as a whole agreed that the minority opinion be submitted to other parties in the government so Kupat Holim could be assisted by them in receipt of economic support from the government through other channels.

In a Kupat Holim directorate report from the year 1931, Kenivsky-Kenev wrote concerning the commission's work:

> So we took a step towards government legislation for workers' health insurance. The matter is not easy to implement in a backward country, but we have to carry on until we succeed at it.[30]

Kenivsky-Kenev also praised the thorough work of the committee on the health insurance issue, which he said was straightforward and free of political calculations, noting the rare but admirable collaboration and unanimity between Jewish and Arab representatives on this important issue.

In mid-1932 the commission closed its hearings without any results. The Kupat Holim proposal for compulsory health insurance legislation did not win enough support, and the Mandate government accepted the recommendations of the majority, and rejected the proposal.

In fact, the commission's deliberations did little to advance Kupat Holim's demands for comprehensive legislation in the health domain (parallel tax and compulsory health insurance). But despite the meager outcome, in practical terms, Kupat Holim remained optimistic, and pleased with what was viewed as a political breakthrough. The very fact that an official commission of the government had addressed the issue had advanced their cause and enhanced chances that such a law would eventually be passed.

In January 1933, Perlson and Kenivsky-Kenev turned to the executive committee of the Federation of Labor, seeking to launch a concerted and coordinated effort by all the Yishuv's institutions on behalf of legislation. They argued:

> If the Federation of Labor on one hand and the political department of the Jewish agency on the other will not undertake vigorous action toward the government an opportunity will be lost....We suggest that the Federation request a discussion with the [high] commissioner concerning its demands in the matter of insurance in the event of illness and assistance to Kupat Holim.[31]

An official reply to Perlson and Kenivsky-Kenev's petition was not found, but in the margin of a Kupat Holim letter—in handwriting—the secretariat had written:

> We affirm receipt of your letter. The executive committee will take into account the matter of insurance and assistance to Kupat Holim in discussion which the Federation plans to request with the [high] commissioner.[32]

There was no talk of vigorous action, nor collaboration with the Jewish Agency as Kupat Holim had requested, but rather, the same attitude of "business as usual" that had characterized the Federation of Labor's behavior in response to Kupat Holim requests in the past. The fact that no discussion was held at the Federation following Kupat Holim's appeal only amplifies this impression; no one even took the time to evaluate the chances that such a tactic would succeed.

Along with its appeal to the Federation of Labor, spurred on by the belief that only a joint effort could bring change, Kupat Holim also approached Dr. Katznelson from the secretariat for health matters at the National Committee, and Dr. Chaim Arlosoroff, head of the political section of the Jewish Agency. In his letters to all parties, Perlson called for them "to make an unconcealed action against Colonel Herron by the National Committee, [for] exchange of letters will not profit the matter.[33]

Perlson calculated that Colonel Herron was the primary obstacle to legislation of compulsory health insurance and financial assistance for Kupat Holim. Only circumvention of his authority and a direct appeal to the British high commissioner, Sir Arthur Wauchope, would help. During the months that followed, Kupat Holim did not let the question of financial assistance from the government and the health insurance issue drop from the pubic agenda. This question stood at the heart of deliberations at the third convention of Kupat Holim, held on April 12 that year. A Kupat Holim initiative also led the eighteenth Zionist congress, that convened in mid-1933, to call upon the Mandate government to legislate a compulsory health insurance law and provide regular backing for Kupat Holim's work.

In June 1933, Dr. Chaim Arlosoroff was murdered, sparking tremendous social and political tensions that split the Jewish community of Palestine into hostile factions. The assassination had an impact on Kupat Holim as well. Arlosoroff had been one of the activists working on behalf of legislation of compulsory health insurance and had good ties with the high commissioner, so his death was a loss to Kupat Holim in its endeavors to advance passage of the law. As a matter of course, Kupat Holim turned to his successor in the political department, Moshe Sharret, requesting that Sharret champion Kupat Holim's interests, but things did not return to the way they had been prior to Arlosoroff's death. Political tumult in the wake of the murder dominated the public agenda for nearly a year, particularly among Labor Federation leadership and the Zionist executive. Thus, Kupat Holim's problems were thrust onto the sidelines of public debate for over a year, with no initiatives taken.

In the wake of Arlosoroff's death and disappointment with the performance of Moshe Sharret and Dov Hos, Yitzhak Kenivsky in 1934 decided to turn directly to David Ben-Gurion:

> Kupat Holim appeals to you regarding an issue that is most vital to [the Fund]. We know how busy you are, and up to now we have not bothered you, but now we cannot refrain from requesting your assistance....Although within the Jewish Agency leadership there are several of our important comrades [e.g., Moshe Sharret] we have not [found] that Kupat Holim matters which have outstanding importance for the working public in general have received deserving treatment in their hands. Among these matters we would stress in particular the question of a health insurance law, or participation of the government in Kupat Holim expenditures.[34]

The Kupat Holim letter to Ben-Gurion is the first evidence that the heads of Kupat Holim were pessimistic about the chances for legislation. For the first time, they suggested an alternative to legislation, namely, government participation in Kupat Holim expenditures. It seems that the health fund's leaders judged that the chance of receiving financial backing without legislation was better than the chance of passage of a compulsory health insurance law. The letter went on to request Ben-Gurion's good services in influencing the British high commission to meet with a delegation led by Ben-Gurion himself, with the participation of Dr. Beilenson, Yosef Baratz, Golda Meirson, and one of the members of the Kupat Holim directorate. Kupat Holim reiterated here a request sent to Ben-Gurion in 1928—six years earlier—asking that he personally intervene in forwarding the proposal for compulsory health insurance legislation. This time as well, David Ben-Gurion delayed his response. On January 7, Kenivsky-Kenev wrote a response to Dov Hos: "Already on November 29, 1934, we appealed to Ben-Gurion regarding his efforts with the High Commissioner...but unfortunately he did not even see fit to answer us." He asked Dos Hos "to apply [your] influence on comrade Ben-Gurion to take the role upon himself."[35]

Hos, indeed, approached Ben-Gurion, urging him to answer Kupat Holim, and in a curt letter that did not mention the subject at hand directly, Ben-Gurion requested that Kenivsky-Kenev send him details on the health fund: the number of members and employees, the scope of the budget, assets, and so forth. Kupat Holim quickly replied, and within four days a detailed report was submitted to Ben-Gurion with all the data he requested. But again, Ben-Gurion's reply failed to materialize. A month later, Kenivsky-Kenev again approached Dov Hos: "We did not receive from you a reply regarding action toward the government via comrade Ben-Gurion [in the matter of Kupat Holim]."[36]

Again, Dov Hos interceded with Ben-Gurion, and while Ben-Gurion did not reply officially, he sent Hos a remark in his writing: "When you are in Jerusalem raise this question in the political department."[37]

After a week, Hos raised Ben-Gurion's request before Moshe Sharret in the political department of the Jewish Agency in Jerusalem, suggesting in a letter that a meeting between the Kupat Holim delegation and the high commissioner be arranged. Sharret was even asked to take upon himself to lead the delegation that the health fund hoped would be headed by Ben-Gurion himself. Dov Hos closed his letter to Sharret by stressing the importance of the issue: "I would request that you place this matter among the series of matters that demand urgent attention."[38]

Thus, David Ben-Gurion declined to deal personally with the question of health insurance legislation and passed responsibility on to Sharret. It is hard to understand Ben-Gurion's motivations, for he does not explain them explicitly in either his personal diary or his correspondence. His attitude toward Kupat Holim's legislative initiatives probably derive from priorities as to where he must invest his time, and subjective questions of political pragmatism.

Political events certainly overshadowed his work. Ben-Gurion was occupied with a host of more burning questions that required his leadership in 1934–1935. First came his personal involvement in attempts to unite Zionist leadership, split in the aftermath of the Arlosoroff murder, and his occupation with other aspects of internal Zionist politics, such as upcoming elections for the Zionist executive and the Jewish Agency. Second, the rise of Hitler to power in Germany precipitated an influx of mass Jewish immigration to Palestine, mainly from Germany, that challenged the absorption capabilities of the Jewish community and further amplified growing tension with Palestinian Arabs over Zionist aspirations. Thus, Kupat

Holim's difficulties and initiatives on behalf of social legislation were not a burning priority under prevailing circumstances.

At the same time, there were other factors at play: As the secretary of the Federation of Labor, the parent organization of Kupat Holim, Ben-Gurion was presumably not eager to support social legislation on a nation-wide basis for practical, political reasons. While he refrained from publicly going on record against the legislation initiative, one can assume from his behavior and indirect references to the subject, that Ben-Gurion feared ramifications of such legislation in the political sphere. He considered Kupat Holim a valued asset to the Labor movement's "political arsenal." Thus it is logical to assume that he would ignore any attempts to mobilize his prestige and influence for a move that might challenge the Labor Federation's exclusive organizational control over Kupat Holim and thus weaken the political and social hegemony of the Labor Federation—that is, a move such as the transfer of control of health services to British Mandate authorities in the wake of such enlightened social legislation.

Following Ben-Gurion's failure to respond favorably to Kupat Holim's request for his personal assistance in gaining passage of a health insurance law, the issue of legislation was finally dropped from the health fund's agenda. No further direct attempts were made to press for passage of a compulsory health insurance law under the British Mandate, although there was still some discussion in the press and parenthetical discussion in the 1936 Royal Inquiry Commission, appointed to find a solution to the Jewish-Arab conflict in Eretz Israel.[39]

The Royal Inquiry Commission was appointed following the outbreak of Arab hostilities (the 1936–1939 "Arab Revolt") against British authority and in protest of Zionist aspirations and Jewish immigration. In the course of its hearings, evidence from both parties—Arab and Jewish—was presented on a variety of issues related to British rule. Kupat Holim seized the opportunity to, again, raise the issue of compulsory health insurance with influential figures in government, but to no avail. Kupat Holim's appeal to the Royal Inquiry Commission was the last attempt by Kupat Holim to bring about realization of a compulsory health insurance under British rule.

After a more than ten-year battle for compulsory health insurance legislation, the heads of Kupat Holim finally came to the conclusion that there was no chance of realizing such a goal, and energies should focus on endeavors to find financial backing, even ad hoc, from the Mandate government.

Efforts on behalf of a health insurance law were renewed only after the establishment of the state of Israel, in 1948, in the framework of a planning committee established by the Federation of Labor's social research institute which formulated the first program for social insurance and government health insurance for the state. Not until 1995, however—fifty years after the establishment of the state of Israel—was a compulsory health insurance law finally passed as the basis for a major reform of the health system.

The Kupat Holim Budget and the Mandate Government

Between 1935 and 1937, Kupat Holim concentrated its efforts on obtaining financial assistance and temporary budgeting from the Mandate government. While regular budgetary backing was not forthcoming, from time to time the government granted various ad-hoc allocations, for the most part for building hospitals, housing for hospital staff, and so forth. Granting Kupat Holim financial support of a regular budget would have required Mandate authorities to do the same for other health institutions, and British authorities sought to avoid any such precedent. In April 1936, the Kupat Holim directorate submitted an annual report on monetary assistance provided by the Mandate government for the building of a hospital for the agricultural villages in Judea (what would become the Beilenson Hospital, and today the Rabin Medical Center in Petach Tikva). A separate sum was granted for building housing for staff, and others for participation in underwriting the establishment of a laboratory and pharmacy at the Emek Hospital and for building rural clinics for the health fund.

The entire Mandate health budget in 1936 was 250,000 Eretz Israel pounds, and the overall assistance received by Kupat Holim that year was a mere 2.5–3 percent of the total budget.[40] Government allocations to Kupat Holim, after years of struggle, were tiny compared to the overall budget, ridiculous in scope if one takes into account that, at the time, Kupat Holim was providing medical services to 25 percent of the Jewish population, including some of the weakest segments of the Jewish population, such as laborers and new immigrants. Governmental assistance was designed merely to "buy quit," that is, to mitigate public criticism and meet Kupat Holim's demands with the absolute minimum possible.

10

KUPAT HOLIM AND THE FEDERATION OF LABOR: RECIPROCAL MEMBERSHIP AND JOINT DUES

THE MEMBERSHIP ISSUE IN THE 1920S

A HEALTH FUND FOR WORKERS ONLY

The first health funds were established with the mission of meeting the health needs of Jewish agricultural workers in Eretz Israel, and the agricultural laborer played a core role in shaping Kupat Holim's "process of becoming." The ordinances and resolutions set forth by the Judea Worker's Health Fund stipulated that "workers and crafts persons who work by themselves will [also] be accepted"[1] as members.

The intention was agricultural workers only. This rule was also at the foundation of the health funds established by workers in the Galilee and Samaria between 1912 and 1915. Class distinction was an important pillar in the organization of the first health funds; in essence, the fact that a person was an agricultural laborer, even if unemployed, was more important than any other factor. The first funds took upon themselves care of the agricultural workers wherever the individual was, whatever his or her economic circumstances. Due to the centrality of a single occupation to the working of the health funds, laborers in the city (welders, construction workers, metal workers, and so forth) organized separately, in a health fund of their own. But the division between rural and urban proletariats did not continue for long, and in the first years of the First World War, the first agreements were signed between the urban workers' brotherhoods and the health funds.

The issue of membership for crafts persons in the health fund was more complex. The definition first adopted by the health fund in its ordinances—"a craftsperson who works by himself"—was insufficient for defining entitlement to join the fund. (For instance, if a craftsperson was assisted by his wife and children, was he considered one who "works by himself"?) Final decision on acceptance of a person or a brotherhood into the ranks of health fund members was taken on an individual basis and not necessarily according to the ordinances. Members of the Federation of Labor who were crafts persons in Petach Tikva—who for two years tried to gain entrance to the Judea Workers' Health Fund—complained in a letter to the secretary of the health fund about the fund's disregard of the request, stressing: "Our federation has about 30 members, all working independently."[2]

In the closing stages of the First World War, when the regional health funds reorganized on the basis of political party affiliation, workers in agriculture still held priority over laborers in the city in terms of eligibility for membership in the fund. The Hapoel Hatzair health fund's office even stipulated with the reorganization of the fund: "This fund, for the time being, is only for agricultural workers and not for urban laborers."[3]

Only after many urban laborers, members of the Hapoel Hatzair party in Jerusalem, asked to become members of the health fund was the membership clause amended to include all laborers.

RECIPROCAL MEMBERSHIP IN KUPAT HOLIM AND THE FEDERATION OF LABOR

In December 1920 the General Federation of Labor was founded, and with it, local health funds were amalgamated into one General Health Fund—Kupat Holim. Membership in the Federation of Labor was defined as encompassing all the Hebrew (i.e., Jewish) workers in Eretz Israel. The question of membership in the Federation—from which membership in the health fund would be derived—was settled soon after the founding convention. In November 1921, the first council (i.e., the first convention) of the Federation of Labor set forth that "all members of the Federation must be members of Kupat

Holim" and Federation institutions (that is, Kupat Holim, Hamashbir, and others) would care "only for members of the Federation who have membership cards and pay dues."

Thus, Kupat Holim also set forth that "only members of the Federation could be received into their ranks, and laborers who were not members were accepted only with the consent of the [Federation's] executive committee." This ordinance allowed Kupat Holim to provide medical assistance to Arab laborers who were not eligible for membership in the Federation.

While the ordinances clarified the linkage in principle between membership in the Federation and membership in Kupat Holim, they did not set forth binding rules for enforcing the principle, particularly what should happen to a member of the Federation of Labor who refused to join Kupat Holim. Thus, in essence, the first resolution of the Federation of Labor's council was solely a recommendation, and the tie between membership in the Federation and membership in Kupat Holim became a one-way street: Members of Kupat Holim were required to be members of the Federation (unless they received special dispensations), but members of the Federation were not required (in practice) to be members of Kupat Holim. Now, the key factor in the question of membership was no longer a person's occupation—whether he was a laborer or a craftsperson working on his own—but rather, his organizational affiliation with the Federation of Labor.

Historian Shabtai Tevet believes David Ben-Gurion was behind this change.[4] Ben-Gurion viewed Kupat Holim as a source of organization power of the first order, and therefore sought to couple it to binding membership in the Federation of Labor. At the outset, the Federation for its part did not tie itself to a binding reciprocal relationship with Kupat Holim, fearing that such a requirement would discourage many workers from jointing the Federation. Thus, in the first years of Kupat Holim, the membership in the health fund was 30 percent less than membership in the Federation of Labor.[5] Hopes among heads of Kupat Holim that all members of the Federation of Labor would join the health fund of their own volition soon proved to be unfounded.

In a 1924 article entitled "Kupat Holim and the Composition of Its Members," Yitzhak Kenivsky-Kenev complained that all members of the Federation did not consider it a duty to join Kupat Holim, noting the "lopsided" composition of Kupat Holim rosters:

> The overwhelming majority of those members [live] in bad conditions that cause much illness…while members of the Federation [live] in more or less good conditions…on better salaries, [although] their numbers in our institution are very small."[6]

This state of affairs caused Kenivsky-Kenev to believe that the economic capabilities of the fund as well as its moral basis were being impaired—that evasion of membership in Kupat Holim on the part of Federation of Labor members whose economic circumstances were good was no less than shirking responsibility and a digression from the moral and ideological foundations of the Federation as a whole. While he was well aware why the Federation declined to enforce the principle, he nevertheless called upon the upcoming meeting of the council in 1925 to affirm

> as a matter of law, that all members among the members of the Federation must be also a member of our primary institution of mutual assistance, Kupat Holim. This ordinance may reduce a known number of Federation members, but will cure the atmosphere in the Federation…and perhaps also increase the number of Kupat Holim members and increase the capability of its medical work.[7]

Kenivsky-Kenev's appeal that the Federation of Labor begin to enforce the dual-membership clause would not be honored until 1936.

In plants and other workplaces where the management provided medical assistance to laborers, there was no room for Kupat Holim, and its penetration of such places of employment was liable to undermine the employees' rights and free the management from responsibility for medical care of their employees. When the issue of membership for workers in the Rishon le-Zion winery in the Federation of Labor and Kupat Holim was raised, the executive committee of the Federation demanded that Kupat Holim waive membership in the health fund because the medical assistance provided by the management of the winery was better than that provided by Kupat Holim. The executive committee also feared that the workers at the winery would choose not to join the Federation if doing so hinged on joining Kupat Holim as well. The Federation argued that increasing the number of Federation members by accepting unorganized workers was of primary importance, while widening the circle of Kupat Holim's membership was secondary. When a strike broke out at the winery and the Federation was called in to mediate between the management and the workers, Federation representatives were quick to give in on the question of Kupat Holim and even agreed that medical assistance provided by the winery management be tacked onto overall wages stipulated in the salary contract signed by the parties, rather than being anchored in a separate entitlement clause.

From 1922, Kupat Holim sought to expand its membership to encompass unorganized laborers as well. In the proposed ordinances submitted by Kupat Holim for ratification by the Federation of Labor's second council (1922) a clause was added concerning membership for those who were not members of the Federation of Labor. Membership was made conditional on the consent of the executive committee and a medical examination.

In its efforts to bring new members into the ranks, Kupat Holim did not hesitate to apply pressure on workers' committees and demand that all employees without exception be obliged to join the fund; if this were not done, Kupat Holim would refrain from extending medical assistance to their laborers who were already members of the fund. In a letter sent by the Kupat Holim directorate to the workers' committee of the Gorlisky-Krinitzy Factory, a producer of construction elements and furniture, Reuven Shenkar wrote:

> Until it will be arranged that all members of the Federation of Labor in the factory will enter Kupat Holim, we will not be able to provide medical aid to the 24 members listed that you submitted to us.[8]

The Federation objected to such tactics on the part of Kupat Holim. The executive committee announced that Kupat Holim was not permitted to require workers in a private factory to join en bloc (based on a collective framework of obligations, as was the case with the cooperative agricultural farms). Each worker should be allowed to receive medical assistance as an individual urban laborer in his or her place of residence. When Kupat Holim demanded that the federation of clerical workers not issue membership cards to clerks who did not join Kupat Holim, they were told: "There is no obligation on the part of the United Clerks Federation to be members of Kupat Holim."

The request that the clerks receive a discount in membership dues as a condition for jointing was rejected by Kupat Holim:

> We cannot agree that at a time that thousands of workers carry the burden of the institution, there will be clerks whose [financial] circumstances are better who are exempt from this obligation.[9]

In its efforts to broaden its ranks, Kupat Holim was forced to accommodate its own interests to the interests of the Federation of Labor. Yet, from a host of standpoints, the interests of the Federation served to block the growth of Kupat Holim. In December 1925, a short time prior to the convention of the first Kupat Holim council, Kenivsky-Kenev complained about the conflict of interests that stymied efforts on the part of Kupat Holim to increase the number of members in the health fund. He said that the Federation did not prevent issuance of membership cards to those who had yet to join Kupat Holim, despite a request on the part of the fund's directorate to do so, and eligibility to vote in the general convention was not withheld from those who failed to join Kupat Holim. Kenivsky-Kenev complained that the Federation did not honor in practice its own resolutions taken by the Federation's first council "that all members of the Federation must be members of Kupat Holim." And in practice:

> Those making a decent wage and living under good conditions…will continue to be loyal members of our Federation without carrying the burden of duties toward this one [i.e., Kupat Holim].[10]

This was the core of Kupat Holim's complaint against the Federation of Labor in the years that the health fund, burdened by growing deficits, sought to extricate itself from financial distress by broadening its membership base.

WHO DID KUPAT HOLIM WANT TO JOIN ITS RANKS?

An August 1925 memorandum from the Kupat Holim directorate raised the issue of groups and organizations that were not organized by the Federation but were attractive as potential members of the health fund. Among the list of candidates for Kupat Holim in Jerusalem were members of the teachers' federation, clerical workers, printers, butchers, employees of Hadassah, nurses in hospitals, and people from "Eastern ethnic groups" (Jews originating from Arab lands). The memorandum went on to list groups of workers who should not be accepted for membership and the reasons. Yitzhak Kenivsky-Kenev, for instance, opposed attempts to mobilize new members from among "Eastern ethnic groups" claiming:

> This is human material that is not capable of participating in an institution for mutual aid but affords itself of philanthropic institutions which are plentiful in Jerusalem. Their entrance into Kupat Holim will only put us at a deficit.[11]

On the other hand, Kenivsky-Kenev was seeking the membership of clerks, teachers, and single laborers. Kupat Holim was not willing to accept just anyone, and particularly not individuals who were liable to exacerbate its existing financial distress.

In deliberations conducted following the memorandum, it was recommended that various incentives be offered to clerical workers and employees of Hadassah in order to convince them to join Kupat Holim. Among the possible benefits raised were discounts on membership and special services, such as home delivery of medications, paid "rest & recuperation" in the summer, treatment without queuing for services, home visits, and other "upgrades" in services rendered. Kupat Holim was prepared to adopt such steps—exceptions that undermined its lofty principles of equality—out of its desperate need to attract members from among the more established classes of the Yishuv to improve its own floundering finances—and perhaps to demonstrate to Hadassah that even its own employees were in need of Kupat Holim.

Despite vigorous steps by Kupat Holim to attract such groups, the breakthrough that was destined to transform the fund's framework came from an entirely different direction: In 1927, the first agreement was signed between Kupat Holim and the Hapoel Hamizrachi Federation, bringing members of Hamizrachi, religious labor Zionists, under the coverage of Kupat Holim.

KUPAT HOLIM AND THE HAPOEL HAMIZRACHI

The first ties between the Hapoel Hamizrachi Federation and Kupat Holim were established in the early 1920s. Hapoel Hamizrachi, a federation of religiously observant but pro-Zionist laborers, was founded in Jerusalem in 1922 with the purpose of being a proletarian wing of the World Hamizrachi Movement.[12] From the beginning, the movement had sought to establish its own independent network of institutions, organization, and settlements. In November 1923, the Hapoel Hamizrachi Federation demanded a separate budget from the Zionist executive in order to establish its own independent health fund, claiming that religious patients had special needs (maintenance of Jewish dietary laws, observance of the Sabbath, and so forth). Yosef Sprinzak, the Federation of Labor's delegate on the Zionist executive, responded to this demand, suggesting that Kupat Holim commit itself to maintain kashrut and meet the special needs of Hapoel Hamizrachi members. However, the members of Hapoel Hamizrachi—some five-hundred strong—decided nevertheless to organize their own health fund that would avail itself of the services of Hadassah and Kupat Holim. Consequently, the Zionist executive allocated a separate budget for operation of a special health fund for members of Hapoel Hamizrachi.

In 1923–1924 attempts were made to integrate Hapoel Hamizrachi into the Federation of Labor, as part of the Federation's policy of seeking to amalgamate all the working class in Eretz Israel under one root organization controlled by the Federation of Labor. In October 1924, after negotiations accompanied by labor unrest and strikes organized by the Federation, the Hapoel Hamizrachi Federation decided to join the Federation of Labor[13]—opening the door for members of Hapoel Hamizrachi to join Kupat Holim as well. At the close of 1924 Kupat Holim had 8,100 members (approximately 15,000 with dependents) and the influx of 500 new members was significant. Moreover, the Hapoel Hamizrachi Federation had a separate budget from the Zionist executive for its own medical aid—a "dowry" the Federation of Labor expected Hamizrachi members would bring with them to the union.

The Zionist executive in Eretz Israel was the party who pushed for Hapoel Hamizrachi's integration into Kupat Holim, as a matter of economy: The existence of two separate health budgets was a needless burden. Moreover, Hapoel Hamizrachi found it difficult to provide its members with suitable services. In June 1924, the Zionist executive announced the merger of the two budgets, and called on the two health funds to unite. In October 1924, the union was ratified by the conventions of the Hapoel Hamizrachi Federation, and the Hapoel Hamizrachi joined the Federation of Labor.

There was, however, opposition to the merger, particularly on the part of the World Hamizrachi Movement, which refused to transfer the budget for medical assistance to Kupat Holim, as called for by the union. Professor Chaim Pik, the Hapoel Hamizrachi representative on the Zionist executive, announced that the budget was the Hamizrachi Federation's and threatened that Hamizrachi delegates to the Zionist Congress would take counter measures (the movement had seventy delegates). As a compromise the Zionist executive suggested that the budget be split proportionally, according to the number of Hamizrachi members in each health fund. In order to prevent attempts to inflate numbers (by registering new immigrants and so forth) Dr. Arieh Behem, who was appointed by the Zionist executive to investigate the matter, proposed that allocation be based only on the five hundred members of Hapoel Hamizrachi that were registered at the time of the merger.

The budgeting conflict with Hapoel Hamizrachi was settled at the Fifteenth Zionist Congress that convened in Basel in August 1927, where the union of the Kupat Holim and the Hamizrachi Health fund was ratified. The health budget of the Zionist executive to Hapoel Hamizrachi was calculated according to the number of members in the organization and embodied as a part of the Zionist executive's general budget to Kupat Holim. In July 1927, a month prior to ratification of the union, the Kupat Holim directorate and the Hapoel Hamizrachi Health Fund had signed an agreement to put the merger in effect.

Within the framework of the agreement the following terms were agreed upon. The branches of the Hapoel Hamizrachi Health Fund in their agricultural settlements were transferred to Kupat Holim. Kupat Holim committed itself to observe the laws of the Jewish Sabbath and maintain kashrut in its sick rooms and convalescence homes, under the supervision of Hapoel Hamizrachi rabbis. A special clerk was appointed to deal with questions of Jewish religious law (Halacha) that might arise regarding Kupat Holim's operation. It was agreed that Hapoel Hamizrachi employers would be integrated into the Kupat Holim organizational machinery (primarily in the kitchens). It was also agreed that should differences of opinion arise between Kupat Holim and Hapoel Hamizrachi, the parties would settle the question through arbitration. It was clarified that Kupat Holim was not responsible for the debts of Hapoel Hamizrachi accrued prior to the signing of the merger agreement. A special clause in the agreement left Hapoel Hamizrachi the option to nullify the agreement at any time, and Kupat Holim committed itself to return all assets it had received as a result of the merger (equipment and sick rooms), should Hapoel Hamizrachi employ the option. Nevertheless, it was agreed that members of Hapoel Hamizrachi would be registered separately within their own binding operative framework, would carry membership cards that were different from the rest of the membership, and would maintain their political identity within the Kupat Holim framework. Kupat Holim committed itself to accept all registered members of Hapoel Hamizrachi without any restrictions, and to maintain all their rights.

The agreement remained in effect throughout the Mandate period. Over time, Kupat Holim learned that its hopes to build itself up from an organizational and fiscal standpoint as a result of the accord were unrealistic. The number of Hapoel Hamizrachi members who sought to join Kupat Holim dropped over the years (up to the establishment of the state of Israel in 1948) and the relative weight of Hapoel Hamizrachi from a budgetary standpoint dwindled. In October 1931, Eliezer Perlson wrote that the number of Hapoel Hamizrachi members registered with Kupat Holim was only 148 members. Perlson noted with concern

> the indifference of members of Hapoel Hamizrachi regarding their membership in Kupat Holim. If this matter will not be rectified, it will force us to raise this question on the agenda of the supervisory committee of Kupat Holim.[14]

In the end, the matter was not raised, although the contribution of the Hapoel Hamizrachi Federation continued to steadily drop.

Only in 1956, when Hapoel Hamizrachi merged with Hamizrachi into the National Religious Party (NRP), were Kupat Holim services expanded to encompass any members of the NRP who wished to join, on the basis of the unification agreement of 1927. The agreement, which provided medical care to members of the NRP within the framework of Kupat Holim, remained in force up until 1995 when a compulsory health insurance system was established. While the tie between politics and health care was severed by this health reform—for *both* federations—even under the new national system most of the elements instituted by the old agreement, from maintenance of kashrut to separate colored membership cards, remain.

THE THIRD FEDERATION OF LABOR CONVENTION

On 5 July 1927, in the presence of 201 delegates and some 800 guests, the third convention of the Federation of Labor was opened in Tel Aviv. The convention was overshadowed by the economic recession that had hit the Yishuv in 1925–1926 and by the impending bankruptcy of Solel Boneh, a key Federation asset. On July 11, a week after the convention opened, the Investigative Commission appointed by the Zionist executive to examine the functioning and organization of Kupat Holim announced its conclusions, and the heads of Kupat Holim expected that the state of Kupat Holim would be on the convention's agenda. The Kupat Holim directorate called for discussion of the proposal that a supervisory committee for Kupat Holim be established to serve as a supreme administrative body (i.e., a board of directors), leaving the directorate to concentrate solely on functional aspects of Kupat Holim's operation. A far more burning question that the heads of Kupat Holim hoped to raise was enforcement of the duty of Federation of Labor members to join Kupat Holim.

The question was not a simple matter. From the time of its founding in 1920 to the days of its third convention, the Federation of Labor had striven to widen the circle of its membership among employees in all sectors of the economy. The heads of the Federation, primarily David Ben-Gurion, were well aware of the difficulty of enforcing membership in Kupat Holim on workers who agreed to join the Federation—fearing that a requirement of dual-membership would jade willingness to join, thus undermining the interests of the Federation. Despite the resolution in principle taken by the first Federation council requiring all members of the Federation to be members of Kupat Holim, the Federation refrained from enforcing membership in the health fund on those of its members who refused to do so. Consequently, the gap between the scope of membership in the Federation of Labor and the scope of membership in Kupat Holim reached 30 percent, and in Jerusalem, 40 percent.[15]

In a report on "Setting-Right Kupat Holim" in preparation for the third convention, the Federation evaded the question. The account dealt primarily with preparing the background for convention deliberations, and only briefly with Kupat Holim ordinances, the question of the parallel tax, and the basket of services the health fund granted members. Clause B of the report—"Membership"—noted that "As a member in Kupat Holim only one who is a member of the Federation of Labor is accepted," but it did not stipulate that members of the Federation must be members of Kupat Holim.

Kupat Holim did not plan to give in on its demands and was determined to raise the issue. The third Federation of Labor convention took place in the shadow of crisis in Solel Boneh and the political tensions it created, and the attention of the convention delegates being riveted on this issue, the health fund's demand to address the issue received only a brief hearing. The demands were accepted "as is," after brief discussion and no special thought. The resolution stated simply:

> All members of the Federation of Labor must be members of Kupat Holim. The convention imposes on the Federation's institutions to actualize this resolution within half a year.[16]

The resolution did not, however, say how the Federation's institutions were to treat someone who refused to join Kupat Holim. In essence, the convention paid lip service to the principle, skimming over the issue without providing any avenues for making the decision binding or enforceable. In retrospect, evasion of the issue would be the source of protracted conflicts between the Federation and the Kupat Holim. More than once the health fund would demand that Federation members who failed to abide by the decision be expelled from the Federation of Labor, a step that the Federation refused to take.

In January 1928, the convention's resolution concerning dual membership was first put to the test. The Kupat Holim directorate launched a registration campaign among all members of the Federation who were not members of Kupat Holim, designed to implement the convention's decision. In a letter that preceded the enlistment campaign Eliezer Perlson and Yitzhak Kenivsky-Kenev appealed to the Federation's executive committee, raising the issue directly:

> If it is the duty of all Federation members to be members in Kupat Holim its implication is one who departs from this duty cannot be a member of the Federation, for if this duty continues to have solely a declarative character, then there is no logic at all in this enlistment endeavor.[17]

The executive committee of the Federation of Labor was caught on the horns of a dilemma. On one hand it was duty-bound to implement the decisions of its own convention, on the other hand it feared that such a move would lead many to cancel their membership in the Federation of Labor, a loss in both financial terms and political clout. The reply of the executive committee serves to explain the background to the convention's decision. They replied: "Membership in the Federation of Labor should not be viewed from a solely fiscal standpoint of Kupat Holim." Each case, the Federation clarified, should be dealt with separately before taken a grave step and removing a person from the Federation.

The third convention's decision regarding dual membership was, therefore, merely a recommendation, not a binding resolution. Strengthening Kupat Holim and broadening its membership by allowing it to open its ranks to any and all who wished to join, and enforcing membership on members of the Federation, *both* stood in contradiction to "forging [Kupat Holim] as an organizational tool." Thus, the Federation was not about to allow Kupat Holim to operate as it wished—that is, requiring members of the Federation to join its ranks. It was in the interests of the Federation to prevent Kupat Holim from becoming too strong or too independent if it was to remain an organizational tool, subject to the needs of the Federation. In April 1929, the question of dual membership again surfaced when Kupat Holim demanded that the laborers in Zichron Yaakov village be required to be members of health fund, or be expelled from the Federation. Ben-Gurion replied:

> [It is] the duty of every member of the Federation to be a member of Kupat Holim, but a member should not be removed from the Federation due to lack of membership in Kupat Holim, and his membership card should not be withheld.[18]

The interests of the Federation of Labor outweighed all others, and enforcement of membership in Kupat Holim was postponed to a later juncture.

WHO IS ENTITLED TO JOIN KUPAT HOLIM?

The placement of Federation interests above all others was also expressed in the response of the executive committee to a Kupat Holim request to accept nonmembers of the Federation into the health fund. The executive committee stood behind its demand that it be the sole judge of who had the right to join Kupat Holim and who did not, and refused to give Kupat Holim any rein in this matter. Thus, Kupat Holim was required to submit to the Federation's executive committee all requests to join the fund, including the candidacy of individuals. Thus was the case of David Elimelach, a laborer from Nes Ziona village whose candidacy for membership in Kupat Holim was rejected because he was not a member of the Federation. Likewise, members of the craftspersons' association in Haifa and "butchers and [real estate] brokers" from Afula city who asked to join were accepted only on a partial basis (without the right to vote or be represented), despite the fact that they were willing to join the Federation of Labor. The executive committee was asked to consider Kupat Holim membership not only for laborers who were not members of the Federation of Labor, but also individuals and groups who were not laborers but hailed from the ranks of "exploiters of labor," in the parlance of the day. The interests of Kupat Holim dictated acceptance of such persons into the health fund, not only because of their economic contribution as dues-paying members, but also in light of the social philosophy that began to gain acceptance within the leadership of Kupat Holim—that the health fund should be a national institution serving the entire Yishuv, not a partisan body belonging solely to the Federation of Labor. Thus, while prevailing opinions in Kupat Holim believed that membership should be open to all, members of the executive committee of the Federation of Labor stood in opposition, holding that:

> a shopkeeper cannot be a member of the Federation, and if such foundations would be accepted, the pioneering foundations of the Federation of Labor would be

> impaired, and such a step would bring about ongoing erosion of Federation principles.[19]

Throughout 1928, Kupat Holim badgered the Federation of Labor, keeping the question of membership constantly on the agenda of the executive committee. This tactic was designed to clarify prevailing circumstances in preparing the groundwork for Kupat Holim's general convention, scheduled to be held in 1929. In January 1928, the Kupat Holim directorate demanded that the Federation's executive committee formulate its position prior to the launch of Kupat Holim's campaign to enlist members of the Federation in the health fund that was to begin in February. In June, September, and October of the same year, after the executive committee failed to respond with a coherent statement of policy as requested, Kupat Holim's supervisory committee again demanded that a date be set to discuss the matter. In October 1928, the Kupat Holim directorate threatened to take any workers' council that failed to uphold the third convention's resolution regarding dual membership to court and announced that it was considering unilaterally withholding medical assistance from those who failed to honor the third convention's resolution.

Despite the threats and the tension, the executive committee again refused to address the issue. Additional appeals in March 1929 were to no avail, and the executive committee continued to drag its feet on taking a stand. Only on 9 May 1929, on the eve of Kupat Holim's second convention, was the issue discussed. At the time, Kupat Holim had 15,000 members, 500 of them nonmembers of the Federation of Labor, while there were about 3000 Federation of Labor members who were not members of Kupat Holim. In a meeting between members of the executive committee of the Federation of Labor and members of the Kupat Holim directorate, it was stipulated that

> Laborers who are not members of the Federation of Labor, whether individuals or communal settlements, will be accepted only with the approval of the executive committee of the General Federation of Labor....A member of the Federation will not be removed [from the Federation] due to non-affiliation with Kupat Holim.[20]

In the joint meeting the two questions had been discussed separately, and a decision in the matter was not easily reached among the participants.

In regard to the need for executive committee approval for Kupat Holim membership, Dr. Beilenson argued that rules should be relaxed regarding admittance of individuals and groups who were not members of the Federation, and they should be granted the right of representation in Kupat Holim. Thus, Kupat Holim would be able to maintain its hegemony and prevent the establishment of rival medical institutions, while at the same time improving the financial state of the fund. Such a step would also lead to an increase in the budget that the health fund received from the Zionist executive, who already had recommended in the past that Kupat Holim broaden its framework. Dr. Beilenson even called for placing this decision in the hands of the supervisory committee and the Kupat Holim directorate. The executive committee, however, could not agree to this demand. Among the staunchest opponents was David Ben-Gurion, who believed Kupat Holim had to remain under the thumb of the Federation. Ben-Gurion argued that if the right to decide resided with Kupat Holim, it would give preference to economic considerations and would not take into account the good of the Federation in accepting new members. This was liable to impair the very character of the Federation of Labor as a whole. Thus, deliberations of the right to decide came back to the point of departure. In the end, the executive committee of the Federation of Labor continued to control the right to decide who would be accepted for membership in Kupat Holim among those who were not members of the Federation, and every request would be discussed separately in accordance with parameters set solely by the Federation, separate from issues of economic benefit to the fund. Kupat Holim had failed to achieve its goals.

In the second issue, retraction of membership in the Federation from those who did not join Kupat Holim, the Federation also had the upper hand. Members of the executive committee rejected Kupat Holim's claim that if they were not allowed to expand the framework of the health fund by accepting those who were not members of the Federation, they should be compensated by enforcing membership in the fund on all members of the Federation. The executive committee held that Kupat Holim was a body subject to the Federation's authority and had no right to demand reciprocity in membership. Therefore the executive committee rejected Kupat Holim's appeal to eject members who refused to join Kupat Holim, and limited themselves to calling for employment of "promulgation and informational ploys" only to urge members to join of their own volition. Kupat Holim lost the battle on this front as well.

Kupat Holim's reaction was swift. Dr. Moshe Beilenson spoke before the second Kupat Holim convention that convened a week after deliberations at the executive committee. He publicly called upon the Federation of Labor to enforce membership in Kupat Holim on Federation members, while stressing the national mission of Kupat Holim and the need to open its doors to all. He again demanded legislation of a compulsory health insurance law that would lead to transformation of Kupat Holim into a national body serving all. Between the lines, Dr. Beilenson's address carried hints of a broader significance. A compulsory health insurance scheme would not only have enhanced the stature and economic circumstances of the fund, but also reduce Kupat Holim's dependence on the Federation of Labor.

His words were echoed in those of Dr. Yosef Meir, the medical director of Kupat Holim, published in *Davar* on 9 June 1929 under the heading "About the Kupat Holim Convention." Dr. Meir sought to alleviate apprehensions within the Federation of loss of control, citing the example of members of the Teacher's Federation whose acceptance as members of Kupat Holim had had nonegative impact on the close tie between the Federation and the health fund.

Dr. Avraham Katznelson-Nissan was even more candid. In a piece published in *Davar* on 6 June 1929 he took to task those who viewed Kupat Holim in a narrow prospective, seeking to restrict Kupat Holim to

> a certain circle belonging to a [particular] political organization or fixed social class—[from which] stems the demand for the organization's title to the [sick] fund, which is nothing less than sectorial in its assistance to members in time of illness.

Katznelson-Nissan believed that the root of the problem was the way in which the Federation perceived the standing and mission of Kupat Holim—as a body that was designed to serve its own self-interests and not as a body with its own independent raison d'être and national goals going beyond the jurisdiction of the Federation of Labor. Only if a new independent perception would be formulated vis-à-vis Kupat Holim's operation and authority, and management turned over to its own auspices, could one expect an improvement in Kupat Holim's performance on the road to realizing its mission.

Kupat Holim as a Political Instrument in the 1930s

Politics and Membership in Kupat Holim: The Mapai Party

In January 1930, the two leading labor parties in Eretz Israel—Achdut Haavodah and Hapoel Hatzair—merged to form the Eretz Israel Workers' Party, or Mapai. The establishment of Mapai changed the political balance of power within the Federation of Labor. Eighty percent of all Federation members were members of the new body, and there was no longer a need for coalitions or the fear of loss of control. The Federation encompassed 21,000 members of whom 18,000 were members of Kupat Holim. Kupat Holim at this point provided medical coverage for 35,000 Jews—19 percent of the Yishuv in Eretz Israel.[21] Mapai had complete control of the Federation, and in essence, the ideological composition and the vested interests of the leadership of the two bodies—the Federation's executive committee and Mapai's secretariat—were almost identical in nature.

The establishment of Mapai and its hegemony over the Federation of Labor had an immediate negative impact on the number joining Kupat Holim among those who had not been members of the Federation beforehand. Organizations of various trades such as the Farmers' Association and bodies with a nonproletarian/socialist political orientation (the revisionists-right wingers and others) were hesitant to join Kupat Holim, fearing such a move would draw them into a "bear hug" of the Federation of Labor and Mapai. The number of requests for membership in Kupat Holim among non-Federation factions ceased almost entirely, and some members left the health fund and began establishing alternative frameworks for health insurance that would not be politically dependent. The words of warning voiced by Dr. Beilenson in May 1929 in the joint meeting of Kupat Holim with the executive committee—that if the partisan character of Kupat Holim was not mitigated, allowing the health fund to become an institution of the Yishuv as a whole, it was liable to lead to the establishment of rivals to Kupat Holim—began to materialize, sparked by a move (the merger) that had only amplified Kupat Holim's political mantle.

In March 1931, Dr. Reuven Katznelson, member of the Hadassah management, called for the establishment of a "popular" health fund under Hadassah auspices—the "Ammamit" Health Fund—that would provide health services in the agricultural villages to those who did not wish to be members of Kupat Holim. The proposal received the immediate support of the Farmers' Association, whose leaders had previously considered joining Kupat Holim. In November 1931, the Ammamit Health Fund received approval of the Yishuv's health committee and the parameters of its operation were defined. Within a short time, the new health fund established branches in most of the agricultural villages where Hadassah had operated previously, and even offered services to other villages such as Yavniel, Ein-Ganin, and Pardes Hana where Kupat Holim had been operating. Competition and rivalry broke out between the two funds, leading to an appeal by the Kupat Holim directorate to the Ammamit Health Fund, suggesting that the two rivals establish a modus operandi—an agreed-upon division of "territory" between the two funds. After prolonged negotiations that lasted more than a year, an accord was worked out. On 4 December 1931, the two sides drew up a list of agricultural villages where one of the funds would have exclusivity, and a list of villages where the two funds would operate side-by-side, all according to the wishes of the residents. It was further decided that in the cities each individual would be free to choose the health fund of his or her choice, without any limitations. This clause was included despite the objections of Kupat Holim, which sought, unsuccessfully, to curtail the operation of the Ammamit Health Fund in proletarian sectors.

In order to prevent defections and block the expansion of the Ammamit Health Fund at its own expense, Kupat Holim turned to the executive committee even before conclusion of the accord, requesting that the Federation relinquish its rigid control and

> ease admission of members among non-members of the Federation of Labor. To refer decisions on acceptance of members of this category to Kupat Holim committees. To these committees we will also transfer the right to remove members of this type. To invite the chariperson of the Manufacturers' Association to participate in the supervisory commitee of Kupat Holim . . . . It's enough that we were late by two years due to this conservatism in the decision to accept in Kupat Holim non-members of the Federation,

> and now we have troubles and difficulties that would not have been at all, had the supervisory committee and the executive committee known two years ago to make this decision."[22]

Perlson even tried to force the issue of acceptance of those who were not members of the Federation in Afula (shopkeepers, butchers, and brokers) but the local Afula workers' council opposed the move and refused to accept them as members.

In October 1931, the Kupat Holim director approached the Federation's executive committee with a new proposal: To bring into Kupat Holim the 3,000 members of the Federation who were not members of the fund to date. But, since the executive committee refused to eject members from the Federation for failing to join Kupat Holim, Kupat Holim suggested that the Federation adopt administrative sanctions against those who refused to comply willingly. This time the executive committee responded positively to Kupat Holim's request, and even added a stipulation of its own: "Evasion of membership in Kupat Holim can be cause for removing a worker from his work at a Federation institution."

Historian Shabtai Tevet believes that this change of heart on the part of the executive committee concerning membership in Kupat Holim was the upshot of organizational changes that the Yishuv was undergoing.[23] Labor legislation had been formulated, and the labor exchange that had been the primary power base of the Federation became a general labor exchange and not solely one open to Federation members. Moreover, the economic situation had improved and workers were less dependent on the Federation as a source of employment and union protection. At the same time, the importance of Kupat Holim in both the Federation and the Yishuv had grown. Workers were far less fearful that their employment in a Federation facility would be terminated, but the threat of loss of medical insurance still carried great weight. Tevet believes that Kupat Holim became a "significant almost singular organizational tool" for the Federation of Labor. Thus, the Federation of Labor itself now had a vested interest in expansion of the health fund's ranks, for growth of Kupat Holim was translated into political power. This change in the Federation of Labor's attitude brought about an easing of terms of eligibility for membership among those who were not members of the Federation of Labor.

The only question remaining was whether the *political* identity of the applicants should still be a factor. This issue broke out in all its ferocity when laborers associated with the Revisionist movement sought to join Kupat Holim.

KUPAT HOLIM AND THE REVISIONIST WORKERS

The Revisionist Zionist movement headed by Zeev Jabotinsky was established in 1925 in response to the moderate political line adopted by the Zionist leadership toward the Mandate government and the Arabs. The Revisionists demanded a "revision" in the consolatory policies of the president of the World Zionist movement, Chaim Weizmann, and other Zionist leaders, in favor of political militancy even at the price of an open clash with the British. The Revisionists also championed changes in the economic and social orientation of the Zionist movement away from a centralized socialist outlook, and toward protection of private capital and support of private initiative, focus on realization of Zionist goals rather than class struggle, and improvement of the lot of the proletariat, including opposition to the use of strikes in labor disputes. The power of the Revisionists had risen from 7% in elections to the 1929 Zionist congress to 21% in elections to the 1931 congress, while the labor movement controlled 29% of the delegates.[24] The Revisionists constituted a clear and present threat to the hegemony of the labor movement. The resulting political constellation was rife with tensions between the sides, but it also compelled Mapai, the Federation of Labor, and Kupat Holim to review and revise their own rigid attitudes toward admission of Revisionists to Kupat Holim.

In January 1932, Hadassah asked Kupat Holim if it was willing to accept Revisionist-affiliated workers into the health fund. The heads of Hadassah believed that if the Revisionists would be eligible for Kupat Holim membership, they would drop their own preparations to establish their own health fund. In the deliberations that followed, David Ben-Gurion, Eliezer Perlson, David Remez, Dr. Moshe Beilenson, and Eliezer Kaplan took part—all of them leaders of the first order in Mapai and the Federation of Labor, a clear sign of the importance assigned this question. Dr. Meir (whose position was presented by Perlson) and Perlson himself believed that Revisionist workers should be admitted in order to take the wind out of the sails of those in Betar who were pushing for a separate health fund that ultimately would compete with Kupat Holim. Dr. Beilinson also supported admitting Revisionists, arguing that they should not have to declare any political allegiances that would set them apart from other members. If this would be the case, he argued, there was a good chance that the Revisionists could be assimilated into the fund without its having a negative political impact, as had been the case with Hapoel Hamizrachi and Hapoel Hatzair when they joined Kupat Holim. The primary reservation came from Ben-Gurion. He demanded that the Revisionists be accepted only on condition that "strike breaking, undercutting wages and such things would not be done by them." In the end, Ben-Gurion's conditions were accepted and it was resolved that membership of Revisionists would be contingent on these stipulations. Yet, it is interesting to note the wording of the reply by Perlson to Hadassah regarding the decision. In response to the Hadassah initiative Perlson did not cite the restrictive clause agreed upon on Ben-Gurion's insistence, but rather:

> Our general posture is that if, in terms of social composition, members of the above mentioned organization are suitable to be members of Kupat Holim of the workers, we are prepared to conduct negotiations with them regarding their entrance into Kupat Holim.[25]

Perlson knew it would seem that detailing the terms of eligibility adopted would cause the Revisionists to recoil from any thoughts of joining the fund, and he preferred to leave discussion of provisos to the negotiation stage.

In November 1932 the question arose again, when the Betar group in Hadera requested to join Kupat Holim en bloc. The importance of the question grew all the more acute when it was learned that the local group had made its request in defiance of Betar headquarters, and that members of the group had already turned down a proposal to join the Ammamit Health Fund under better terms. In a discussion of the question, Ben-Gurion again raised his previous reservations—that they be accepted on a conditional basis. The idea was not undisputed and feelings of some were far from amiable: Ada Fishman-Maimon, who also participated in the deliberations, argued: "Foes such as these I don't want to admit to Kupat Holim."[26]

Neta Harpaz, a member of the executive committee, said: "They have one line—to appear as strike-breakers, and as such I am against it to accept them."

In the end, Kupat Holim recommended that the Revisionists be accepted, with Ben-Gurion's stipulation. Again, Perlson did not mention the conditionals for Betar's acceptance openly in his reply, hiding them between the lines. The difficult state of Kupat Holim in accepting the Revisionists is clearly evidenced in Perlson's behavior. On one hand, Kupat Holim could not ignore the political rivalries over the future character of the Yishuv that set the Revisionists apart from Mapai and the Federation of Labor; on the other hand Kupat Holim could not close its eyes to the competition and the dire need of the health fund to broaden its membership base within the working public, regardless of the political philosophy of consumers of its health services.

THE ESTABLISHMENT OF THE LEUMIT HEALTH FUND

In June 1933 Dr. Chaim Arlosoroff, head of the political department of the Jewish Agency, was murdered while walking along the Tel Aviv beachfront. The murder generated a storm in the Yishuv and amplified tensions between right and left factions, as members of the right-wing Revisionist movement were accused of being the perpetrators. During Passover, just two months prior to the murder, violent clashes had broken out between Revisionists and other laborers and the camps had accused each other of being responsible. After further violence on the last day of Passover, Betar's leadership publicly accused Kupat Holim of playing a part in the riots, claiming that "Kupat Holim's headquarters served as a storehouse for bricks and rocks rained on the heads of girls and boys."[27]

Perlson denied the charges and an inquiry commission appointed by the Tel Aviv municipality announced that "no proof or evidence was found to substantiate that there was an assault from the Kupat Holim directorate."[28]

Betar, however, continued to stand behind its version of events. Kupat Holim, which only a short time prior had decided to accept laborers who were members of Betar into its ranks, found itself facing a full-blown crisis. How should they deal with Revisionist workers and their supporters among the ranks of Kupat Holim and the

Federation of Labor? The arguments raised by Ben-Gurion a year earlier regarding a particular political orientation necessitated by membership in Kupat Holim arose in all its fury. In the wake of the controversy over the murder and the polarization of the political arena, Revisionist members and their supporters—including members of Betar from Hadera and laborers from Benyamina villages—dropped out of Kupat Holim. Before Kupat Holim had time to formulate a policy of how to deal with the Revisionists within the fold, those that had picked up and left began organizing their own health fund.

In November 1933, four months after the murder, a group of thirty-five members of the Revisionist movement meeting at the home of Dr. Y. Weinschel declared the establishment of the National Workers' Health Fund, or Leumit Health Fund. A short time later branches were opened in Haifa and Ramat Gan (a city near Tel Aviv), and by the end of 1933, the Leumit Health Fund already had 206 members. A year later the new Leumit Health Fund boasted a membership of 786 members throughout the country—close to a thousand insurees including dependents.[29] Due to budgetary constraints, it was decided that services would be provided by private doctors in their own clinics, according to the choice of the member, and the fund would pay for the doctor's service fee directly. In this manner the fund circumvented the necessity of establishing its own clinics. Hospitalization services were provided in municipal and government hospitals and Hadassah institutions. Other services such as x-ray and physiotherapy were provided via private institutes and medications dispensed via commercial pharmacies. Thus, circumstances forged a new model of health services in Eretz Israel.

The early days of the Leumit Health Fund were marked by three outstanding characteristics. First, the mission of the fund was to serve "nationalist workers"—that is, those who were not members of the Federation of Labor but who were oriented toward a proletariat engaged in a world-wide class struggle, rather than focusing solely on nationalist aspirations of Zionism. Second, unlike Kupat Holim, the Leumit Health Fund admitted any member of the Yishuv without any political strings attached. The fund not only declared this policy in their ordinance, but also stressed this fact in their promotional literature, which protested the politicization of Kupat Holim. Third, the fund promised its member annual rest and recuperation, as did Kupat Holim. This reflects the importance that labor organizations and the working public assigned to this entitlement; both funds viewed annual "rest & recuperation" for the well, not the sick, as an integral part of the minimal basket of services that a member should be entitled to.

The Leumit Health Fund had been established a mere three years after the Ammamit Health Fund, an event further aggravated by the political turmoil that accompanied it. Both, however, were a "wake-up" call for Kupat Holim, which was forced by events to formulate new policies to meet the challenge of growing competition and to maintain its position. Since the competition between the health funds was political, not economic, most of the steps taken by Kupat Holim against the Leumit Health Fund were of a purely political nature. In 1933–1935, Kupat Holim fired workers—doctors and laboratory workers—who declared openly their support of the Revisionists and opposition to the Federation of Labor. Kupat Holim did not conceal the political motive of the dismissals.

When the Leumit Health Fund turned to the Zionist Congress requesting official recognition and economic aid from the Jewish Agency, it was met by fierce opposition on the part of Kupat Holim. Kupat Holim's opposition was based on the decision of the fourteenth Zionist congress in 1925 that "in Eretz Israel there is room for only one health fund" and on other resolutions taken by subsequent congresses that also promised Kupat Holim exclusivity. In 1935 and 1937, Kupat Holim fought tooth and nail against transferring Jewish Agency monies to the Leumit Health Fund for doctors' treatment of new immigrants, and granting the Leumit Health Fund a place on the Yishuv's health committee and the Zionist executive in Eretz Israel. When Kupat Holim learned that the Leumit Health Fund had reached a secret agreement with the Ammamit Health Fund, whereby the latter undertook responsibility for new immigrants in the Leumit Health Fund, in order to receive the Jewish Agency budget, Kupat Holim waged a war against *both* its competitors together. Kupat Holim applied all of its political clout to prevent transfer of funding; even bringing the "arrangement" to the attention of the health committee hoping exposure would block implementation.

In order to block the expansion of the Leumit Health Fund in the urban sector—particularly among independent professionals, most of them new immigrants from Germany—Kupat Holim adopted a new tactic, a special dues-payment system for those planning to immigrate to Israel: payment of dues a year in advance. German Jews, who encountered difficulties transferring their assets to Eretz Israel because of limitations set forth in the Nuremberg Laws, could now pay for medical coverage for when they immigrated, while still in Germany. These agreements were formulated within the framework of the "transfer agreements" that the Jewish Agency had worked out with Germany that eased transfer of money and assets of immigrants to Eretz Israel. In this manner, Kupat Holim succeeded in attracting many immigrants to its ranks who would probably not have joined Kupat Holim after their arrival in the country.

In June 1936, Kupat Holim learned that the Leumit Health Fund was fundraising among members of the British Jewish community, while misleading the donors. The Leumit Health Fund had not clarified its political identity to the donors, using the general term "health fund" that most of the audience assumed to be Kupat Holim. Kupat Holim embarked on a campaign abroad to "educate" potential donors, distributing brochures, leaflets, and other promotional material in which the differences between the various health funds in Eretz Israel was explained.

Competitions between Kupat Holim and the Leumit Health Fund spread to the industrial sector of Eretz Israel as well, opening up another front where Kupat Holim began to employ a host of tactics to protect its standing and keep the competition at bay. It was not rare for Kupat Holim to pressure workers' committees and the management of plants in order to withhold medical assistance from groups of Revisionist laborers, even threatening to withhold medical assistance from the plant as a whole if its wishes were not obeyed. One such case was the Dead Sea Works. Kupat Holim pressured the phosphate plant to submit a list of Revisionist workers at the plant with the objective of withholding medical assistance from them—in clear violation of the terms of the agreement signed by Kupat Holim with the Dead Sea Works management in which Kupat Holim had committed itself to provide medical services to *all* the plant's employees.

Kupat Holim's actions designed to block the growth of the Leumit Health Fund were only partially successful, despite the unbridled political and organizational power applied by Kupat Holim in its attempts to overwhelm its competitor. The reasons were factors beyond the control of Kupat Holim or the Federation of Labor: The mid-1930s brought far-reaching political, social and economic change that transformed the "playing field."

THE CRISIS OF THE FIFTH ALIYAH

On 1 December 1935, an amendment to the Mandate government's "Practice of Medicine Ordinance" took affect. The amendment allowed the director of the Mandate government's health department to limit the number of licenses to practice medicine, without right of appeal. The legal action was designed to halt the great wave of immigration from Germany that included countless doctors who had begun immigrating to Eretz Israel following Hitler's rise to power in 1933. Mandate authorities feared that the influx of so many doctors and the surplus it would create would lead to fierce competition and unemployment, degrade level of medical services, and undermine professional ethics. However, when plans to legislate such a step were publicized, another four hundred physicians accelerated their immigration plans and came immediately, hoping to arrive before the law came into effect. Historian Yoav Gelber says this led to the serious crisis in the medical profession that followed—a crisis that only subsided at the height of the Second World War.

The influx of countless Jewish physicians from Germany brought about a tremendous growth in the number of doctors in the Yishuv. From 447 licensed physicians in 1929 (the year marking the end of the Fourth Aliyah and the beginning of the Fifth Aliyah), the medical community ballooned to 1,961 physicians in 1936. This figure does not even include an unknown number of doctors who entered the country illegally by various means without immigration visas[30] while many others were already in the country waiting to receive a license to practice medicine. In 1942 there were 2,015 licensed physicians practicing medicine—five times the number a decade earlier—and an unprecedented doctor-patient ratio by any standard (1:140). The employment situation for doctors became more and more aggravated as the number of doctors swelled, and by the mid-1930s it was clear that the medical community was in the throes of a major crisis. Hadassah employed 60 physicians, full- and part-time, and in all the health funds together there were 200 doctors, 170 of them in Kupat Holim.[31] Most of the Kupat Holim doctors worked part-time, for it was Kupat Holim's policy to assist in absorbing as many doctors as possible, but even then the supply of positions was small compared to the scope of immigration, and most of the physicians were forced to engage in private practice. Due to the fierce competition, doctors fees dropped and many private medical institutions were opened up—clinics, diagnostic and treatment institutes, private hospitals, and so forth.

Under such market conditions, Kupat Holim did not have much of a chance of increasing its membership to any great extent, for medical services on the private market were cheaper and more accessible, and the demand for Kupat Holim services dropped. Due to the large increase in doctors, the competitive edge of the other health funds—Leumit and Ammamit—was enhanced, and they expanded their services, offering them at lower fees than Kupat Holim's. When Kupat Holim's Beilenson Hospital was opened in 1936, most of the medical staff were specialists from among the German immigrants. The Emek Hospital was expanded as well—doubling Kupat Holim's hospitalization capacity and raising the level of professionalism considerably—but the number of Kupat Holim members did not grow by much.

Due to the large number of specialists who came with the Fifth Aliyah and worked within the framework of Kupat Holim, ideological clashes also emerged within the profession. Besides the knowledge they carried with them and the latest professional procedures they instituted, the newcomers also sought to introduce changes in the organizational structure of Kupat Holim, in accordance with standards current in central Europe: private practice integrated with public service, the right of the patient to choose his or her physician, and maintenance of the professional freedom for the physician. The immigrant doctors also sought to transfer authority for medical decisions from the hands of Kupat Holim functionaries to medical professionals and improve the working conditions of medical staff. Kupat Holim, however, refused to change the centralist-collectivist structure of the health fund, rejecting all initiatives for change. Thus, the quality of doctors and medicine in Kupat Holim rose rapidly thanks to the integration of the physicians from Germany, while the organizational structure of Kupat Holim remained antiquated and frozen as it had been at the beginning of the 1920s.

THE "MAS ACHID" (JOINT DUES)

In January 1936, there were 64,000 members of the Federation of Labor out of 322,000 inhabitants of the Yishuv in Eretz Israel. Only

42,000 Federation members, however, were members of Kupat Holim. In addition there were another 2,500 insurees who were not members of the Federation—1,500 from Hapoel Hamizrachi and 1000 additional members from places of employment with group medical coverage for employees, contracted from Kupat Holim. Census data indicate that out of 4,500 members of the Hanoar Haoved (Working Youth movement) only 1500 were members of Kupat Holim (some under their parents' policy).[32] Among the membership of Kupat Holim, 50 percent lived in rural communities, most paying minimal dues on the progressive scale due to their economic straits. Among Kupat Holim members in urban communities, only 30 percent were in occupations that paid full dues to the health fund.[33]

Due to the large gap between the scope of membership in the Federation and the scope of membership in Kupat Holim (approximately 22,000) and the difficulty of competing with other health-service providers in the Yishuv (private health services, the other health funds, and so forth), at the outset of 1936 Kupat Holim sought to renew its struggle to enforce reciprocal membership between the Federation of Labor and Kupat Holim.

A host of steps were taken in this direction. Local governing councils were requested to use their influence to get laborers who were members of the Federation of Labor to join the health fund. Lists of job candidates for Federation institutions were examined in order to force upon them membership in Kupat Holim as a proviso for being chosen (according to a resolution dating back to 1932). Advertisements were published in the daily press calling upon members of the Federation of Labor to join the ranks of Kupat Holim as an act of moral and ideological solidarity. Warning letters were sent to those who were not members of Kupat Holim in which members were urged to hurry to sign up to forestall any diminution of their rights in the Federation of Labor (primarily loss of entitlements to use the Federation's "loan fund," and access to credit). Groups of Federation members—working women, members of the Working Youth movement and Hapoel Hamizrachi—were scrutinized to prevent evasion of dues and to mobilize members of such groups to "sell" the idea of Kupat Holim to members of their families.

Together with these steps, a new modus *operandi* was instituted: unification of dues collection for Kupat Holim and dues to the Federation, and unification of membership in the two institutions. A member received one membership card that covered entitlements of membership in both the Federation and Kupat Holim. Thus the duty of membership in both the Federation and Kupat Holim—passed by the third convention of the Federation of Labor in 1927—was finally instituted in practice. Two of the main architects of the formula labeled "Joint Dues" (Mas Achid) were Eliezer Perlson and Yitzhak Kenivsky-Kenev, members of the Kupat Holim directorate. And this time, David Remez, secretary of the Federation of Labor (who had replaced Ben-Gurion in 1935 when the latter had become the chairperson of the Jewish Agency), approved the proposal. At the beginning of 1936, the first meeting was called to discuss the proposal.

Attending the gathering were David Remez as head of the Federation of Labor, Aharon Beker, secretary of the Tel Aviv workers' council, Melech Noistadt (Noi), head of the Federation of Labor's "membership dues bureau," and Eliezer Perlson and Yitzhak Kenivsky-Kenev as representatives of the Kupat Holim directorate. David Remez suggested establishment of a committee "to clarify ways of managing a joint dues for the Federation and Kupat Holim" and crystallization of a framework for joint dues. Remez even suggested that three committee members go on a learning tour of European nations where a joint dues system had already been instituted between labor unions and health funds, in order to study the various organizational methods employed in collecting dues.

In February 1936 the first circular was sent from the Kupat Holim directorate to the health funds' branches about merging the dues as a step in instituting the duty of dual membership. In October of the same year, a comprehensive discussion was held at the executive committee of the Federation of Labor on unification of dues administration, and a plan of action was formulated: Kupat Holim dues and Federation dues were to be merged into one payment, called "joint dues." The Federation's dues bureau would be called the "central membership dues bureau" and dues collected would be divided between the two institutions. The Federation's unemployment fund would pay the joint dues of unemployed members. If a member of the Federation died, his family would receive a monetary grant. One membership card, in which stamps would be pasted to serve as certification of payment, would serve both institutions.

Putting the plan into effect, however, encountered numerous difficulties. Some delegates feared that the joint tax would be too heavy a burden for those of limited means and would deter others from joining. Members of Kupat Holim feared that the fund would be discriminated against in allocation of the joint dues and demanded that budgetary calculations be clarified prior to launching the plan. Others claimed that the plan would enhance bureaucracy and shrink the ability of members to influence improvements in service, particularly in Kupat Holim. As one of the members put it:

> Up until today I could leave Kupat Holim if I was treated unjustly, and with that still remain in the Federation of Labor. With institution of the joint dues I will be forced to suffer all the harsh treatment from Kupat Holim or have to leave the Federation.[34]

The executive committee finally approved the plan and set a date for launching the joint tax: January 1937. Aharon Beker noted that in approving the plan, the possibility that hundreds of members would leave the Federation of Labor was taken into account, but in the end the organizational advantages of the merger would become apparent, and that therefore it was decided to go forward. In November 1936, Kupat Holim's supervisory committee convened to discuss the proposal for joint dues. They decided to adopt the executive committee's proposal in principle, but with several reservations that dealt primarily with payment for medical care for the disabled. In December 1936, nine members of the central membership dues bureau were elected and began to crystallize arrangement for joint collection of dues.

The district directors of Kupat Holim, who convened in a separate meeting, claimed that merging dues would curtail the scope of dues-paying to Kupat Holim, which was higher than dues-paying to the Federation of Labor: 92 percent in Kupat Holim compared to 77 percent in the Federation of Labor. They again expressed apprehensions that the high dues would deter those of limited means, and would cause many to leave the Federation and Kupat Holim together. The district directors criticized the decision to transfer dues collection to the dues bureau, for the central membership dues bureau's overhead would be greater than that of Kupat Holim, thus the high cost of administration was liable to become a burden on the overall budget. Furthermore, they claimed that the Federation's dues-collection system suffered from a delay in updating dues levels (which were calculated on a progressive scale by income), preventing levies from truly reflecting actual wages. Yet despite all the misgivings, the majority favored merging the dues frameworks as a way to achieve Kupat Holim's core objective for over seventeen years—enforcing reciprocal membership between the Federation of Labor and Kupat Holim. It was estimated that 22,000 new members would join Kupat Holim as a result of the merger, that revenues would increase and the fiscal state of the health fund would improve, and that the health of members would rest on the shoulders of the Federation of Labor, not solely on Kupat Holim.

Deliberations on institution of the joint dues was also discussed at the thirty-fifth council of the Federation of Labor that convened in February 1937. Opponents were headed by the "Poel Zion Left" faction that called for reducing dues while also petitioning the Mandate government and the municipalities to participate in underwriting health budgets of Kupat Holim. In the end, the Federation's council approved the plan by a majority, without reservations. The joint dues—and with it the duty of duel membership in both institutions—became a fact of life.

This was the last step in the organization of Kupat Holim as an integral part of the Federation of Labor. The framework of joint dues as formulated by the Federation's council in 1937 continued to operate for the next five and a half decades. In 1993, the first steps were taken to inaugurate a compulsory health insurance system that would severe the bond between the Federation of Labor and Kupat Holim, making Kupat Holim one of four health funds in a non-partisan apolitical national health system.

Twice during those five and a half decades serious questions arose concerning the method of collecting dues. On the first occasion, in 1954, a secret Federation of Labor committee considered collection of dues for Kupat Holim through the auspices of the National Insurance Institute, Israel's social security system. This proposal was part of a broader agenda championed by David Ben-Gurion that sought to de-politicize all national institutions, including the army, education, and public health and welfare functions. The idea of transferring Kupat Holim dues collection to the National Insurance Institute in lieu of the joint dues was part of several unsuccessful attempts to introduce legislation for compulsory health insurance made in 1955, 1957, 1958, 1967, and 1973—an effort finally crowned with success in 1995.[35]

The second occasion came forty years later, in the wake of findings by the 1990 Netanyahu Commission, a state inquiry commission appointed by the government to "examine the function and efficiency of the health system" at a time that Kupat Holim was afflicted by severe economic and social crisis that endangered the organization's very existence. The findings of the commission—the twelfth official state inquiry commission appointed to examine the health system and the issue of compulsory health insurance first raised in 1925—led Minister of Health Chaim Ramon in 1993 to transfer collection of dues from the Federation's central membership dues bureau to the National Insurance Institute, Israel's social security machinery, as part of a government bail-out of Kupat Holim, which was on the verge of collapse. This move culminated in passage of the compulsory health insurance law in 1995.

KUPAT HOLIM, THE FEDERATION OF LABOR, AND THE JOINT DUES

Did the amalgamation of dues achieve its objectives?

In September 1937, Kupat Holim conducted a "first summary on the outcome of joint dues," and, after receiving the preliminary data from the branches, met to discuss several questions: Did the merger indeed bring about reciprocal membership in practice? What was the scope of dues-paying compared to prior to the merger? What was the cost of dues collection? To what extent was the commitment to pay membership dues of the unemployed and the disabled from the Federation's unemployment fund carried through? In addition, the gathering discussed the difficulties and special expenditures involved in absorbing all members of the Federation in the health system, and the tie between the insuree and the health fund before and after the merger.

The data demonstrated that the primary objective of the merger was achieved: 18,000 members of the Federation of Labor joined Kupat Holim as a result of joint dues. However, the rate of dues-paying declined while expenditures on dues-collection rose, particularly since Kupat Holim was required to participate in the establishment of dues bureaus in agricultural settlements where dues collection had previously been in the hands of the suck fund. Administrative costs also grew due to the task of registering members, issuing membership cards, filling-in and processing questionnaires and patient records—outlays that Kupat Holim had to help cover. The promise of dues payment for those out of work from the Federation's unemployment fund was not honored, and the addition of these new members was a burden on Kupat Holim. The report noted the difficulty in absorbing thousands of members of the Sfardi communities in Jerusalem and Tiberias, a large percentage of them in very poor health. As for the fiscal balance, the report noted that there had been no improvement despite a significant increase in the number of members. The authors of the report expressed their concern that the growth in the bureaucracy brought about by the establishment of a central dues-payment bureau had made the bureau a very powerful body in itself, far removed from the daily hardships and ongoing needs of Kupat Holim:

> Little by little the fact we were so apprehensive about has materialized, that merger of dues administration in the Federation of Labor would create a new institution, a solely financial institution, that as a matter of nature—due to the fact that it will have only revenues, not responsibly for expenditures—will not be concerned about its own expenditures, while Kupat Holim's machinery [while it has] been freed of direct responsibility for these revenues… is now dependent on the general dues administration of the Federation of Labor.[36]

The report called for taking action based on the findings—to work to remedy them—but the call fell on deaf ears. The power of Kupat Holim in the new organizational setup had been weakened. Indeed, it had gained thousands of new members, but its financial straits were worse than they had been before, while as a result of the merger Kupat Holim had also lost its independence.

Thousands of unemployed members who joined the fund "for free," with no one picking up the bill as promised, neutralized any benefit brought by dues payment by more established members. In many respects Kupat Holim came out of the merger at a loss. Indeed, the accuracy of the report is reflected in the fact that most of the flaws in the system that were recognized immediately after the joint dues system was inaugurated were destined to impact and burden Kupat Holim's operation for the next forty-six years. The flaws were not only discussed in a series of investigative commissions that scrutinized Kupat Holim's performance over the years; the same flaws became apparent to Kenivsky-Kenev and his colleagues immediately after the merger. Ultimately they led to the loss of Kupat Holim as a core Federation asset in the mid-1990 bail-out.

In the introduction to the report written by Yitzhak Kenivsky-Kenev at the time, one can sense between the lines the tremendous disappointment in the meager gains from the joint dues. It seems that Kupat Holim's devotion for so many years to the mission of actualizing, at almost any cost, the dream of reciprocal membership had led the fund to ignore or make light of the many drawbacks of joint dues. In years to come, Kupat Holim would pay a heavy price for its dogged pursuit and ultimate "success" in bringing about a joint dues arrangement in the framework forged in 1937.

What motivated the Federation to agree to a merger of dues, as proposed by Kupat Holim? What caused the change in attitude toward reciprocal membership it had patently avoided for so many years?

One possible factor was personnel changes at the Federation of Labor. David Ben-Gurion had been adamant and consistent in his opposition to reciprocal membership. In March of 1923 he wrote in his diary:

> We won't have the power to decree that all members of the Federation [be members of Kupat Holim], and if we will try to decree [it], we will bring about the foundation of another Federation…and it would be better from the beginning not to create a fabrication.[37]

In the end, David Ben-Gurion left the leadership of the Federation of Labor to become head of the Jewish Agency and the dominant leader of the Zionist movement as a whole. In his stead, David Remez was appointed head of the Federation of Labor. Remez—who had served as the head of Solel Boneh in the crisis years of the institution (1926–1927) and was a rival of Ben-Gurion—sought to show he was as able as his predecessor. Under his leadership, the Federation grew in size and power to the extent that it was able to fulfill promises it could not "deliver" in the past, or had chosen to evade.

The Federation's motivations were clearly in a detailed article in *Davar*, 28 December 1936. According to Y. Kinamon, a Kupat Holim activist, the Federation found itself in financial difficulties in the mid-1930s. Many of its members knew how to demand entitlements but evaded paying dues. The decision passed in the days of Ben-Gurion that a member would not receive services without a membership card was not executed in practice. Even when cases of evasion were uncovered, no significant steps were taken against the offenders. The Federation of Labor's own operation branched out to become the largest organized power base in the Yishuv, but the growth of revenues as a result of the growth in membership was insufficient to cover expenditures. Separated from Kupat Holim, the Federation could not count on the fund for collecting dues (exploiting Kupat Holim as an instrument for enhancing its own dues-collection); since not all members of Kupat Holim were members of the Federation, it could not mobilize Kupat Holim for its own needs. Kupat Holim also refrained from applying sanctions against members of the Federation of Labor who paid their dues to the health fund but were behind in paying their dues to the Federation. The two bodies operated parallel to one another and could not combine their power and their assets. When the number of "non-Federation members" of Kupat Holim grew, the Federation feared the growth in the health fund's power was liable to diminish the Federation's dominion over Kupat Holim. The heads of the Federation worried that Kupat Holim would become a consumer institution in lieu of a mutual assistance institution. According to Kinimon, this fear—of losing control of Kupat Holim—was what motivated the Federation of Labor to implement reciprocal membership by merging dues-collection, thus bringing Kupat Holim back under its control while ensuring that the principle of mutual assistance would be maintained. Integration of Kupat Holim within the Federation of Labor was supposed to enhance the Federation's power, and allow it to oblige all its members to share the burden of responsibility for Kupat Holim's operation.

Along with all these considerations, one should add the pressure applied by workers' councils, particularly in Tel Aviv. The councils found themselves in serious financial difficulties and viewed the merger of dues-paying as an avenue to improve their finances. That same year, Revisionists in Tel Aviv were negotiating for the establishment of a joint labor exchange for workers. The political tensions between the sides had diminished a bit, but at the same time apprehension that the Federation was losing control of its members and that there was a need to strengthen its ties had grown. Institution of dual membership with Kupat Holim was seen as a vehicle for achieving this objective under changing circumstances.

What conclusions did the Federation of Labor reach concerning the merger, once it was inaugurated? Did it fulfill expectations?

In December 1937, the Federation of Labor published a report evaluating the first eight months of the joint dues arrangement. The report viewed operation of the joint dues as a great success. The scope of dues-collection was better than what the Federation deemed acceptable prior to the merger. Fears of mass desertions of members had not materialized. The revenues of workers' councils grew, as did revenues to the Federation's unemployment fund, the disability fund, and a fund earmarked for survivor benefits in cases of death. The report noted the improvement in assistance that a Federation member could now enjoy. There was not one mention of a flaw, not one oversight or shortcoming in the wake of the joint dues format. Indeed, from the Federation of Labor's standpoint, the arrangement was a huge success, both organizationally and financially. The joint dues enhanced the stature of the Federation in the economy and amplified its economic power. Not surprisingly, the Federation refused in the years that followed, particularly after the establishment of the state, to allow re-discussion of the joint dues format. For years to come the heads of the Federation also opposed any suggestion that a compulsory health insurance system be legislated and operated via the National Insurance Institute, for it was clear to them that an end to the joint dues framework would weaken the Federation and undermine its position as the strongest organized body in the Israeli economy.

THE PUBLIC AND THE JOINT TAX

The February 1935 decision to institute joint dues was echoed in the labor press in a host of features and articles published even during the deliberations. Most of the writers sought to analyze the advantages and drawbacks of the new method, and many addressed the question of whether the Federation of Labor and Kupat Holim had the moral right to make a member join another institution. Most viewed establishment of the new dues framework favorably and argued that the institutions indeed had the moral right to take such a step, which emanated from the principle of mutual assistance. Ada Fishman-Maimon even viewed the new dues system as an achievement for working mothers, for the women would now enjoy equal status with their husbands: The setup involved introduction of individual membership cards—not one "family card" issued to the head of the family, thus the joint dues would be registered in the cards of both spouses, entitling each to equal services.

An editorial in *Davar* on 12 January 1937 claimed that the new joint dues framework was better than all parallel insurance frameworks of labor organizations abroad, due to the principle of mutual assistance to which it was anchored.

A series of letters from members in *Davar* throughout January 1937 endorsed the new method of dues collecting, although there was criticism of a number of areas—for example, apprehensions that the level of dues would constitute a burden for working families. Some expressed doubts whether the Federation of Labor would be able to carry through on its promise of "maximum services, minimum dues" that champions of the joint dues format promised on a number of occasions. From the letters of Federation and Kupat Holim members published in the press, it is evident that most of the rank-and-file were familiar with the pros and cons of the joint dues, but nevertheless supported the concept on the assumption that it would be a positive move for both the Federation and Kupat Holim—ultimately improving indirectly the situation of the members.

The decision to institute the joint dues framework required members of Hapoel Hamizrachi to reexamine their association with the health fund after a decade of collaboration (since 1927) during which they had enjoyed the services of Kupat Holim. The Federation decided to "take advantage of the moment" to bring Hapoel Hamizrachi in as members of the Federation of Labor, by putting heavy pressure on Hapoel Hamizrachi to acquiesce to such a move. The Federation actually discriminated against the members of Hapoel Hamizrachi in terms of services, while at the same time saddling them with dues higher than that of the Federation members. In response to a Hapoel Hamizrachi complaint, the Federation claimed that it was investing additional monies from its budget to cover Kupat Holim's deficit, and that members of Hapoel Hamizrachi were only being asked to add their proportional share over and above regular dues ("despite the fact that in the original contract, Kupat Holim had specified it was not liable for the Hapoel Hamizrachi Health Fund's prior debts").[38] Moreover, the Federation argued that most of the Hapoel Hamizrachi members in Kupat Holim came from the lower classes and were paying minimum dues, while the more established members of Hapoel

Hamizrachi had yet to join Kupat Holim. Thus, the full burden of care for Hapoel Hamizrachi members fell on the shoulders of Kupat Holim and the Federation of Labor, while Hapoel Hamizrachi enjoyed high revenues and did not participate in the real expenses incurred by its own members.

The executive committee of the Hapoel Hamizrachi Federation ultimately decided by a majority vote to join the joint dues framework—that is, to require all members of the Hapoel Hamizrachi movement to join the Federation of Labor *and* Kupat Holim together. Members of the Hapoel Hamizrachi leadership stressed that this move would strengthen the status of Hapoel Hamizrachi in Kupat Holim and the Federation of Labor, and in the last analysis would profit the entire movement, without any negative impact on the social security and medical coverage of the members—an objective of ideological importance in its own right. In late 1938, a new contract was signed between Hapoel Hamizrachi and the Federation of Labor for the enrollment of Hapoel Hamizrachi members under the joint dues framework. The contract was an exact copy of the agreement signed in 1927, except for an additional clause that stipulated that collection of dues and registration would be carried out henceforth by Kupat Holim, while the Federation of Labor would take steps to equalize the entitlements of Hapoel Hamizrachi members with those of others.[39] As a result of the accord, 80 percent of all the members of Hapoel Hamizrachi joined the new agreement, and the number of Hapoel Hamizrachi members in Kupat Holim and the Federation of Labor rose from 1,500 to 2,600—3.4 percent of the health fund's membership that year (76,000).[40] Due to the agreement between the Federation of Labor, Kupat Holim, and Hapoel Hamizrachi, collaboration among the three organizations was renewed, and lasted until the introduction of health reform in 1995.

The entrance of Hapoel Hamizrachi's members into the framework of the joint dues was the last step in completing enforcement of reciprocal membership between the Federation of Labor and Kupat Holim. Only a few hundred members of the Federation of Labor were left who refused to accept the new framework, and those were forced to leave both the Federation and Kupat Holim. Among them was a group from the Macabi Sports Federation, who refused to bow to the political authority of Mapai, or to be in the same organization with their rival, the Hapoel Sports Federation, opposing obligatory membership in the Federation of Labor now forced upon all members of Kupat Holim. The group left Kupat Holim, and established in 1940 the Macabi Health Fund, which sixty years later constituted the second largest health fund in the state of Israel, and Kupat Holim's biggest rival.[41]

THE JOINT DUES CRISIS

In October 1937, five months after the joint dues format began to operate, Kupat Holim initiated a review of the subject. The move was the outcome of disappointment with the joint dues' meager contribution to improving the economic state of the health fund, and the demand by the Federation's executive committee that Kupat Holim shoulder part of the executive committee's budget. Actually, Kupat Holim did not rule out the joint dues, only the manner in which it was being collected. Kupat Holim sought to change pay arrangements between the health fund and the executive committee—the main issue being a demand to update deductions from its budget as the health fund's part in the expenditures of the executive committee—but, all requests for a review were totally rejected. The executive committee claimed that its own financial troubles were equal to the financial troubles of Kupat Holim, and there was no reason to change the prevailing system.

Because of the executive committee failure to respond to Kupat Holim's financial distress, the health fund's directorate decided to seek changes in the arrangement for collecting the joint dues. In May 1938 the Kupat Holim directorate submitted a proposal to the Federation's executive committee calling for "organization of collection of the joint dues and allocation of expenditures."[42] In a long and detailed memorandum, the heads of Kupat Holim stressed that their aim was not to withdraw from the principle of duel membership in both organizations, nor did they seek to retreat from the principle of joint Kupat Holim-Federation dues. They merely objected to the way collection was being carried out. The primary objection was the lack of a tie between the provider of service (Kupat Holim) and the insuring agent (the central membership dues bureau)—a structure that had been seriously detrimental to the quality of medical service, led to great waste, and caused difficulties in organizing the work of the health fund. As an example, the memorandum claimed that despite merging of dues collection and amalgamation of the dues bureaus of the health fund and the Federation, not only had the move *not* curtailed administrative costs, but the costs had *grown*. Kupat Holim believed that the root of the problem was the central dues collection bureau. According to the memorandum, the expenditures of the dues collection machinery had grown by 4.5 percent more than collection costs in Kupat Holim prior to the merger. Thus, Kupat Holim had been forced to allocate a larger percentage of its budget for administrative costs at the expense of medical services. Administrative costs had risen without any proportion to the rise in dues collection —by some 14 percent. Moreover, the number of employees in the new dues collection bureaus had also grown without any proportion to revenues and number of members. Too many parties were involved in collection, wasting money, time, and energy and creating an ungainly and costly system. The heads of Kupat Holim charged that

> the lack of direct dependence of the bureaus on the financial needs of the institutions, and the fact that the burden of caring for maintenance of institutions does not rest on [the bureaus]—free the employees of the bureaus psychologically from worrying about curtailing expenditures and economy.[43]

The Kupat Holim directorate even uncovered an atmosphere of irresponsibility among the bureaus who accepted members without a preliminary check, solely in order to increase the number of members in the Federation of Labor, noting the additional burden on Kupat Holim and its budget:

> These elements that have no tie to the Federation of Labor, including merely the needy and beggars in need of social welfare that have no background in the workplace.[44]

The health fund placed the blame on the isolation of the central membership dues bureaus from any responsibility for the operation of Kupat Holim. Therefore, the health fund called for abolishment of the bureau in its present form and for placing dues-gathering of the joint dues in the hands of Kupat Holim. The fund would transfer the funds it collected to their destination, and would in this way enhance countrywide dispersion of collection points to all points of settlement in the Yishuv. As an alternative, Kupat Holim proposed that centralized collection of the joint dues be abolished and that each institution collect joint dues by itself and transfer the required sum to the Federation of Labor. The heads of Kupat Holim warned:

> Separation of the role of [dues] collection and its expenditures, from the general role of maintaining an institution and providing services to members—is one of the most serious dangers for a special collection institution.[45]

But recognition of the pitfalls of the new system had come too late. The executive committee rejected all Kupat Holim's proposals. The central membership dues bureaus had become a *fait accompli* and an integral part of Kupat Holim. They continued to operate in their original form for another fifty-eight years, "set in granite" by the joint dues agreement signed in February 1937.

It was only in January 1995 when the Compulsory Health Insurance Law came into effect that the Gordian knot that bound Kupat Holim to the Federation of Labor was finally severed and collection of dues for medical services from Kupat Holim (and from the Macabi, Leumit, and Ammamit health funds) was transferred to the auspices of the National Insurance Institute.

Epilogue

Summary and Conclusions

The history of Kupat Holim reveals a singular experiment, the work of members of the Second Aliyah who founded a health organization that embodied in its founding principle prescripts for a health insurance plan and social values of justice and equality as the members of the Second Aliyah perceived them.

The first health funds for workers were established in order to remedy the poor state of health of agricultural workers and remedy the lack of health services accessible to all. At the outset, the health funds had to find an immediate solution to burning health problems and only afterwards were able to formulate an ideological posture. Pragmatism preceded ideology. Consequently, the first health funds adopted a dynamic and flexible mode of operation according to changing needs of the day and did not fetter themselves in permanent work and organizational norms. Sick rooms were established as needed; paramedics and caretakers were sent to sites blighted by illness, and the members themselves were required to participate in providing medical assistance, to fulfill the duty of "linah" by attending to sick comrades. The flexibility of the first health funds to respond to changing health needs was characteristic of their operation in the First World War, when the funds took upon themselves to organize medical assistance for the entire Jewish Yishuv, not solely for laborers, and even established the necessary logistic infrastructure for this purpose: sick rooms and mobile services, collection of capital from every possible source, import of medications from abroad, and so forth. Flexibility, dynamism, and response to changing needs continued to be pillars of Kupat Holim operations even after the establishment of the Federation of Labor in 1920 that brought about unification of the health funds. This characteristic is clearly evidence in the goals that Kupat Holim established for itself.

The ideological positions of Kupat Holim crystallized within the same flexible mindset and dynamism that characterized its operation. Due to the flexibility of Kupat Holim's founders on the practical level, its ideological platform reflected awakening needs of the membership. When the primary need was for primary care for laborers, Kupat Holim established permanent clinics in most of the points of agricultural settlement and hired paramedics and nurses to work in them on a regular basis. When the number of laborers in the city grew, Kupat Holim clinics were established in working class neighborhoods and primary care was expanded to cover medical care in general. After relations with Hadassah soured due to disagreements over financial matters, and hospitalization of settlers from the Jezreel Valley in Hadassah hospitals was disrupted, Kupat Holim initiated establishment of the Emek Hospital to liberate itself from total dependence on Hadassah for hospitalization services, taking responsibility for the ongoing operation of the Jezreel Valley hospital. Thus, services that Kupat Holim provided its members developed according to the needs of the hour, not according to a long-range planning, yet from stage to stage as Kupat Holim evolved, the principle of equality among members was maintained.

The centrality of the laborer as a member of Kupat Holim was emphasized from the outset, not only in provision of medical services but also in the "management culture" that administrated the fund. Representatives of the members were those who ran Kupat Holim branches and occupied its management positions, while medical professionals did not hold positions of power and influence. Thus, Kupat Holim was a workers' organization *for* workers and run *by* workers under their own management. Even when the health fund began to employ physicians in its services, the doctors' stature was equal to that of all other salaried personnel, and they did not enjoy any special standing.

Flexibility and pragmatism, however, did not hold up when the health funds had to settle their relationship vis-a-vis the political system in Eretz Israel. The workers of the Second Aliyah could not separate politics from daily needs. The first health funds were drawn into the political maelstrom that accompanied the mergers and schisms of the Zionist labor movement in 1918–1920, and from this point forward, politics and health went hand in hand. The capitulation of the first health funds to being used to serve political goals—applying the need for medical coverage by newcomers as a ploy for gaining new members to a particular political party, and later Kupat Holim's acquiescence to being used as a tool to impose the organizational authority of the Federation of Labor (for instance, in the Ein-Harod episode and the disagreement with Tel Chai)—became the source of the political orientation and organizational-political obligation Kupat Holim carried through most of its years.

Kupat Holim's ideal of mutual assistance has roots both in Jewish tradition and in the nineteenth-century European belief that regimes were responsible for the health of their subjects. The founders of health funds for workers in Eretz Israel adopted the idea of health insurance that had already won a place in Europe, and combined it with the foundations of Jewish tradition such as "bikur holim" and "linat tzedek"—visiting the sick and attending to the sick at night—part of a network of mutual assistance that characterized the life of Jewish communities for generations. The need to integrate Jewish social-service foundations developed because the structure of health funds in Europe that sprung up in an urban and industrial setting was not suitable to the rural lifestyle of new Zionist settlement. Consequently, in Eretz Israel health funds emerged that viewed their primary duty as providing first aid to agricultural workers isolated from medical centers and hospitalization facilities, who needed medical assistance available near their place of work. Ensuring medical assistance in the vicinity of the workplace required that the first health funds alter their original identity as insurance companies, and become medical-service providers. The health funds formulated a system that brought about the establishment of first aid stations and sick rooms, employment of paramedics in villages and encampments, local supply and distribution of medications, and all this on the basis of the principle of mutual assistance. Mutual assistance was the avenue through which members of the Second Aliyah coped with the difficulties they encountered in their first years in the country in order to overcome unemployment and economic distress. The communal kitchens, organization in groups as contractors for public works projects, and the first kibbutzim were expressions of the principle of mutual assistance that members of the Second Aliyah enshrined in the motto, "Each according to his ability, each according to his need." But the principle did not only reflect the Second Aliyah's sense of social justice. Without it, they could not have operated.

From its formative days, Kupat Holim perceived its role in a broad national context, aspiring to expand and increase its membership rolls to embrace all workers in the Yishuv, to forge a network of institutions and services that would provide social insurance and health insurance for its members from first aid to hospitalization and rest and recuperation. In this manner Kupat Holim sought to become a key body in the constellation of health services in Eretz Israel, also working on behalf of broad social legislation, particularly passage of a compulsory health insurance law, and seeking to involve the regime in underwriting health services and their development for the Jewish Yishuv as a whole.

This broad perspective of a national mission was primarily ideological. From a practical standpoint, however, Kupat Holim did not have the ability to realize its goals. The same gap between ideals and capabilities to realize them can be found in the early operations of the Federation of Labor, whose own economic institutions stood on the verge of bankruptcy and could not provide the services they promised. Nevertheless, this outlook served as a primer and stimulus for broadening frameworks, making a supreme effort to strive toward realization of national goals.

Political loyalty and obligations to the labor movement stood at the foundations of Kupat Holim's relationship with the Federation of Labor. What was true for David Ben-Gurion in 1921—that Kupat Holim was "one institution that gave power to the Federation"—remained essentially true until the mid-1990s. From the outset, the relationship between the two bodies was complex, a mixture of contrasting and complementary forces, support and loyalty together with clashing interests, struggles for independence versus devotion to political duty, initiatives and submission to dictates, and a complex array of "reciprocities" that in fact lacked any semblance of equality or balance and that consequently served as a seedbed for discontent, tension, and crisis. The close tie between Kupat Holim and the workers' organization was set forth with the foundation of the first health funds. Members of the agricultural workers' federation participated in the management of health fund branches from the start, and these management posts gave party functionaries a power base and an influential position in the fund itself—and through it, power within the working public as a whole.

From the Federation of Labor's standpoint Kupat Holim was a source of organizational power of the first magnitude, designed first and foremost to serve the vested interests of the Federation itself, and only secondly the interests of the fund and its membership. Thus was the case when Kupat Holim was instructed to cut off medical aid to Ein-Harod in 1923, in order to pressure members of the kibbutz to give in to Federation demands on an issue that had nothing to do with health matters. Thus was the case in 1924–1927 when Kupat Holim was forced to waive payments from cooperative settlements and other debtors in accordance with the demands of the Federation's leadership. Thus was the case in 1930–1933, when the Federation postponed requests to join Kupat Holim by workers who were not members of the Federation, out of fear that it would weaken Federation control of Kupat Holim. And this was the case again, in 1924–1926, when the Federation curtailed mobilization of donations from abroad that had been initiated by Kupat Holim.

The Federation of Labor's actions, designed to foster its own vested interests at the expense of Kupat Holim, were also geared to restrain the growth and strengthening of the health fund, out of fear that Kupat Holim would eventually liberate itself from Federation control. Consequently, the Federation at first sought to evade assisting the health fund in its attempts to bring about legislation of a compulsory health insurance law, then refrained from coming to Kupat Holim's aid when the health fund found itself in the midst of economic crisis—even demanding that all monies owed the Federation be paid on time, totally ignoring the objective difficulties facing Kupat Holim.

The health and medical assistance issue was not a central issue for the Federation of Labor. Kupat Holim issues were considered of marginal importance, in second or third place on a packed agenda if they were raised at all. Matters of work, education, and culture were more important than health, and one can find, for instance, comprehensive discussions at the Federation's conventions concerning the Ohel theatre or the literary contribution of the Hebrew poet Chaim Nachman Bialik, while Kupat Holim matters enjoyed at best a brief hearing. The secondary importance assigned health matters is also reflected in the identity of the Federation's executive committee appointees to Kupat Holim governing bodies—the directorate and the supervisory committee. Most were personalities of secondary importance whose political standing in the Federation of Labor was relatively low. None were members of the inner circle, the frontline leadership of the Federation at the time. The Agricultural directorate, Hamashbir, and Solel Boneh were considered far more important appointments.

The terms of membership between Kupat Holim and the Federation of Labor were set forth in the ordinances of the first Federation council in November 1921, at which it was resolved that all members of the Federation would be members of Kupat Holim. For more than sixteen years the Federation avoided realization of this obligation, only because such a step would likely be detrimental to its own vested interests.

Between 1920 and 1937, membership in Kupat Holim was 30 percent lower that in the Federation of Labor, a state of affairs that had a negative impact on the growth and the revenues of the health fund and overshadowed relationships with the Federation. The Federation of Labor feared that many members would be lost if Federation members were forced to join Kupat Holim. Moreover, the avowed position of Ben-Gurion—a dominant figure and often domineering leader most were hesitant to cross—was that one should not compel Federation members to be members of the health fund. Only in 1935 after Ben-Gurion left the leadership of the Federation of Labor to take up the position of head of the Jewish Agency, and after Kupat Holim proposed to unite collection of dues for the Federation and Kupat Holim, did the Federation see its way to requiring all members join Kupat Holim. After a short time, when it became evident to the health fund that the new arrangement was detrimental to Kupat Holim and the heads of the health fund suggested that collection of joint dues be transferred to Kupat Holim, reform of the "system" was flatly rejected by the Federation, which preferred to protect its own best interests, while Kupat Holim, again, capitulated, agreeing to honor the original arrangement despite its major drawbacks. When issues arose in which there was a conflict of interests between Kupat Holim and the Federation of Labor, it was always Kupat Holim that gave in on its demands—due both to its own political and organizational commitments to the Federation, and to its own relative weakness compared to the overwhelming superior force of the Federation's machinery. Kupat Holim had no choice but to maneuver and try to "engineer" things to its advantage, such as was the case in its championship of a compulsory health law, discussions over the amount of joint dues, and other issues.

Economic crises accompanied Kupat Holim from the outset, particularly because dues of insurees covered only half of its expenditures. The arduous financial straits of the Federation of Labor—Kupat Holim's "parent organization"—prevented the fund from receiving assistance from internal sources and required Kupat Holim "to knock on doors with hat in hand" for many years. Already in the 1920s, economic crises brought about the establishment of an inquiry commission by Zionist institutions in an attempt to find an organizational solution and fiscal formula that would allow Kupat Holim to continue to operate. The primary source of the problem was twofold: first, the class identity of Kupat Holim members, most of them laborers from the lower classes, day workers, members of cooperative settlements, unemployed, and new immigrants, making for a very narrow tax base founded on a population with meager or no means; the second, a closed economic structure and centralized organization by which the fund managed itself in its first years (in keeping with the Federation model and management style). The first inquiry committee had already concluded that Kupat Holim had to carry out far-reaching changes in its *modus operandi*, grant autonomy to districts, curtail the scope of its administrative personnel, and more tightly supervise professional consultations and referrals to specialists. Despite the clear directives of the inquiry commission, almost none of its conclusions were applied throughout the entire Mandate period, primarily because the financing and political clout required to do so were unavailable.

Kupat Holim was caught from its first days of existence between its social commitments to ensure the health and well-being of the working class and the cost of services. For a long time the fund struggled with the question of how it should operate, "according to needs or according to abilities." The fiscal crises and chronic deficit dictated adoption of makeshift ad-hoc management culture in lieu of straightforward work norms, and prevented long-range planning. Investments in infrastructure were ad-hoc, the building of clinics and hospitals were made possible only when donors could be found, there was no possibility of investing in preventive medicine or health education, and most of the fund's capital was expended on immediate needs: first aid, fighting epidemics, malaria, and TB, and so forth. Due to the daily struggle to find funding, Kupat Holim was open to political pressures on one hand, and engaged in chronic conflict with the Zionist executive, the Mandate government, and the Federation of

Labor on the other. Throughout most of its years of operation, Kupat Holim was unsuccessful in obtaining regular budgeting either from the Zionist executive or from the Mandate government.

Despite all this, Kupat Holim continued constantly to expand its services from 1920 to 1937, and during this period the scope of Kupat Holim's outreach in the Jewish community grew from 5% to 40% coverage of the overall population of the Yishuv in Eretz Israel.

Two core factors were in Kupat Holim's favor: The first was the dogged devotion of key members of Kupat Holim's own management—Eliezer Perlson, Yitzhak Kenivsky, Reuven Shenkar, and Dr. Moshe Beilenson—who were propelled by a deep-seated belief in the national mission of Kupat Holim and viewed the health fund as an integral part of realization of the Zionist idea. This approach was what allowed the health fund to steadfastly continuing to answer the needs of its members, expanding "against all economic logic."[1]

The second factor was the growth and expansion of the Federation of Labor, whose transformation into a powerful almost hegemonic political and economic factor in the Jewish Yishuv impacted positively on Kupat Holim as well. The Federation paved the way for Kupat Holim and even served as a source of support. The Federation's exploitation of Kupat Holim for its own needs as an organizational tool in fact *accelerated* the expansion of the health fund and consolidated Kupat Holim's stature among the workers and subsequently among all members of the Federation. Even after introduction of the joint dues formula and the health fund's loss of economic independence, Kupat Holim continued to grow in stature as the exclusive health insuring body for members of the Federation of Labor.

Throughout its history, Kupat Holim struggled with a dilemma over principles: Whether it was possible over time to sustain an ideological stance in matters of health and society and political and national issues under the constant pressure of economic constraints and without a solid financial base for such activity. Kupat Holim aspired to broaden its health services and become a body that dealt not only with mutual assistance and health insurance alone, but to provide services to all classes of society, to harness health services and make them a political tool in the hands of the Federation so the Federation could realize its socialist vision, and to become a major player in the medical field in Eretz Israel. It was clear that a comprehensive program such as this required tremendous economic resources, but such sums were not available.

In the issue of "needs or abilities," the "needs" were manifested across the board in all areas of the ambitious program that Kupat Holim had taken upon itself, while "ability" hinged on finding the needed funding. In actuality, no one was prepared to carry the burden of bridging the tremendous gap between needs and abilities—not the members of the health fund, the recipients of Kupat Holim's services; not the Federation of Labor; not national Zionist institutions. Many members and groups enrolled in Kupat Holim were unwilling to pay full dues; the Federation did not come forward with its part in contributing toward the development of Kupat Holim's services and even saddled the fund with organizational and political roles that had nothing to do with health; and national Zionist institutions were unwilling to assist Kupat Holim to transform itself into a core national body in the health service domain. The gap between economic abilities and social and political ideology of the labor movement in Eretz Israel runs through the history of Kupat Holim from its beginnings to this day.[2]

One cannot, however understand the behavior of the labor movement in Eretz Israel, its struggles and successes, without taking into account the powerful beliefs that propelled its members forward, and the role they assumed for themselves as social architects destined to lead the entire Jewish People, both toward a "new day" as part of a Socialist revolution, and towards national revitalization as part of the Zionist revolution. These long-range visions were not verbalized clearly from an ideological standpoint and were for the most part vague yearnings, while in practice the "dreamers" focused their energies and resources on realizing concrete, short-term goals, moving step-by-step on the road to their lofty aspirations—behavior epitomized in the Zionist slogan, *"dunam po ve dunam sham"* (acre here and acre there, acre follows acre). Yet, national and social aspirations served as a justification for striving and for existing, under objectively arduous circumstances.

The growth and shaping of Kupat Holim into a core organization in the Yishuv evolved over a period of twenty-six years. During these years, a framework for health work was forged (local clinics, hospitals, salaried physicians, a basket of services, and more), relationships between Kupat Holim and the Federation of Labor and the Zionist executive were hammered out, culminating in complete unification of membership in Kupat Holim and membership in the Federation, and Kupat Holim formulated for itself a clear corporate vision and mission for the future. Although it did not assume its final form until 1937, it is this framework that has guided the operation of Kupat Holim for more than eighty years of its existence.

NOTES

NOTES TO INTRODUCTION

1. M. I. Roemer, *National Health Systems of the World,* Vol. I (Oxford University Press, 1991), 422-23.

NOTES TO CHAPTER ONE

1. The Jewish community in Israel during the Ottoman and the British periods had been called by the Jewish community's people "Yishuv," which means in Hebrew a place or a settlement. This term is used throughout the book as equivalent to the term "Jewish community."
2. The geographical region of the present state of Israel has been called in the past one hundred years by several names: The Jerusalem Region during the Ottoman period until 1918; Palestine during the British mandate years 1918–1948; and Eretz Israel (the biblical name of the Holy Land) by the Jewish communities in Israel and abroad. For simplicity, the common name Eretz Israel is used through out the book, both for the Ottoman and for the British periods. For explanations of other persons, places, and organizations named in this book, see the Glossary.
3. M. Eliav, *Eretz Israel ve-Yishuvah ba-Meah ha-19* (Eretz Israel and its settlement in the 19th century) (Jerusalem, 1978), 498, for table showing the growth of the Jewish Yishuv in Eretz Israel in the 19th Century.
4. Ibid., 195, 168–67; G. Fein, *Eetot Sufa* (Stormy time) (Jerusalem, 1980), 339–28.
5. N. Levi, "Doctor Shimon Frankel (1809–1880) ha-Rofe ha-Ivri ha-Rishon be-Eretz Israel" (Dr. Shimon Frankel [1809–1880], the first Jewish doctor in Eretz Israel), *Harefuah*, 118 (1990): 490.
6. Shifra Shvarts, "Eidatiut, Dat ve-Politika be-Hakamat Batei ha-Cholim ha-Yehudiim ba-Yerushaliyim ba-Meah ha-19" (Ethnicity, religion and politics in establishment of hospitals in Jerusalem in the 19th century), *Korot*, 9 (1988): 235.
7. Yehoshua Leibowitz, *The History of Jewish Hospitals in Jerusalem* (Jerusalem, 1981).
8. Eliav, *Eretz Israel ve-Yishuvah ba-Meah ha-19*, 498.
9. The father of Edmond de Rothschild, who came to be called "the renowned benefactor" within the Yishuv, due to his massive support of Zionist settlement.

10. The agricultural community's salaried physician provided medical care gratis solely to the farmer-landowners, not to Jewish Socialist pioneers who worked as farm hands for them.
11. The goals of the World Zionist Organization were set forth in the Basel Program: "Zionism seeks to establish a home for the Jewish people in Palestine, secured under public law." Since its foundation the WZO has established companies and institutions to carry out its policies.
12. The Baron's central role underwriting Zionist endeavors gave birth to the unique Hebrew phraseology "the Baron's villages," "the Baron's administrators," and "the renowned benefactor" in Zionist lore, the last to this day embedded in the Hebrew title of the Rothschild Foundation in Israel, Yad HaNadiv (The Benefactor's Memorial Fund).
13. R. Aaronson, *ha-Baron veha-Moshavot* (The Baron and the villages) (Jerusalem, 1990), 141 n. 21.
14. Z. Saliternik, "Reminiscences of the History of Malaria Eradication in Palestine and Israel," *Israel Journal of Medical Sciences*, 14 (1978): 518–20.
15. This is an expression from the Bible, Numbers 13:32.
16. Saliternik, "Reminiscences of the History of Malaria Eradication in Palestine and Israel," 518–20.
17. H. Yafe, *Dor ha-Maapilim* (The generation of clandestine immigration) (Tel Aviv, 1939), 13.
18. Aaronson, *ha-Baron veha-Moshavot*, 141 n. 21.
19. Y. Ben Artzi, *ha-Moshava ha-Ivrit ba-Nof Eretz Israel 1882-1914* (The Hebrew village on the Eretz Israel landscape 1882-1914) (Jerusalem, 1988), 176, table 3.
20. "A key aim of Zionism, and particularly labor Zionism was to rebuild Jewish employment patterns by nurturing a Jewish working class—farmers and laborers—as the foundation for building a healthy, self-sustaining society." For a comprehensive overview of the history of Zionism see W. Laqueur, *A History of Zionism* (London: Weidenfeld & Nicolson, 1972).
21. Aaronson, *ha-Baron veha-Moshavot*, 298.
22. Ibid.
23. Eliav, *Eretz Israel ve-Yishuvah ba-Meah ha-19*, 498.
24. Yafe, *Dor ha-Maapilim*, 312–15. Dr. Hillel Yafe wrote in his diary that in Jaffa 300 Arabs died, in Gaza 3,000 died out of a population of 20,000, and in Lod 700 died out of a population of 4,000.
25. *Hashkafa*, 4th year, No. 86 (1904).
26. Yafe, *Dor ha-Maapilim*, 314–15.

Notes to Chapter Two

1. The Kishnev Pogrom refers to anti-Semitic riots in 1903 in Kishnev, Moldavia, supported by the Russian authorities, in which 47 Jews were killed and 92 wounded. The pogrom caused an international outcry and led to formation of Jewish self-defense leagues and immigration.
2. The Jewish Defense Group from Hommel (in Byelorussia) was founded in 1904–5 following the Hommel pogrom.
3. M. Eliav, *Eretz Israel ve-Yishuva be-Mea ha-19* (Eretz Israel and its settlement in the 19th Century) (Jerusalem, 1978), 335.
4. Tel Aviv was founded in 1909 as the "first Hebrew city" on the sand dunes north of Jaffa.
5. Z. Tzachor, *ba-Deresh le-Hanhagat ha-Yishuv* (On the way to leading the Yishuv) (Jerusalem, 1982), 16–18.
6. Y. Gorny, "Shinuim ba-Mivneh ha-Chevrati veha-Politi shel ha-Aliayah ha-Shniya" (Changes in the social and political structure of the Second Aliyah), *Hatzionut* (Zionism), A (1970): 5, 205–28.
7. Petach Tikva was the first Jewish agricultural settlement in Eretz Israel, established northeast from Jaffa in 1878.
8. *Hapoel Hatzair* (The young worker), 1908, No. 3; quoted in Yosef Shapira, *Avodah ve-Adama* (Toil and soil) (Tel Aviv, 1961), 240.
9. Bracha Havas, ed., *Sefer ha-Aliya ha-Shniya* (The Second Aliyah book) (Tel Aviv, 1947), 186.
10. Shapira, *Avodah ve-Adama*, 240–41.
11. M. Reicher, *ha-Telem ha-Acharon* (The last furrow) (Beit Neta, 1966), 54–55.
12. Tzachor, *ba-Deresh le-Hanhagat ha-Yishuv*, 11.
13. A. Monchik, "Lifnei 'Bereshit Kupat Holim" (Before Kupat Holim was created), ALM, IV–243–1–56.
14. A. Kosovsky, "Tikei Merkaz Kupat Holim" (Portfolio of Kupat Holim directorate), ALM, IV–243–1–56.
15. *Hapoel Hatzair*, 1908, No. 3.
16. Y. Ori, "be-Tzaadei Bereishit" (In the steps of creation), ALM, IV–243–1–56.
17. Ibid.
18. Ibid.
19. B. Freiber, "Tikei Merkaz Kupat Holim" (Portfolio of the Kupat Holim directorate), ALM, IV-243-1-56.
20. Luntz, Luach *Eretz Israel le-Shnat 1910–11* (Eretz Israel calendar for the year 1910–11) (private publication, Jerusalem), 10.
21. Reicher, *ha-Telem ha-Acharon*, 54.
22. Yet even Katznelson did not work for the actualization of the resolution, despite his decisive role in passage of the motion. This was typical

of Katznelson, and not due to any withdrawal of support for the original idea or its importance. Historian Anita Shapira notes in her biography of Katznelson his tendency "to refrain from taking responsibility that required firmness and commitment," a characteristic that impacted both on his personal life and his behavior as a public figure. Anita Shapira, *Berl,* Part I (Tel Aviv, 1983), 87.

23. Ibid.
24. "Chronika" (Chronicles) *HeAchdut*, No. 28 (April–May 1911).
25. See chapter 1 on the young socialist pioneers' objection to such "parasitic" existence.
26. N. Harpaz, "Reshita shel Kupat Holim ba-Yamei ha-Aliyah ha-Shniya" (Beginnings of Kupat Holim in the days of the Second Aliyah), ALM, IV–243–1–56.
27. "Al Davar Kupat Holim" (Regarding Kupat Holim), *HeAchdut,* No. 42 (1911).
28. *HeAchdut*, No. 42 (1911).
29. Takanot ve-Hachlatot Kupat Holim (Ordinances and resolutions of Kupat Holim) (Jaffa, Shavuot, 1912), ALM, IV–243–1–56.
30. The Yemenite people suffered mainly of malnutrition, malaria, and trachoma and lacked the modern knowledge of the importance of personal and environmental hygiene.
31. *Hapoel Hatzair*, No. 35 (1911).
32. Freiber, "Tikei Merkaz Kupat Holim."
33. Ibid., 3.
34. Ibid., 7.
35. In the history of Kupat Holim, the advantage was not a "one way street." In the decades prior to enactment of the Compulsory Health Insurance Law in 1995, the obligation worked in reverse, inflating membership in the Federation of Labor, and improving its situation.
36. However, institution of universal coverage under the 1995 National Compulsory Health Insurance Law left Kupat Holim intact and functioning as an health-provider organization, allowing it to compete for members alongside three other smaller health funds on a "level playing field" that severed Kupat Holim's status as a Federation of Labor asset. This was accompanied by nationalization of dues-collecting, which was turned over to a non-partisan independent public authority—the National Insurance Institute (i.e., Israel's social security system). Stripped both of financial independence and the ability to funnel part of health fund dues to other issues on the Federation agenda, today Kupat Holim and the other three smaller health-provider organizations in the national compulsory health insurance system receive funding on a proportional basis, by size of membership.

37. In Hebrew the word "tzdaka" (charity) does not carry Christian overtones of benevolence or compassion or "giving out of good will"; the word stems from the Hebrew root z-d-k or "justice".
38. *Mishna*, Zera'im (seeds order), Pea 7-8.
39. S. Kottek, "The Essenes and Medicine," *Clio Medica*, 18 (1983): 93.
40. Ch. Harpaz, "Bituch Briut me-B'chna Historit Kalkalit" (Health insurance from a historical economic standpoint), *Dapim Refuim* (1959): 247.
41. H. R. Shryock, *The Development of Modern Medicine* (Madison: University of Wisconsin Press, 1979), 387.
42. Harpaz "Reshita shel Kupat Holim ba-Yamei ha-Aliyah ha-Shniya."
43. "be-Machaneh ha-Sotzialim" (In the socialist camp), *HeAchdut*, 12 (1912): 16.
44. "le-Shealat Kupat Holim" (On the question of Kupat Holim), *Hapoel Hatzair,* Year 13 (1916–17), No. 15, 4.
45. M. Grey, "Poverty, Politics and Health: The Farm Security Administration Medical Care Program, 1935–1945," *Journal of the History of Medicine and Allied Sciences*, 44 (1989): 320–50.

Notes to Chapter Three

1. M. Sherman, "The Jewish Physicians in Gaza," *Harefua* [Medicine], 52 (1957): 382–91.
2. Ibid.
3. Y. Aphter, *Kupat Holim shel Poalei Yehuda be-Milchemet ha-Olam ha-Rishona* (The Judea Workers' Health fund in the First World War), *be-Sha'ah Zu* (At this hour), A (1916): 33–40.
4. Ibid.
5. *Hapoel Hatzair*, 18 (1915).
6. Ibid.
7. A. Kosovsky, Kupat Holim Files, ALM IV–243–1–56.
8. Y. Aphter, *Kupat Holim shel Poalei Yehuda be-Milchemet ha-Olam ha-Rishona* (The Judea Workers' Health fund in the First World War), *be-Sha'ah Zu* (At this hour), A (1916): 33–40.
9. Ibid.
10. Ibid.
11. Ibid.
12. N. Efrati, *me-Mashbare le-Tikva , ha-Yishuv ha-Yehudi ba-Eretz Israel be-Milchemet ha-Olam ha-Rishona* (From crisis to hope: The Jewish Yishuv in Eretz Israel in the First World War) (Jerusalem, 1991), 267.
13. B. Katznelson, *Igrot 1915–1918* (Letters 1915–1918) (Tel Aviv, 1961), 13.
14. Aphter, *Kupat Holim shel Poalei Yehuda be-Milchemet ha-Olam ha-Rishona*, *be-Sha'ah Zu* , 33–40.

15. Ibid.
16. Katznelson, *Igrot 1915–1918*, 16.
17. Z. Tzahor, *On the Road to 'Yishuv' Leadership* (Jerusalem, 1981), 75.
18. The Balfour Declaration was the British declaration of sympathy with Zionist aspirations. The official statement took the form of a letter to Lord Rothschild on 2 November 1917 by the British foreign secretary, Arthur James Balfour, declaring that the British government favored the "establishemnt in Palestine of a national homeland for the Jewish people."

Notes to Chapter Four

1. Carol B. Kutcher, "The Early Years of Hadassah, 1912-1921" (Ph.D. diss., Brandeis University, 1976), 123–216.
2. Ibid.
3. Donald Miller, "A History of Hadassah 1912-1935" (Ph.D. diss., New York University, 1986).
4. Hadassah Medical Federation, *Esrim Shnot Sherut Refu'I be-Eretz Israel 1918–1938* (Twenty years of medical service in Eretz Israel 1918–1936) (Jerusalem, 1939), 1–25.
5. Ibid.
6. B. Dinburg (Dinur), "Eretz Israel be-Shnot Tarpag" (Eretz Israel in the year 1922–23), *me-Shanah le-Shanah*, 294–97, Government of Palestine Report, July 1920–Dec. 1921 (His Majesty Stationary Office, London, 1922).
7. Hadassah Medical Federation, *Esrim Shnot Sherut Refu'I be-Eretz Israel 1918–1938*, 19–20.
8. Letter from Dr. A. Katznelson to the Political Department of the Jewish Agency, 16 Feb. 1937, Central Zionist Archives (CZA), Jerusalem, S370–25.
9. Hadassah Medical Federation, *Esrim Shnot Sherut Refu'I be-Eretz Israel 1918–1938*, 18.
10. N. Levi, *The History of Medicine in the Holy Land* (Tel Aviv, 1998), 197–208.
11. Y. Slutzky, *Mavo le-Toldot Tnuat ha-Avodah ha-Yisraelit* (Introduction to the history of the Israeli labor movement) (Tel Aviv, 1983), 286–88.
12. *Hapoel Hatzair*, issue 15 (1920): 4.
13. Hapoel Hatzair Health fund portfolios, Lavon Institute: Labor Movement Archive (hereafter ALM), IV–402–8, clause 16, Ordinance 1.
14. Hapoel Hatzair Health fund portfolios, ALM, IV–402–8, pp. 33–35.
15. Hadassah Medical Federation, *Esrim Shnot Sherut Refu'I be-Eretz Israel 1918–1938*.

16. *Hapoel Hatzair*, issue 15 (1920): 4–5
17. The work was carried out by Jewish labor gangs organized by members of the Third Aliyah's Labor Battalion who I believe contracted to do the work.
18. Hadassah Medical Federation, *Esrim Shnot Sherut Refu'I be-Eretz Israel 1918–1938*, 17–18.
19. *Contras*, booklet 71 (1920): 10.
20. Achdut Haavodah portfolios, ALM, IV-404-41, pp. 1-7; Ch. Golan (ed.), ha-Protokolim shel ha-Vaad ha-Poel, ha-Moetza veha-Viedah, December 1919 – December 1920 (The Protocols of the Executive Committee, the Council and the Convention, December 1919 – December 1920) , Socialist Zionist Federation of Eretz Israel Workers Achdut Haavodah, Yad Tabenkin (no date), pp. 39-40.
21. Kupat Holim portfolios, ALM, IV–243–55.
22. *Ha-Administratzia shel Hapoel Hatzair, Jaffa, Eretz Israel, Cheshbon Ha'avarat Kupat Holim le-Tarap* (Administration of Hapoel Hatzair, Jaffa, Eretz Israel: Bill transfer of Kupat Holim to 1920), comparison of a bill sent to the Committee of Delegates up until 1920, Hapoel Hatzair portfolios, directorate, ALM, IV–402–119.
23. M. I. Roemer, *Health Care Systems in World Perspective* (Ann Arbor, MI, 1976), 5–10.
24. Hapoel Hatzair portfolios, Central Committee, ALM, IV–402–8.
25. *Hapoel Hatzair*, issue 24 (1919): 7.
26. Hapoel Hatzair portfolios, directorate, ALM, IV–402–119
27. *Contras*, booklet 14 (1919): 21.
28. *Contras*, booklet 71 (1920): 12.

Notes to Chapter Five

1. T. Even Shoshan, *Toldot Tnuat ha-Poalim be-Eretz Israel* (History of the labor movement in Eretz Israel) (Tel Aviv, 1963), 446.
2. Z. Tzachor, *ba-Deresh le-Hanhagat ha-Yishuv* (On the road to leadership of the Yishuv) (Jerusalem, 1982), 134.
3. Sh. Tevet, *Kin'at David* (David's envy), vol. 2 (Jerusalem and Tel Aviv, 1980), 156.
4. Ibid., 495.
5. Kupat Holim portfolios, Lavon Institute: Labor Movement Archive (hereafter ALM), IV–243–1–56.
6. Idit Zartal, *Yamim oo-Maasim* (Days and deeds) (Tel Aviv, 1975), 42–43.
7. Kupat Holim portfolios, ALM, IV–243–1–55.
8. *Davar* (newspaper), 4 April 1961, 4.
9. Kupat Holim portfolios, ALM, IV–243–1–55.

10. Zartal, *Yamim oo-Maasim*, 48.
11. D. Ben-Gurion, *Hapoel ha-Ivri ve-Histadruteno* (The Hebrew worker and his federation), 2nd ed. (Tel Aviv, 1964), 122; "Protokol ha-Veida [convention] Shniya shel ha-Histadrut ha-Klalit shel ha-Ovdim ha-Ivriim be-Eretz Israel" (Protocols of the 2nd Convention of the General Federation of Hebrew Laborers in Eretz Israel) (Tel Aviv, 1922–23), 25; Tevet, *Kin'at David,* 157.
12. Zartal, *Yamim oo-Maasim*, 48.
13. "Protokol ha-Vaadah [committee] ha-Shniyah," 25.
14. Y. Kenev (Kenivsky), *ha-Bituach ha-Sotziali be-Eretz Israel, Hesegav oo-Biyotav* (Social insurance in Eretz Israel: Its achievements and problems) (Tel Aviv, 1941–1942), 280–81.
15. "Protokol ha-Vaadah ha-Shniyah," 166, clause 2.
16. Kenev, *ha-Bituach ha-Sotziali be-Eretz Israel, Hesegav oo-Biyotav*, 293.
17. Zartal, *Yamim oo-Maasim*, 49–50; D. Nadav, "Inyan shel Chaim ve-Mavet" (A matter of life and death), *BaGilboa*, 172 (Nov.1989): 33. According to Nadav, there were thirty-two beds.
18. Reuven Shenkar Report, Kupat Holim Files, ALM IV–208–1–38.
19. Ibid.
20. Executive Committee of the Federation of Labor portfolios, Secretariat, ALM, IV–208–1–38.
21. *Mechiyenu* [Our lives], issue 40, special publication (11 June 1923), 144 (author unknown).
22. Nadav, "Inyan shel Chaim ve-Mavet," 32.
23. Executive Committee of the Federation of Labor portfolios, Secretariat, ALM, IV–208–1–38.
24. Ibid.
25. *Mechiyanu*, 145.
26. *Pinkas*, 2, issue 9 (1923): 134.
27. Nadav, "Inyan shel Chaim ve-Mavet," 33.

Notes to Chapter Six

1. This issue remained central to Kupat Holim up to the point in 1995 when the fund became solely an executive arm in a legislated compulsory medical insurance system, which then disassociated Kupat Holim from the Federation of Labor, making it one of four independent public health-service providers for the state of Israel.
2. D. Giladi, *ha-Yishuv ba-Tkufat ha-Aliya ha-Reviet* (The Yishuv in the period of the Fourth Aliyah) (Tel Aviv, 1973), 38.
3. Y. Kenev (Kenivsky), *ha-Bituch ha-Sotziali ba-Eretz Israel, Hesegav oo-Biyotav* (Social Insurance in Eretz Israel: Its achievements and problems), (Tel Aviv, 1941–42), 156–67.

4. Eliezer Perlson, *Briut Haoved* (The health of the worker), (Kupat Holim directorate: Tel Aviv, 1924), 37–40.
5. Reuven Shenkar, *Briut Haoved*, 37–40; Kenev, *ha-Bituch ha-Sotziali ba-Eretz Israel*, 266–67, 280–81.
6. Shenkar, Report to the Secretriat of the Federation of Labor executive committee, June 1923, Portfolio of the executive committee of the Federation of Labor, Secretariat, ALM, IV–208–1–38.
7. Portfolio of the executive committee of the Federation of Labor, Secretariat, ALM, IV–208–1–38.
8. *Pinkas* [booklet], 7, Supplement July–August (Jerusalem, 1923), 10–11.
9. Portfolio of the executive committee of the Federation of Labor, Secretariat, ALM, IV–208–1–38.
10. Ibid.
11. Ibid.
12. Ibid.
13. Ibid.
14. Ibid.
15. Tevet, *Kin'at David* (David's envy), (Jerusalem and Tel Aviv, 1982), 495.
16. Portfolio of the executive committee of the Federation of Labor, Secretariat, ALM, IV–208–1–97A.
17. *Davar*, 9 Feb. 1925, 3.
18. *Briut Haoved*, 37–40.
19. Ibid., 28.
20. Portfolio of the executive committee of the Federation of Labor, Secretariat, ALM, IV–208–1–38.
21. Ibid.
22. Ibid.
23. Ibid.
24. Tamtzit ha-Din ve-Cheshbon shel ha-Vaada le-Chakirat Matzav Kupat Holim me-Yom 10 be-Mai 1927 (Abstract of the account of the Inquiry Commission into the state of Kupat Holim from the 10th of May 1927), Portfolio of the executive committee of the Federation of Labor, Secretariat, ALM, IV–208–1–97.
25. Ibid.
26. Ibid.
27. Ibid.
28. Ibid.
29. *Davar*, 25 May 1927, 3.
30. Ibid.
31. Ibid.
32. Ibid.
33. Ibid.
34. *Davar* 24 August 1927, 3.

35. *Davar*, 6 January 1927, 2.
36. Portfolio of the Health Committee of the Jewish Community, CZA, S/25/6632.
37. The World Zionist Organization Papers, Resolutions of the 15th Zionist Congress, Basel 1927, General Office of the Zionist Organization (London, 1928), 33–34.
38. Ibid, 1.
39. National Board statement on Reorganization of Health Work in Palestine, Portfolio of the Health Committee of the Jewish Community,CZA S/25/6632, 1–7.
40. The "disturbances" refers to four waves of violence during the British Mandate period. In the 1921 disturbances seventeen people were killed in the neighborhood of Jaffa, and Jewish defense was organized to repel the attackers. The response of the authorities was vigorous, but they concurrently introduced a conciliatory policy toward the Arabs and as a first step temporarily suspended further Jewish immigration to Palestine.
41. Kupat Holim Portfolio, ALM 243–2–10B.
42. A. Mendelberg, "Kupat Holim's Roles," *Britut Haoved*, Kupat Holim directorate (Tel Aviv, 1924–1925), 22.
43. Ibid.
44. Ibid.
45. Ibid.
46. Perlson, *Briut Haoved,* 22-25.
47. *Davar*, 5 November 1925, p. 3. The term "Kupat Holim council" was replaced after 1927 by the term "Kupat Holim convention." Thus, council in 1925 was, in fact, the first Convention of the fund, although not labeled as such.
48. *Hapoel Hatzair*, Year 19, pamphlet 12–13 (1925): 18.
49. *Davar*, 13 Dec. 1925, p. 000.
50. Ibid.
51. *Hapoel Hatzair*, Year 19, pamplet 12–13 (1925):18.
52. *Contras,* 12, pamphlet 232 (1925)**,** 9.
53. Ibid.
54. Ibid.
55. Yosef Baratz, "On the Issue of Kupat Holim,," *Hapoel Hatzair*, Year 21, 27–28 (1928), 2.
56. I. Kanievsky-Kanev, The Roles of Kupat Holim, *Davar*, 4 (June, 1928): 2.
57. Doch ha-Veida ha-Shniya shel Kupat Holim (Report of the Second Convention of Kupat Holim), p. 2, portfolio of the executive committee of the Federation of Labor, Secretariat, ALM, IV–208–572.
58. *Hapel Hatzair*, Year 21, 6 (1928):12.

59. *Davar,* 4 March 1929, 2.
60. Henrietta Szold, Opening Welcomes, 6, Portfolio of the executive committee of the Federation of Labor, Secretariat, ALM, IV–208–1-572A.
61. Dr. M. Beilinson, The Social Mission of Kupat Holim, 5, Portfolio of the executive committee of the Federation of Labor, Secretariat, ALM, IV–208–1-572A.
62. Ibid.
63. Y. Kanev-Kanievsky, Protocols of the 2nd Kupat Hpolim Convention, Portfolio of the executive committee of the Federation of Labor, Secretariat, ALM, IV–208–1-572A, 1–26.
64. Ibid.
65. Z. Tzahor, *Israel Political Roots* (Tel Aviv, 1987), 64–65..
66. A. Shapira, *Berl,* vol. 1 (Tel Aviv, 1983), 284–88.
67. *Hapoel Hatzair*, Year 26, 23 (1933): n.p.

Notes to Chapter Seven

1. D. Netherland, Hashpaat ha-Rofim ha-Olim me-Germania al Hitpatchut ha-Refua ba-Aretz ba-Shanim 1933–1948 (The impact of immigrant doctors from Germany on the development of medicine in Eretz Israel in the years 1933–1948), *Cathedra*, 30 (1983): 114–15.
2. Hapoel Hatzair Central Committee portfolio, ALM, IV–402–119.
3. Ibid.
4. Kupat Holim portfolio, ALM IV–122–15.
5. *Contras*, 14 July 1919, 21.
6. Blumenfeld Report, 24 Nov. 1919, BGA.
7. *Hapoel Hatzair*, Year 13, 2 (1919): 1.
8. *Contras*, 71: 3 (1920): 25–26.
9. Hapoel Hatzair portfolio, ALM, IV–402–119.
10. Donald Miller, "A History of Hadassah, 1912–1935" (Ph.D. diss., New York Univ., 1968), 322–32.
11. D. Netherland, *Cathedra*, 30 (1983): 114–15.
12. *Pinkas*, 7, supplement (1923): 15–17.
13. Henrietta Szold, *Esrim Shnot Hadassah be-Eretz Israel* (Twenty years of Hadassah in Eretz Israel), (Hadassah Medical Federation: Jerusalem 1939), 17–18.
14. Heskem Kupat Holim-Hadassah (Kupat Holim-Hadassah accord), Kupat Holim portfolio, directorate, ALM, IC–243–1; *Pinkas*, 7, supplement (1923): 15.
15. *Pinkas*, 7, supplement (1923): 15.
16. Kupat Holim portfolio, ALM, IV–243–26.
17. *Hapoel Hatzair*, Year 16 (1923), 19.

18. S. Shvarts, T. Brown. "Kupat Holim, Dr. Isaac Max Rubinow and the American Zionist Medical Unit's Experiment to Establish Health Care Services in Palestine 1918–1923," *Bulletin of the History of Medicine*, 72: 1 (1998).
19. "Hachlatot Asayfat ha-Mecha'a neged Hadassah" (Decisions of the protest meeting against Hadassah), *Hapoel Hatzair*, Year 20, pamphlet 14 (Jan., 1927): 15.
20. Hadassah-Kupat Holim portfolio, ALM IV–243–22B.
21. Ibid.

Notes to Chapter Eight

1. *Davar,* 9 December 1925, p.1–2.
2. Health Committee portfolio, CZA, S25/397.
3. Ibid.
4. Kupat Holim Center portfolio, ALM, IV–243–2–3A.
5. Kupat Holim Center portfolio, ALM, IV–243–1–16.
6. Harry Sacker letter to E. Perlson, 18 July 1927, ALM, IV–208–146B.
7. The Federation of Labor Secretariat Portfolio, ALM, IV–208–97C.
8. Health Committee portfolio, CZA S25/397.
9. Ibid.
10. In the disturbances of 1929 a total of 133 Jews were killed and 339 injured in Jerusalem, Safed, and Hebron (which was abandoned by Jews until the early 1970s). Rural settlements throughout Palestine were attacked and some abandoned. The British authorities were demonstrably passive during the riots.
11. Health Comittee potfolio, CZA, S25/368.
12. Ibid.
13. Health Committee portfolio, CZA, S25/397.
14. E. Zartal, Yamim Umaassim (Days and deeds), (Tel Aviv, 1975), 68.
15. Health Committee portfolio, CZA, S25/397.
16. Ibid.
17. Ibid.
18. Ibid.
19. Ibid.
20. Ibid.
21. Ibid.
22. The Federation of Labor Secretariat portfolio, ALM, IV–208–1–572B.

Notes to Chapter Nine

1. David Ben-Gurion, *Hapoel ha-Ivri ve-Histadruto* (The Hebrew worker and his Federation), 2nd ed. (Tarbut ve-Chinuch [Culture and Education],

Tel Aviv, 1964), 22; Protokol ha-Veida ha-Shniya shel ha-Histadrut ha-Klalit shel ha-Ovdim be-E"Y (Protocols of the 2nd Convention of the General Federation of Labor in Eretz Israel), (Tel Aviv, 1923), 25.

2. Ramsay MacDonald was British Prime Minister and Labor Party leader in the 1930s.
3. *Hapoel Hatzair*, 12–13 (1925): 18–19.
4. *Briut Haoved* (1924): 37–40.
5. "Kupat Holim, Peuloteha ve-Hitpatchuta" (Kupat Holim, its operations and development), Din ve-Cheshbon Merkaz Kupat Holim (Kupat Holim directorate Report), ALM, IV–208–572, A, portfolio NN/4/1.
6. M. I. Roemer, *Health Care Systems in World Perspective* (Ann Arbor, MI, 1976), 104–105.
7. *Briut Haoved* (1925): 17.
8. Yitzhak Kenivsky, *ha-Bituch ha-Sotziali be-Eretz Israel ve-Hesegav oo-Biyotav* (Social insurance in Eretz Israel, its achievements and problems), (Tel Aviv, 1941–42), 343.
9. Letter from Yitzhak Kenivsky to the Federation of Labor executive committee, 21 November 1928, ALM, IV–208–146, A.
10. Ibid.
11. Ibid.
12. *Davar*, 4 June 1928, 2.
13. *Davar*, 10 April 1929, 13.
14. "Kupat Holim, Peuloteha ve-Hitpatchuta be-Shnat 1929–1930" (Kupat Holim, its operations and development 1929–1930), Din ve-Cheshbon shel Merkaz Kupat Holim (Kupat Holim directorate report), ALM, IV–208–1–572, 17-19.
15. Ibid., 19.
16. Ibid., 26.
17. Letter (in Hebrew) from the Kupat Holim directorate to the chief secretary of the Mandate government in Eretz Israel, 20 January 1930, p. 1, ALM, IV–208–163A; the same letter, in English, from Kupat Holim directorate to the High Commissioner the Lord Chancellor, 20 January 1930, Health Committee portfolio, CZA, S25/6632.
18. Ibid., ALM, IV–208–163A.
19. Letter from the acting chief secretary of the Mandate government in Eretz Israel to the secretary of the Federation of Labor executive committee, February 1930, Health Committee portfolio, CZA, S25/6632.
20. Letter from Henrietta Szold to Colonel Kisch, 18 March 1920, Health Committee portfolio, CZA, S25/6632.
21. Ibid.
22. Hachlatot Asefat ha-Nivcharim shel Knesset Israel be-Inyanei Briut ve-Ezra Sotzialit (Decisions of the representative assembly of Knesset Israel on health matters and social welfare), December 1930, Health Committee portfolio, CZA, S25/6632.

23. Ibid.
24. Ibid.
25. Ibid.
26. Letter from Yitzhak Kenivsky to Dov Hos, 10 February 1931, ALM, IV–243–2–16.
27. Letter from Yitzhak Kenivsky to Dov Hos, 2 June 1931, ALM, IV–2701–208–B.
28. Letter from Yitzhak Kenivsky to Dr. Chaim Arlosoroff, 4 September 1931, Health Committee portfolio, CZA, S25/368.
29. Ibid.
30. Kupat Holim directorate Report 1931, ALM, IV–243–1–117.
31. Letter from Yitzhak Kenivsky and Eliezer Perlson to the Federation of Labor executive committee, 13 January 1933, ALM, IV–208–1–572A. Copy of letter also sent to Dr. Chaim Arlosoroff and Dov Hos.
32. Ibid., remark in handwriting in the margin, without signature.
33. Letter from Eliezer Perlson to Dr. Avraham Katznelson, 2 February 1933, CZA, S25/368.
34. Letter from Yitzhak Kenivsky to David Ben-Gurion, 29 November, 1934, ALM, IV–208–1–966.
35. Letter from Yitzhak Kenivsky to Dov Hos, 7 January 1935, ALM, IV–208–1–966.
36. Letter from Yitzhak Kenivsky to Dov Hos, 3 February 1935, ALM, IV–208–1–966, portfolio NN/4//1.
37. Ibid., remark by Ben-Gurion in the margin of the letter.
38. Letter from Dov Hos to Moshe Sharret, 18 February 1935, Ben-Gurion Heritage Institute Archives.
39. All mention of proposals for a health insurance law were entered into the appendix and assigned secondary importance in the framework of Kupat Holim requests for financial assistance from the Mandate government; see *Davar,* 16 December 1935, 3; 17 December 1935, 3; 12 January 1936, 3; letter from Yitzhak Kenivsky to Golda Meirson and Dov Hos, 17 December 1936, ALM IV–208–969; letter from Yitzhak Kenivsky to Dr. Avraham Katznelson-Nissan, 17 December 1936, ALM, IV–208–0060; letter from Yitzhak Kenivsky to Dov Hos, 1 June 1937, ALM, IV–243–3–167/22.
40. Tochnit le-Peulat Kupat Holim be-Yachas le-Memshela (Kupat Holim working plan vis-à-vis the government), 17 November 1937, CZA, S25/370; *Davar*, 16 December 1935, 3.

Notes to Chapter Ten

1. ALM, IV–243–53.
2. Kupat Holim of the Judea Workers portfolio, ALM, IV–243–53.

3. Kupat Holim of the Hapoel Hatzair portfolio, ALM, IV–402–119.
4. Shabtai Tevet, *Kinat David* (David's Envy), II (Tel Aviv and Jerusalem, 1982), 495.
5. *Briut Haoved*, A (1924): 30.
6. Ibid.
7. Ibid., 31.
8. Shenkar letter, 18 March 1926, ALM, IV–208–97B.
9. The Federation of Labor Secretariat portfolio, ALM, IV–208–97C.
10. Ibid.
11. Kupat Holim Secretariat potfolio, ALM IV–243–1–17.
12. The orthodox Jewish community was split between those who vehemently opposed Zionism as a form of blasphemy, an attempt to "rush the End of Days" when Jews would return to their Homeland, and religiously observant Jews who were Zionists, such as the Hamizrachi Movement and Federation.
13. Not all members of Hapoel Hamizrachi joined the Federation of Labor; those who did not established the Federation of Mizrachi Workers that became a part of the World Mizrachi movement. D. Giladi*, ha-Yishuv be-Tkufat ha-Aliyah ha-Rivi'it* (The Yishuv in the period of the Fourth Aliyah), (Tel Aviv, 1973), 90, 150, 225.
14. Perlson letter to the Federation of Labor Executive Committee, 8 October 1931, ALM IV–208–1–270B/4/NN.
15. The portfolios of the Kupat Holim directorate, ALM, IV–243–1–17. Kupat Holim directorate report from 25 August 1931 on the entrance of all members of the Federation in Jerusalem into Kupat Holim; *Briut Haoved*, A (1924): 30.
16. Decisions of the 3rd Convention (1927), Ben-Gurion Heritage Institute Archive, 21.
17. Federation of Labor Secretariat portfolio, ALM, IV–208–143B.
18. Tevet, *Kin'at David*, 496.
19. Ibid., 497.
20. Portfolio of Kupat Holim Secretariat, ALM–IV–243–2–12/70A.
21. Tevet, *Kin'at David*, 490.
22. Decisions of the Federation of Labor Executive Committee, 14 September 1931, ALM, IV–208–1–270/4NN.
23. Tevet, *Kin'at David*, 499.
24. Z. Tzachor, *Shorshei ha-Politika ha-Yisraelit* (The roots of Israeli politics), (Hakibbutz Hameuchad and Ben-Gurion University, 1987), 72–73.
25. ALM, IV–208–1–270C/4NN.
26. Ibid.
27. *Doar Hayom* (Daily Mail), 16 August 1933.
28. Ibid.
29. Histadrut ha-Ovdim ha-Leumi'im be-Eretz Israel, Kupat Holim le-Ovdim Leumi'im (The National Workers Federation in Eretz Israel:

Health fund for national workers), The Executive Report (April 1935): 1; ALM, IV–432–4.

30. Some immigrated illegally on ships running a British blockade, and hundreds came to participate in the Macabi Games and simply didn't go back.
31. Y. Gelber, *Moledet Hadasha* (New homeland), (Jerusalem, 1990), 437, 440.
32. The number of Federation and Kupat Holim members on 1 January 1936. See ALM IV–20–1–970, portfolio 1/4/NN; *Davar*, 30 December 1935, 4.
33. *Davar*, 2 October 1935, 3; 20 January 1936, 4.
34. A. Becker, *Im Hazman Ubnei Hador* (Of time and men), (Tel Aviv 1982), 62.
35. Shifra Shvarts, "Health Reform in Israel: Seventy Years of Struggle," *Social History of Medicine*, 11:1 (1998).
36. Membership Report, 17 Sept. 1937, 1–14, Kupat Holim portfolio, ALM, IV–208–1578.
37. Yoman Ben-Gurion (Ben-Gurion's diary), 25 March 1932, Ben-Gurion Heritage Institute Archive, 78.
38. *Alon Hapoel Hamizrachi* (The Mizrachi Bulletin), 4 April 1937.
39. Hatza'at ha-Poel ha-Mizrachi be-Davar Mas Achid (The proposal of Hapoel Hamizrachi concerning a joint dues), 27 June 1938, ALM, B, IV–208–1505.
40. Helkam shel Hevrei ha-Poel ha-Mizrachi be-Hachnasot ve-Hotzaot Kupat Holim (The portion of members of Hapoel Hamizrachi in revenue and expenditures of Kupat Holim), 1 January 1939, ALM, IV–208–2094; *Davar*, 22 January 1936, 1.
41. In 2002 Kupat Holim's share of members in Israel society is 56% (about 3.6 million members), and Macabi's share is 26% (about 1.5 million members).
42. Memorandum, 24 May 1938. The Federation of Labor Secretariat portfolio, ALM, IV–208–1502B.
43. Ibid.
44. Hozer al Darkei Kabalat Haverim Hadashim le-Histadrut vele-Kupat Holim (Circular on avenues for acceptance of new members to the Federation and Kupat Holim), 10 November 1939, ALM, IV–208–2094.
45. Ibid.

Notes to Epilogue

1. Operating "against all economic logic"—taking a leap of faith on vision alone, or, in Zionist parlance, "to make something out of nothing"—is endemic to Zionist culture. It was a common thread in many Zionist institutions and the mindset of those Jews who opted to go to Eretz Israel when the vast majority of Jews emigrating from Europe were heading for America—the "logical" choice, in economic terms
2. Even under the Compulsory Health Insurance system (enacted 1995), deficits and the inability to collect "dues" from everyone continue to plague the system, which is still caught between "needs" and "abilities"—though now the issue is not political but rather the rising cost of health care and public demand for access to expensive diagnostics and treatments, coupled with the government's inability to enforce the levy in a comprehensive manner or mobilize enough funding from the public to really cover the "basket of services" promised. It is a problem common to all Western health systems.

Glossary

Persons

Ahad Ha'am (Asher Ginsberg, 1856–1927), Hebrew essayist, leader of Lovers of Zion movement, was born in Ukraine and settled in Tel Aviv in 1922. One of the most influential of modern Jewish thinkers, he wrote many works on Judaism, its thoughts and philosophy. He expounded his views in favor of "cultural" rather than "political" Zionism.

Yaakov Aphter (1894–1969), Labor pioneer in Eretz Israel, was born in Kishiniev, and settled in Eretz Israel 1913 as an agricultural worker in kibbutz Degania. One of the founders of Kupat Holim and its first secretary, he was also a member of the Federation of Labor Executive Committee (1921–1930), a leading member in Mapai party, and a member in the National Committee. Aphter was the founder of Hamashbir Company and directed it for many years.

Dr. Chaim Arlosoroff (1899–1933), Zionist labor leader; born in Ukraine, joined Hapoel Hatzair in Germany and soon became one of its leaders. He advocated synthesis of Marxism and Practical Jewish settlement in Eretz Israel, and also believed in cooperation between Arabs and Jewish national movements. He settled in Tel Aviv 1924, and became head of the Jewish Agency political department. He was assassinated by unknown assailants on a Tel Aviv beach in 1933.

Moshe Beilenson (1899–1936), Hebrew writer, journalist, physician, and a chief spokesman for the Labor movement in Eretz Israel, was born in Russia, settled in Tel Aviv in 1924, joined the editorial board of *Davar,* and wrote most of its editorials. He chaired the Kupat Holim Supervisory Committee 1929–1936.

David Ben-Gurion (1886–1973), Israel statesman, born in Plonsk (then Russian Poland), settled in Eretz Israel in 1906. Exiled by the Turks in 1915, he went to the U.S., became active in the formation of the Jewish battalion, and returned to Eretz Israel in 1918 as a soldier in the Jewish Legion. He helped found the Achdut ha-Avoda party (1919), which in 1930 merged with Hapoel ha-Tzair to form the Mapai, which he headed. Ben-Gurion was secretary general of Histadruth 9 (1921–1933), chairman of Jewish Agency Executive (1935–1948), and headed the group that drew up the Biltmore Program in 1942. In April 1948 he headed the

People's Council, which—largely on his initiative— proclaimed the rebirth of the independent Jewish nation on May 14,1948. He was Israel's first prime minister and minister of defense, serving until 1963.

Yitzhak Ben Zvi (1884–1963), labor leader, scholar, second president of Israel (1952–1963), was born in Poltava, Ukraine where, with B. Borochov, founded the Poalei Zion Party. Active in self-defense organization, he settled in Eretz Israel (1907), where he became chairman and president of Vaad Leumi (the National Committee), and founded the Institute of Study of Oriental Jewish Communities in the Middle East (1948), which became the Ben Zvi Institute in 1952.

Ada Fishman-Maimon (1893–1973), was born in Russia, settled in Eretz Israel in 1912, became secretary general of the Women Workers' council (1921–1930), and was a leading authority on women rights in Eretz Israel and, after 1948, in the state of Israel.

Avraham Hartzfeld (1888–1973), was a Labor pioneer in Eretz Israel. Born in Ukraine, he became a member of Russian Socialist Zionist party, sentenced to life imprisonment in Siberia, and escaped to Eretz Israel 1914. A founder of Histadruth, he played a major role in planning the agricultural settlement and personally participated in establishment of almost every new settlement. He was a member of the Mapai Knesset 1949–1959.

Theodore Herzel (1860–1904), father of political Zionism, journalist, and founder of the World Zionist Organization, was born in Budapest and received a Doctor of Law from Vienna in 1884. Spurred by the Dreyfus Case he began Zionist activities in 1895. In 1896 he wrote the pamphlet "The Jewish State" containing his Zionist program. He established the Jewish National Fund and Jewish Colonial Trust, and in 1902 published a utopian novel, *Altneuland* (Old-new land), in which he described the building of a new Jewish State in Palestine. Herzel died while controversy over the Uganda Scheme (see below) still raged. Buried in Vienna, his body was reinterred on Mt. Herzel in Jerusalem, 1949.

Dov Hos (1894–1940), Labor leader in Eretz Israel, he founded Achduth ha Avoda (United Labor) Party in 1919, and was active in Histadruth and Haganah. In 1931 he visited Britain to make contract with the Labor Party. He was Deputy Mayor of Tel Aviv (1935–1940) and brother in law of Moshe Sharett. Hos was killed with his wife and daughter in a road accident.

Zeev Jabotinsky (1880–1940), Zionist leader, soldier, orator and writer, was born in Russia, studied law in Rome, and became correspondent of the Odessa newspaper under the pen name "Altalena." He organized the first self-defense league in Eretz Israel (in the riot of 1920), formed and headed World Zionist Revisionists in 1925, seceded from the Zionist movement (1935), and established a new Zionist organization. He was the ideological leader of the right-wing Revisionist movement (today the Likud party in Israel).

Rose Gell Jacobs (1888–1975), U.S. Zionist leader, was president of Hadassah 1930–1932, 1934–1937, and a member of Executive of Jewish Agency for Palestine 1937–1946.

Dr. Avraham Katznelson-(Nissan) (1888–1956), Labor politician in Eretz Israel, Israel diplomat, and physician, was born in Byelorussia, settled in Eretz Israel in 1924, and directed the health department of the Zionist Executive 1931–1948. He was a member of the Mapai party, and the Israel Minister to Scandinavian countries 1950–1956.

Berl Katznelson (1887–1944), Zionist labor leader, was born in Russia, and settled in Eretz Israel in 1909, where he worked as laborer and became secretary of Council of Judean Farm workers. He served in the Jewish legion 1918–1920. He was instrumental in establishing Histadrut in 1920; in 1925 he founded Histadrut's daily newspaper, *Davar*, of which he was chief editor until his death. In addition, he was a director of the Jewish National Fund, and established Am Oved Publishing house, serving as editor-in-chief.

Yitzhak Kenivsky-Kenev (1896–1979), Zionist labor leader, was born in Russia and settled in Eretz Israel in 1919. He was one of the founders of Hechalutz (Zionist-pioneer) movement, the founder of the Institute for Social Sciences Research of the Federation of Labor, instrumental in establishing Kupat Holim and a member of its board of directors for many years. Kenivsky was a leading authority and activist in Social Security legislation in the pre-state period. He was the founder of the Israel National Security Institute and the power behind the Israel Social Security Act (1954).

Israel Jacob Kleigler (1889–1944), Eretz Israel bacteriologist, was born in Ukraine, settled in Eretz Israel 1920, and became a leading figure in public health and malaria control.

Irma Lindheim-Levy (1886–1975), U. S. Zionist leader, was president of Hadassah 1826–1928. She joined the Labor Zionist group in 1930, and settled in Eretz Israel in 1933 at kibbutz *Mishmar Ha-Emek* (The valley guards).

Judah Leon Magnes (1877–1948), U.S. reform rabbi, communal leader; Eretz Israel educator, was the moving spirit and leading figure of Kehillah of New York. His opposition to U.S. entry into the First World War out of pacifist convictions undermined his leadership in Jewish community.

He was chancellor of Hebrew University in Jerusalem 1925–1935. Believing in establishment of Eretz Israel as bi-national state, he sought accord between Arabs and Jews.

Golda Meirson-Meir (1898–1978), Israel prime minister (1969-1974), Labor leader, was born in Kiev, emigrated to U.S. in 1906, and settled in Eretz Israel in 1921. She was secretary of the women workers' council, a member of the Federation of Labor Executive Committee, a member in the Israeli parliament (1949–1974), Minister of Labor (1949–1956), Minister of Foreign Affairs (1956–1965), and Secretary General of Israel Labor Party .

Sir Moses Montefiore (1784–1885), born in Italy, emigrated to England in 1744. Montefiore visited Palestine seven times, donated money to open schools for girls and workshops for boys, supported special educational programs for poor children, and opened a clinic to provide medical services to the Jewish community in Jerusalem.

Yitzhak Max Rubinow (1875–1936), Russian-born economist, physician, and socialist, concluded his medical studies in New York. He was secretary of B'nai B'rith (1929–1936) and leader of the movement for employee rights and social and health insurance in the United States, and the first director of the Hadassah Medical Unit in Eretz Israel (1918-1922).

Harry Sacker (1881–1971), British Zionist, lawyer, came to Eretz Israel in 1919, served on the Zionist Executive 1927–1931, and returned to England in1932.

Moshe Sharret-Shertok (1894–1965), Zionist leader, second prime minister of Israel, was born in Ukraine and settled in Eretz Israel in 1906. Head of the Jewish Agency's political department (1933–1948), he was also Israel's first foreign minister until 1956, and chairman of the Executive of the Zionist Organization and the Jewish Agency, 1960–1965.

Reuven Shenkar (1896–1965), Labor Federation and Hechalutz movement activist, was born in Russia and settled in Eretz Israel in 1920. He was a member of the Kupat Holim central committee and the treasurer of the fund for many years.

Nachum Sokolov (1859–1936), Hebrew writer, Zionist, journalist, and editor of the Hebrew newspaper Ha-Olam [The world], he was the second secretary-general of World Zionist Organization in 1906. In London in the First World War he was involved in Zionist political activity and efforts to obtain the Balfour Declaration. He was chairman of the Jewish Agency Executive 1929, and president of World Zionist Organization 1931–1935.

Dr. David de Sola-Pool (1885–1970), U.S. rabbi of Sephardic congregation in New York, he founded and directed the Jewish education committee of New York (1922), was president of the Synagogue Council of America (1938–1940), and wrote on U.S. Jewish history and religion.

Captain Joseph Trumpeldor (1880–1920), pioneer, soldier, Zionist, he studied dentistry but volunteered for the Russian army, losing an arm in fighting at Port Arthur 1904–5. He went to Eretz Israel in 1912, but returned to Russia in 1917 to start the Hechalutz movement. He returned to Eretz Israel in 1919, organizing the defense of Jewish settlements in Upper Galilee, and was killed in defense of kibbutz Tel Hai (Israel-Lebanon border). Trumpeldor became the symbol of pioneering and armed defense in Eretz Israel. He is known for his saying "It is good to die for one's country."

Menachem Ussiskin (1863–1941), a Zionist leader born in Russia, became secretary of Lovers of Zion. In one of his pamphlets he laid the foundations for "Synthetic Zionism," which later dominated the Zionist movement. He led opposition to the Uganda Scheme in 1903, represented Russian Jewry at Paris peace conference, settled in Jerusalem 1919, and became a member of the Zionist Executive. From 1923 he chaired the Jewish national Fund, and was responsible for purchasing wide tracts of land, especially in Jezreel Valley.

Dr. Hillel Yafe [Joffe] (1864–1936), Eretz Israel pioneer doctor, was born in Ukraine, studied in Geneva, and settled in Eretz Israel in 1891. He practiced medicine and organized the anti-malaria service; on his advice eucalyptus tress were planted in swamps. He served as chairman of the Lovers of Zion executive committee 1895–1905.

Dr. Chaim Yaski (1896–1948), Ophthalmologist, medical administrator in Eretz Israel, was born in Kishinev and settled in Eretz Israel in 1919 as director of the Hadassah Medical Organization and Hadassah hospital (1931–1948). He was killed by Arabs in the massacre of a Scopus convoy.

Agencies, Movements, and Organizations

Aliya (immigration). Any of five waves of Jewish immigration to Palestine: First (1882–1903), Second (1903–1914), Third (1919–1923), Fourth (1924–1928), Fifth (1933–1939).

Achduth Haavoda (United work). Socialist-Zionist Party established in Palestine in 1919, headed by David Ben-Gurion.

Am Oved (Working nation). The publishing house of the Labor Federation, founded by Berl Katznelson in 1942.

Ammamit Sick Fund. Today the United Sick Fund, the third biggest sick fund in Israel. It was established by the Hadassah Medical Organization in 1930 in order to provide medical aid to the non-socialists sectors such as the landowners/farmers etc.

Bank Hapoalim (The workers' bank). Israel's leading commercial bank, established 1923 by the Federation of Labor.

Betar. Zionist youth movement founded in 1923 by Union of Zionist Revisionists, its ideology based on Revisionism. It established settlements in Eretz Israel and engaged illegal alyia. It also developed the Betar Sports Organization.

Bilu movement. An acronym for "*Beit Ya'akov, lehu venelha*" (O House of Jacob, come, let us go—Isaiah 2:5), *Bilu* was an association founded by young Jews in Kharkov, Russia, after the pogroms of 1881–82. Its members advocated aliya, settlement in Palestine, and revival of the Hebrew language. The first group of thirteen men and one girl reached Jaffa in the summer of 1882 and formed the nucleus of First Alyia.

Bund (General Jewish workers' union). Jewish socialist party in Lithuania, Poland, and Russia, founded in Russia in 1897, and particularly influential in Russia between 1905 and 1920. The Bund was committed to Yiddish autonomism and secular Jewish nationalism, and sharply opposed Zionism and other conceptions of a word-embracing Jewish national identity.

Eretz Israel. The geographical region of the present State of Israel which has been called in the past one-hundred years by several names: The Jerusalem Region during the Ottoman period until 1918; Palestine during the British Mandate years 1918–1948, and Eretz Israel (the biblical name of the Holy Land) by the Jewish communities in Israel and abroad. For simplicity, the common name Eretz Israel is used through out the book, both for the Ottoman and for the British periods.

The Eretz Israel Office (The Palestine office). A Zionist Institution established in Jaffa in 1908, headed by Arthur Rupin. It was a central agency for pro-Zionist settlement activities after the First World War, aiding land purchase and immigration.

Hachalutz (The pioneer). Jewish Zionist Socialist movement, established in the U.S. in 1915 and in Poland in 1917, which organized immigration of young Jews to Palestine with the mission to return to the soil of the Land of Israel, become tillers of the land in the service of the nation, and established settlements and workers' cooperative groups

HaNoar HaOved (The working youth movement). The Federation of Labor's youth movement for boys and girls aged 9–18, founded in 1926. It provided founding groups for forty kibbutzim and was the biggest youth movement in Israel with over 150,000 members.

Hapoel Hamizrachi Federation (The eastern worker). Zionist religious pioneering and labor movement founded 1922 in Jerusalem that established settlements, a sports organization (Elitzur), and the Benei Akiva youth movement. It merged with Mizrachi in 1956 and founded the National Religious Party, MAFDAL.

Hapoel Hatzair (The young worker). Populist party established in Palestine in 1905. It published a paper by the same name.

Histadruth (General federation of Jewish workers in Palestine). A labor organization founded in 1920 that came to embrace almost all Jewish workers in Palestine.

Jewish Colonization Association (JCA). A philanthropic association to assist needy Jews or, in countries of persecution, to help them emigrate and settle elsewhere in productive employment. It was founded by Baron Maurice de Hirsh in 1891, and established agricultural colonies in Eretz Israel.

The Jewish Agency. The executive body and representative of World Zionist Organization. Its authority and functions were the first to be recognized by the British Mandate over Palestine.

The Jewish Legion. A military formation of Jewish volunteers in the First World Watr who fought in the British army for liberation of Eretz Israel .

JOINT (JDC). The American Jewish Joint distribution committee, American Jewry's overseas relief and rehabilitation agency. Established 1914, it carried out rescue and relief work during and after both world wars, especially for Jews in East and Central Europe.

Knesset Israel. The Jewish community assembly during the British Mandate period.

"Linat Tzedek". Free overnight lodging organized by the community for night-watching sick members of the community. Linat Tzedek was an essential institution of Jewish communities since the middle ages.

Lovers of Zion movement. A movement and ideology whose aim was national renaissance of Jews and their return to Eretz Israel. It came into being in Russia in 1882 as a reaction to the 1881 pogroms and flourished mainly in the large Jewish communities of East Europe.

National Committee. The supreme institution of the organized Jewish community in Eretz Israel and the executive body of the elected assembly. The Committee was founded in 1920. Its departments included Health, Education, Welfare Services, Rabbinate, and Political.

Passfield White Paper. A British government statement of policy presented to parliament that played an important part in history of Mandatory Palestine. Six such documents were issued between 1922 and 1939 dealing with British Policy in Eretz Israel. The sixth paper (1939) restricted Jewish immigration and land purchase.

Poalei Zion (Workers of Zion). The Marxist Zionist party, influenced by the thinking of Berr Borochov; established in Russia in 1906 following the October Revolution.

Shaw Commission. One of a number of commissions of inquiry sent to Palestine by the British government during the Mandate period, both to investigate the roots of the conflict between the Jews and the Arabs and to propose guidelines for British policy in Palestine. Most of the commissions were appointed following riots and disturbances. The different commissions and reports were named after their chairs/directors.

Solel Boneh. A Histadruth concern for building, public works, and industry. It played large role in development of the state of Israel, and was also active in construction work in other countries.

The Templers. A German sect that founded settlements in Eretz Israel in the nineteenth and twentieth centuries to realize apocalyptic vision of the prophets. They established residential quarters in Haifa, Jerusalem, and Jaffa as well as in the four colonies. In the First World War they were repatriated to Germany.

Uganda Plan (Uganda Scheme). The name commonly given to the proposal made by the British government to the Zionist organization to establish an autonomous Jewish colony in British East Africa (now Kenya). The scheme was strongly opposed in the Sixth Zionist Congress (1903) when introduced by Herzel, and was finally rejected at the Seventh Congress after Herzel's death in 1904.

World Zionist Organization (WZO). The worldwide official organization of Zionist movement founded on the initiative of Herzel in 1897.

Yishuv. the name given the Jewish community in Israel by its people during the Ottoman and the British periods. "Yishuv" means in Hebrew a place or a settlement. This term is used through out the book as equivalent to the term Jewish Community.

Zionism. A movement founded in Europe in 1897 advocating the return of Jews to Zion (Israel), and working the land (becoming farmers and agricultural workers).

Zionist Congress. The supreme institution and legislature of the World Zionist Organization, which oversees the organization's institutions. It meets every four years to formulate policy and elect officials. It has approximately 600 delegates, 38% Israelis, 29% from the U.S. and 3% from the rest of the world.

Works Cited

Primary and Archival Sources

Ben Gurion Archives, Sede Boker, Israel.
Lavon Institute, Israel Labor Archives, Tel Aviv (ALM).
Central Zionist Archives, Jerusalem (CZA).
Hadassah Archives, New York, N.Y.
Tel Aviv-Jaffa Municipality Historical Archives, Tel Aviv (TJMH).
American Association for Labor Legislation Archives, Cornell University, Ithaca, N.Y.

Books

Aaronson, R. *ha-Baron veha-Moshavot* (The baron and the villages). Jerusalem, 1990.

Atias, M. *Sefer ha-Teudot shel ha-Vaad ha-Leumi* (Book of documents of the National Committee). Jerusalem, 1963.

Becker, A. *Im Hazman Ubnei Hador* (Of time and men). Tel Aviv, 1982.

Ben-Artzi, Y. *ha-Moshava ha-Ivrit ba-Nof Eretz Israel 1882–1914* (The Hebrew village on the Eretz Israel landscape 1882–1914). Jerusalem, 1988.

Ben-Gurion, D. *Hapoel ha-Ivri ve-Histadruteno* (The Hebrew worker and his federation). 2nd ed. Tel Aviv, 1964.

Efrati, N. *me-Mashbare le-Tikva , ha-Yishuv ha-Yehudi ba-Eretz Israel be-Milchemet ha-Olam ha-Rishona* (From crisis to hope: The Jewish Yishuv in Eretz Israel in the First World War). Jerusalem, 1991.

Eliav, M. *Eretz Israel ve-Yishuva be-Mea ha-19* (Eretz Israel and its settlement in the 19th century). Jerusalem, 1978.

Even-Shoshan, T. *Toldot Tnuat ha-Poalim be-Eretz Israel* (History of the labor movement in Eretz Israel). Tel Aviv, 1963.

Fein, G. *Eetot Sufa* (Stormy time). Jerusalem, 1980.

Gelber, Y. *Moledet Hadasha* (homeland). Jerusalem, 1990.

Giladi, D. *ha-Yishuv be-Tkufat ha-Aliyah ha-Rivi'it* (The Yishuv in the period of the Fourth Aliyah). Tel Aviv, 1973.

Hadassah Medical Federation, *Esrim Shnot Hadassah be-Eretz Israel* (Twenty years of Hadassah in Eretz Israel). Jerusalem, 1939.

Havas, B., ed. *Sefer ha-Aliya ha-Shniya* (The Second Aliyah book). Tel Aviv, 1947.

Katznelson, B. *Igrot 1915–1918* (Letters 1915–1918). Tel Aviv, 1961.

Kenivsky-Kenev, Y. *ha-Bituch ha-Sotziali be-Eretz Israel ve-Hesegav oo-Biyotav* (Social insurance in Eretz Israel: Its achievements and problems). Tel Aviv, 1941–42.

Kutcher, C. B. "The Early Years of Hadassah, 1912-1921." Ph.D. diss. Brandeis University, 1976.

Laqueur, W. *A History of Zionism*. London: Weidenfeld & Nicolson, 1972.

Mendelberg, A. *Tafkidey Kupat Holim* (Kupat Holim's roles). Kupat Holim directorate. Tel Aviv, 1924–25.

Miller, Donald. "A History of Hadassah 1912–1935." Ph.D. diss. New York University, 1986.

Slutzky, Y. *Mavo le-Toldot Tnuat ha-Avodah ha-Yisraelit* (Introduction to the history of the Israeli labor movement). Tel Aviv, 1983.

Reicher, M. *ha-Telem ha-Acharon* (The Last furrow). Beit Neta, 1966.

Roemer, M. I. *National Health Systems of the World*. Vol. 1. Ann Arbor: Oxford University Press, 1993.

———. *Health Care Systems in World Perspective*. Ann Arbor, 1976.

Shapira, A. *Berl*. Tel Aviv, 1983.

Shapira, Y. *Avodah ve-Adama* (Toil and soil). Tel Aviv, 1961.

Shryock, H. R. *The Development of Modern Medicine*. Madison: University of Wisconsin Press,1979.

Tevet, S. *Kin'at David* (David's envy). Jerusalem and Tel Aviv, 1982.

Tzachor, Z. *Shorshei ha-Politika ha-Yisraelit* (The roots of Israeli politics). Hakibbutz Hameuchad and Ben-Gurion University, 1987.

———. *ba-Deresh le-Hanhagat ha-Yishuv* (On the road to leadership of the Yishuv). Jerusalem, 1982.

Yafe, H. *Dor ha-Maapilim* (The generation of clandestine immigration). Tel Aviv, 1939.

Zartal, I. *Yamim oo-Maasim* (Days and deeds). Tel Aviv, 1975.

Articles in Periodicals

Aphter, Y. "Kupat Holim shel Poalei Yehuda be-Milchemet ha-Olam ha-Rishona" (The Judea workers' sick fund in the First World War). *be-Sha'ah Zu* (At this hour). A (1916): 33–40.

Dinburg (Dinur), B. "Eretz Israel be-Shnot Tarpag" (Eretz Israel in the year 1922–23). *me-Shanah le-Shanah* (1923):294–97.

Gorny, Y. "Shinuim ba-Mivneh ha-Chevrati veha-Politi shel ha-Aliayah ha-Shniya" (Changes in the social and political structure of the Second Aliyah). *Hatzionut* (Zionism). A (1970): 205–28.

Grey, M. "Poverty, Politics and Health: The Farm Security Administration Medical Care Program, 1935–1945." *Journal of the History of Medicine and Allied Sciences,* 44 (1989): 320–50.

Harpaz, Ch. "Bituch Briut me-B'chna Historit Kalkalit" (Health insurance from a historical economic standpoint). *Dapim Refuim* (1959): 245–51.

Kottek, S. "The Essenes and Medicine." *Clio Medica*, 18 (1983): 93–95.

Levi, N. "Doctor Shimon Frankel (1880–1809) ha-Rofe ha-Ivri ha-Rishon be-Eretz Israel" (Dr. Shimon Frankel [1880–1809]: the first Jewish doctor in Eretz Israel). *Harefuah*, 118 (1990): 490–91.

Nadav, D. "Inyan shel Chaim ve-Mavet" (A matter of life and death). *BaGilboa,* 172 (Nov., 1989): 25–34.

Netherland, D. "Hashpaat ha-Rofim ha-Olim me-Germania al Hitpatchut ha-Refua ba-Aretz ba-Shanim 1933–1948" (The impact of immigrant doctors from Germany on the development of medicine in Eretz Israel in 1933–1948). *Cathedra,* 30 (1983): 111–60.

Shvarts, S. "Eidatiut, Dat ve-Politika be-Hakamat Batei ha-Cholim ha-Yehudiim ba-Yerushaliyim ba-Meah ha-19" (Ethnicity, religion and politics in establishment of hospitals in Jerusalem in the 19th century). *Korot*, 9 (1988): 232–42.

———. "Health Reform in Israel: Seventy Years of Struggle." *Social History of Medicine*, 11:1 (1998): 73–88.

Shvarts, S., T. Brown. "Kupat Holim, Dr. Isaac Max Rubinow and the American Zionist Medical Unit's Experiment to Establish Health Care Services in Palestine 1918–1923." *Bulletin of the History of Medicine*, 72 (1998): 28–46.

Index

A

Achad Ha'am, 19, 319
Achdut Haavodah, 82-8, 91, 93, 96, 98-9, 178-9, 183-5, 266
Acre, 79, 215, 323
Afula, 158, 164, 202, 206, 209-211, 216-7, 262, 268
Aliya (First to Fifth), 13, 17, 19-24, 28, 30, 35, 45, 52-3, 68, 75, 98-9, 105, 113-5, 124, 162-3, 169, 228-9, 275-6, 291-4, 323
America, 53, 71-2, 141-2, 188, 198, 205, 208
American Zionist Medical Aid Unit (AZMU), 73, 75, 87,171, 177, 180-1, 183, 188
see also Hadassah Medical Federation
Ammamit Health Fund, 267, 270, 273, 276, 290, 324
Aphter, Yaakov, 43, 57, 60-4, 66, 84, 90, 94, 96, 101, 184, 319
Arab, 9, 12, 15-6, 18-9, 21, 40, 68, 78-9, 81, 141-2, 160, 201, 213-4, 216, 219-220, 226, 228, 236, 239-240, 242-3, 246-7, 251, 255
Arlosoroff, Chaim, 219, 220-1, 240-1, 244-6, 271, 319
Arza Convalescence, 104, 158
Ashkenazi Jews, 7, 11, 18
Austria, 11, 52, 56
Ayelet Hashachar, 117,118
AZA, 46-7

B

Bader, David, 33, 42
Balforia, 103, 118
Balfour Declaration, 69-70, 226, 306n18
Balfour, Lord, 69-70, 226
Banks (Hapoalim, Anglo-Palestine, Leumi), 126-8, 324
Baratz, Yosef, 134, 151-2, 156, 245
Barshira-Bashrovker, Israel, 225, 232
Basel, 138, 209, 257
Bavli, Eliezer, 128, 131
Beer Sheva, 61, 79, 215
Beer Yaakov, 32
Beilinson, Moshe, 134-5, 140, 153, 156-9, 161-2, 220-2, 233, 245, 264-6, 269-270, 298, 319
Beirut, 8
Beit Alfa, 103, 108, 118, 204, 209
Beit, Kibbutz, 119-120
Beker, Aharon, 278-9
Belkind, Alexandra, 12, 57
Ben Gurion, David, 94-5, 99-100, 102, 105-111, 121-2, 166, 174-5, 179, 188, 199, 227, 232, 245-7, 251, 259, 261, 264, 269-272, 278, 280, 283, 294, 296, 319
Ben-Artzi, Yossi, 16
Ben-Shemen, 28, 31-4, 58
Ben-Zion, Gat, 8
Ben-Zion, Hershovitz, 106, 108, 202-4, 213, 218, 222
Ben-Zvi, Yitzhak, 118, 323

Berginsky, Tzila, 57
Berlin, 46, 140
Berwald, Alexander, 212
Betar, 270-1
Bialik, Chaim Nachman, 295
Bilu movement, 13, 22, 324
Birchiyahu, Chana, 57
Birchiyahu, Mordechai, 57
Bismarck, Auto Von, 49, 51-2, 198
Bismark health plan, 51-2
Bluestone, Efraim, 196-7, 199-201, 205, 207-9, 212
Brandeis, Louis, 71
Britain (U.K.), 69, 139, 208, 226, 229, 239
British (army, Health authorities, Parliament, royal family), 10, 48, 67, 69-70, 73-4, 77, 79-80, 92, 114, 188, 220, 240
see also England
Briut HaOved, 117, 143, 230

C

Carlsbad, 188-9, 194
Carmel, 104, 158
Central Europe, 46, 276
Chancellor, Sir, Robert John, 174, 226
Chenkin, Yehoshua, 98
China, 205
Cholera, 9, 17-9
Christians, 8-9, 57
Cohen, Hugo, 203
Collective general health fund committee, 68
committees (for Afula, of community emissaries, of Delegates, to Ease the Crisis), 9, 56, 70-1, 73-4, 85-6, 88-9, 180-2, 185, 210-1
Contras, newspaper, 83, 91, 148, 178, 182, 184
Convalescence, 14, 36, 84-87, 104, 115, 127, 134, 144, 58, 236
see also Arza and Carmel
Crimean War, 11

D

Davar, newspaper, 123, 132, 134-5, 137, 146-7, 174, 232, 265, 283, 286
Dead Sea, 47, 164, 274
Defoe, Daniel, 49
Degani, Eliyahu, 99, 102
Degani, Yaakov, 184-5
Degania, Kibbutz, 134, 151
Degania-B, Kibbutz, 117
Dentistry Clinics, 73
Disturbances (1921, 1929, 1936-9), 310n40, 312n10
Dizengoff, Meir, 55
Druze, 9
dysentery, 60

E

East Europe, 13, 46-7, 52, 201
Egypt, 9, 56, 77-8, 80, 86
Ein Ganim, 28-9, 40, 267
Ein Gedi, 47
Ein Harod, 98, 101, 103-7, 109-112, 118, 121, 140, 154, 172-3, 193, 202-4, 206, 209-10, 212-3, 216-7, 293, 295
Elbinger, Y., 98
Eliav, Mordechai, 10
Elimelach, David, 262
Elkind, Menachem, 105
England, 9, 47-50, 53, 56, 80, 92
see also British
epidemics (Malaria, Smallpox, Typhus, yellow fever), 8-9, 14, 17-9, 24, 43, 50-1, 60-1, 73, 68, 78-9, 81,

86-7, 90, 104, 106, 112, 136, 179-180, 191, 202, 217-8, 220, 297
Eretz Israel Office, 12, 37-8, 43-4, 58-9, 61-2, 324
Eretzisraeli-Gavrieli, Chaim, 94, 225, 232
Ettinger, Akiva, 59
Europe, 7, 9, 13, 16, 36, 45, 47, 49-50, 52-3, 55, 88, 102, 152, 230, 232, 293
see also East Europe
see also West Europe
Executive Committee, 19, 94-7, 100-1, 103, 105-111, 117-123, 126-7, 134, 136, 138, 151, 165-6, 209, 230-2, 234-5, 237, 243, 251-3, 261-4, 266-8, 271, 278-9, 287-8, 290, 295

F

Farm governing committee, 122-3
Federation of Agricultural Workers, 28, 39, 93
Federation of Labor, 39, 42, 65, 68-9, 92, 94-103, 105, 107-111, 113, 115-6, 119, 124-5, 130, 132, 134-6, 141, 144, 146-7, 149-155, 157, 160-7, 175, 183, 185-6, 193-4, 197-9, 201-2, 204, 209, 224-8, 230-5, 237, 241-5, 247-254, 256-7, 259-269, 271-4, 276-287, 289-290, 292-9
see also Histadruth
First World War, 7, 16, 20, 28, 39, 44, 55, 60-73, 75, 77, 82, 84, 89, 113, 188, 196, 249-250, 291
Fishman-Maimon, Ada, 270, 285, 320
France, 11, 47, 56
Frankel, Shimon, 10
Freiber, Baruch, 28, 31
Froise, Walter, 232
FSA, 45

G

Galilee Agricultural Workers Federation, 29
Galilee Worker's Federation, 65
Galilee, 7, 13, 18, 23, 28, 31, 39, 60, 64-7, 78, 82, 91, 98, 180, 191, 215, 217-8, 249
Gaza, 18, 56-7, 61, 79, 215
Gelber, Yoav, 275
Geneva, 232
Germany, 10, 47, 49-52, 55-6, 203, 229, 246, 273-6
Glicker, 153, 156, 158, 160, 212, 233
Goldberg-Harpaz, Neta, 23, 31, 134, 271
Gorny, Yosef, 20
Governing Committee, 11-2, 16, 18, 21-3
government health department, 214
Gutmann Yunis, Bat Sheva, 12, 57

H

Ha'hashkafa, newspaper, 18
Haaretz, newspaper, 182
Hachalutz movement, 83, 99, 324
Hadassah Medical Federation, 77-8, 171, 188, 200, 207-8, 238
see also American Zionist Medical Aid Unit
Hadassah, 70-3, 76, 85, 100, 104, 114, 116, 121, 131-2, 137-142, 145, 147, 150-1, 153, 156, 159, 162, 164, 177-201, 203-9, 211-2,

216, 222, 224, 227-8, 255-6, 267, 269-270, 272, 275, 292
Hadera, 14, 24, 36, 42, 58, 99, 102, 270, 272
Haifa, 15, 20, 73, 75-6, 78-80, 93, 96, 101, 104, 112, 144, 155, 160, 164, 191, 197, 199-200, 203-4, 206, 210, 215, 217, 233, 262, 272
"Haluka" (Allocation), 8, 31
Hamashbir, 67-8, 96, 106, 127, 251, 296
Hammel, Russia, 20
HaNoar HaOved (Working Youth Movement), 277, 325
Hapoel Hamizrachi, 125, 225, 256-8, 270, 277, 286-7, 325
Hapoel Hatzair, 25-6, 43, 53, 77, 82-5, 88, 90-1, 93, 96, 98-9, 134, 177, 182-4, 250, 266, 270, 325
Hapoel Hatzair, newspaper, 27, 66, 83, 86, 146, 151, 181, 195
Harpaz, Chaim, 47, 48, 52
Hartzfeld, Avraham, 61, 64, 84, 94, 97-8, 104-5, 182, 320
Hashomer, 40
Hasneh, Insurance Company, 146
He'achdut, newspaper, 53
Health Fund (Committee, International Organization, Law, Office, Workers), 25, 27, 30, 33, 42-3, 53, 55, 77, 83, 87, 113, 159, 192, 199, 213
Hebrew (Israel) Medical Federation, 7, 12, 34, 39, 41, 57, 59, 77, 178
Hebrew Doctors Association of America, 205
Hebrew Medical Society in Eretz Israel (Medical Federation), 59
Hebron, 7, 9, 79, 226
Herzel, Theodore, 320
Herron, Colonel G. W., 77-8, 82, 219-220, 227, 238, 240-2, 244
Hewachdut, newspaper, 31-2
Hissin, Haim, 12
Histadruth, 325
Hoffman, 57
Holland, 47
Hope-Simpson, John, 226
Hos, Dov, 239-241, 245-6, 320
Hospital, "Beth David," 196
"Bikur Holim," 11, 46, 52, 75, 293
"Emek," 174, 202, 205, 208-9, 212, 214-8, 220-4, 240, 248, 276, 292
"Ezrat Nashim," 11
"Linat Tzedek," 8, 22, 35, 46, 52-3, 293
"Misgav Ladach," 11, 75
"Mount Sinai," 196
"Shaarei Tzedek," 11, 75
Government, 75, 79-80
Hadassah, 75-6, 85-6, 144, 191-2, 198-9, 201, 204-5, 214, 217, 292
in Acre, 215
in Afula, 164, 206, 217
in Beer-Sheva, 215
in Gaza, 56-7, 215
in Hadera, 24
in Haifa, 73, 75-6, 80, 197, 199-200, 203-4, 206, 215, 217
in Jaffa, 24, 30, 33, 61-2, 75, 215
in Jerusalem, 16, 76, 208
in Jezreel Valley, 76, 101, 140, 158, 201, 204-6, 208, 211, 219, 292
in Kibbutz Ein-Harod, 101, 103-4, 106-7, 109, 111-2, 140, 173, 193, 202-4, 209-210, 212-3
in Nablus, 215
in Petach Tikva (Beilenson), 76, 223, 248, 276
in Safed, 73, 75, 191
in Tel-Aviv, 76, 197, 215

in Tiberias, 73, 75, 191, 195, 205
in Zichron Yaakov, 16, 24, 66-7
Jewish, 75-6
Ophthorities, 80
Rothschild, 11, 73, 75
Shaar Zion Community, 11-2, 17, 25, 29-30, 43, 58, 60, 73, 75, 87
workers, 101, 103-4, 106-7, 109, 111-2, 140, 173, 193, 202-4, 209-210, 212-3
see also Hospital in Kibbutz Ein-Harod
Hulda, 28, 32, 62

I

Insurance (health, compulsory, dis bility, medical, obligatory, social), 36, 39, 45, 51-3, 54, 88-9, 91, 102, 125, 139, 143-4, 147, 149, 152, 158-9, 161-2, 164, 157, 223-6, 228-230, 231-2, 234-246, 248, 259, 265-6, 268, 280-1, 285, 290-1, 293-5, 298, 304n36, 308n1, 314n39, 317n2
International Association of Health Funds, 235
International Labor Office, 231-2, 235, 241
Izakovich, Yitzhak, 40-3, 57, 62, 64, 178

J

Jabotinsky, Zeev, 182, 269, 320
Jacobs, Rose Gel, 142, 320
Jaffa, 7, 11-5, 17-20, 24-5, 29-30, 32-5, 37-8, 41, 43, 58, 60-3, 66-7, 73, 75, 78-9, 83-4, 87, 101, 182-3, 191, 215
Jenin, 79
Jerusalem, 7-11, 14, 16, 18, 20, 33, 37, 41, 57, 69, 72-3, 75-6, 78-81, 83, 85, 87, 101, 104, 106, 109, 119, 129, 142, 158, 178, 182, 184-5, 193, 206-8, 217, 246, 250, 255-6, 260, 282
Jewish Agency, 77, 141, 163, 215-6, 218-9, 222, 238, 240, 243-6, 271, 273-4, 278, 283, 296, 325
Jewish Agricultural Settlements, 12, 16-8, 20, 43, 55, 61, 86, 117, 149, 249
Jewish Colonization Association (JCA), 17-9, 22, 325
Jewish Community, 7, 9-11, 13, 18, 20, 27, 35, 46, 56, 69, 71, 74, 77, 78, 81, 205, 226, 244, 274, 293, 298
Jewish Defense Group, 20-1
Jewish Laborers, 12, 17-8, 21, 25, 27, 31, 43, 47, 55, 65, 90, 92, 180
Jewish Legion, 86, 325
Jewish medical community, 18
Jezreel Valley, 76, 98, 101, 103-5, 112, 140, 158, 172, 174, 180, 191, 201-2, 204-6, 209-211, 213, 218-9, 223, 292
see also Norris Bloc, East Jezreel Valley
Joint-Jewish Distribution Committee, 73, 78, 101, 114, 181, 185, 192, 205-7, 325
Jordan Valley, 211
Judea Worker's Committee, 31
Judea, 7, 13, 24, 28-9, 31, 33, 40, 57-66, 82, 223, 248
Judean Agricultural Workers Federation, 28-9, 32-5, 38-40, 42-3, 58-9

K

Kaminsky, David, 142
Kaplan, Eliezer, 269

Karlsbad, 77, 98
Kass, Amally, 8
Katznelson, Berl, 29-30, 32, 34, 66, 68, 87, 135, 170, 174, 321, 303n22
Katznelson, Reuben, 267
Katznelson-Nissan, Avraham, 77, 134, 146, 149, 155, 214-5, 219-220, 238-9, 241-2, 244, 265, 321
Kegan, Helena, 57
Kenivsky-Kenev, Yitzhak, 99, 103, 114, 121, 137, 144, 150, 152-4, 156, 158-9, 199, 203-4, 207, 225, 229-232, 235, 240-3, 245-6, 251-2, 254-5, 260, 278, 282-3, 298, 321
Kfar Giladi, 108, 118, 120-2, 185
Kfar Saba, 67-8
Kfar Yechezkel (Heftziba), 204, 209
Kinneret, 28, 65, 68, 82, 117-8, 169, 170-1
Kisch, Colonel, 138, 198, 237
Kishnev Pogrom, 20
Kishnev, 20
Kleigler, Israel Jacob, 321
Knesset Israel, 325
Kosovsky, Avraham, 26, 195
Kottek, Shmuel, 46-7
Krakow, 46
Kupat Holim (General Health Fund), 36-7, 39-40, 42, 44-6, 52, 57-8, 69, 76-7, 79, 88-9, 92-167, 170, 175, 177, 185-210, 212-300
Kushta, Constantinople, 59, 61, 77
Kutcher, Carol, 72

L

Labor Movement, 88, 96, 112, 162, 181, 187, 204, 232, 247, 269, 294, 299
Landesman, Berta, 180
Latvia, 47
Lavie, Shlomo, 154
League of Nations, 226
Lebanon, 14-5
Leibowitz, Yehoshua, 9, 46
Leumit Health Fund, 271-4, 276, 290
Levi, Nissim, 8
Levin, Elimeleh, 68
Linat Tzedek, 23, 291, 325
Lindheim-Levy, Irma, 142, 188, 199, 321
Lishansky, Sara, 97
London, 10, 129, 206, 208-9, 237-241
Lovers of Zion, movement, 325
Lucerne, 48

M

Macabi Health Fund, 288, 290
MacDonald, Ramsay, 226, 239
Machanayim, 117-8
Magnes Judah Leib-Leon, 196, 208, 321
Maimonides, 46
Malchin, Shabtai, 87, 97
Mandate Government, 74-5, 77-9, 81, 124-5, 132, 138, 152, 158-161, 164, 188, 204-6, 212, 214-7, 219-223, 225-235, 238-244, 247-8, 269, 275, 280, 297-8
Mandate Health Office, 78-9, 81
Mandatory Health Department, 81
Mapai Party, 266, 269, 271, 287
Marjaiu'n, 15
Mas Achid, 100, 276, 278
Medical Services, 52, 54, 59, 95, 98
Meir, Yosef, 154, 160, 265, 269
Meirson-Meir, Golda, 134, 245, 321

Mendelberg, Abraham, 143-4
Metula, 15
Migdal, 180
Mijallah, Majdida, 15
Miller, Donald, 73, 185
Minucha Ve Nachala Society, 17
Mission (Clinics, Hospital, Christian), 9-11, 30, 57, 76, 199, 227
Monchik-Margalit, Eliyahu, 25-6, 146-7
Montefiore, Moshe-Moses, 9-10, 322
Morgenthau, Henry, 59
Moscow, 111
Moslem, 8, 9, 57
Motza, 134
mount Moreh, 202
mount Scopus, 201
Muhammad, Ali, 8
Mutual Responsibility Fund Against Epidemics, 25

N

Nablus, 79, 215
Nachlat Yehuda, 122-3
Nadav, Daniel, 111
Nahalal, 98, 119, 204
National Civil Association, 210
National Committee, 77, 134, 146, 219, 237-9, 244, 325
National Insurance Institute, 280-1, 285, 290
National Office for Health, 50
National Religious Party (NRP), 258-9
National Workers Health Fund, 272
Nazareth, 79, 104
Nes Ziona, 58, 262
Netherland, Doron, 185
New York, 71, 190, 192, 196-7, 199-200
Newak, 128
Nofach, Miriam, 57
Noistadt-Noi, Melech, 278
Norman, Yaakov, 83
Norris Bloc, East Jezreel Valley, 209-210
Northern German Confederation, 50
Noyman, 212
Nuremberg Laws, 274

O

Organization of American Christian Women, 72-3
Organization of American Zionist Women, 73
Ori, Yaakov, 22, 27, 41, 134
Orthodox, 10, 13, 21, 315n13

P

Pacha, Ibrahim, 8
Palestine Restoration Fund, 181
Parallel Tax, 89, 92, 101-3, 116, 125, 135, 161, 229, 239-240, 243, 260
Pardes Hana, 267
Paris, 11, 19
Passfield White Paper, 226, 326
Passfield, Lord, 226
Pasteur Institute in Jerusalem, 87
Perlson-Peri, Eliezer, 99-103, 106-7, 109, 111, 114-5, 119, 121, 126-7, 131-2, 140, 142, 145, 148, 153-4, 156-7, 161, 188, 193, 198-200, 204-8, 210, 212, 218-9, 222, 229, 243-4, 258, 260, 268-271, 278, 298
Petach Tikva, 21-3, 26, 28-9, 32, 34, 36, 43-4, 58, 61, 63, 76, 82-3, 170, 223, 248, 250

Pik, Chaim, 257
Poalei Zion, 25-7, 82, 326
Pochas, David, 34
Pochovsky, Haim, 57
Poland, 46-7, 105
Preparatory committee of workers in Eretz Israel, 68
Public Health Department, 77

R

Rabin Medical Center, 223, 248
Rabin, Yitzhak, 223, 248
Rabinovitz, Yosef, 94
Ramallah, 79
Ramat Gan, 282
Ramlah, 79
Ramon, Chaim, 281
Rashish, Pinchas, 134
Rechovot, 17, 22-3, 32, 34, 83, 177
Red Cross, 71, 178
Remez, David, 66, 269, 278, 283
Revisionist Movement, 269-272, 274, 284
Rishon Le-Zion governing committee, 62
Rishon Le-Zion, 13, 15, 22, 32, 62, 123, 153, 252
Rokach, Yehuda, 136, 137
Rokeach, Shimon, 25
Romania, 47
Roosevelt, Theodore, 54
Rosental, 193, 213
Rosh Pina, 15, 18
Rotberg, Meir, 33
Rotberg, Yosef, 97
Rothschild, Baron, Edmond, 11-9, 21, 73
Rothschild, family, 11
Rotnoff, Natan, 206
Rozenau, 138
Rubinow, Isaac Max, 73-4, 85-6,171, 177, 179, 181, 183-5, 194, 196, 322
Ruchama, 34
Rupin, Arthur, 61
Russia, 8, 13, 20-1, 25, 47, 53, 55-6, 105

S

Sacker, Harry, 138, 208, 212, 322
Safed, 7-9, 11, 15, 73, 75, 101, 104, 191
Saliternik, Zvi, 14
Salvation Army, 72
Samaria Health Fund Committee, 31
Samaria Worker's Federation, 66
Samaria, 7, 13, 24, 31, 39, 61, 64, 67, 78, 82, 104, 215, 217, 249
Samuel, Herbert, 77
Second World War, 54, 275
Selkind, Alexander, 196
Sfardi Jews, 7, 11, 18, 282
Shapira, Anita, 30, 163
Shapira, Yosef, 180
Sharret- Shertok, Moshe, 244-6, 322
Shenkar, Reuven, 99, 103-4, 109, 115-7, 121, 148-150, 154, 161, 192-4, 199, 210, 223, 229, 253, 298, 322
Sherman, Moshe, 34, 39, 41, 56
Shochat, Mania, 94, 97
Smilansky, Moshe, 56, 182
Smith, Adam, 50-1
Sneh, Nachum, 63, 66-7
Sokolov, Nachum, 127, 322
Sola-Pool, David de, 182, 322
Solel Boneh, 96, 135-6, 150, 230, 259-260, 283, 296, 326

Soroka, Moshe, 99, 101, 204-5, 213
Sprinzak, Yosef, 98, 256
Stein, Mark, 22
Strauss, Nathan, 72
Sweden, 52
Switzerland, 48
Szold, Henrietta, 71-2, 86, 138, 140-2, 156, 179, 186-8, 193-7, 199, 204-6, 208, 212, 216, 237-8, 241

T

Tahon, Yaakov, 62
Tannenbaum, Meshulam, Shimon, 196
TAZ, 47
Technion, 212
Tel Aviv, 20, 55, 60, 67, 76, 96-7, 104, 108, 129, 133, 145, 164, 197, 210, 214-5, 259, 271-2, 278, 284
Tel Chai, 99, 117-8, 120-2, 293
Tel Yosef, 98, 105-6, 108-9, 111, 118, 209
Tevet, Shabtai, 94-5, 109, 121, 166, 231, 251, 268
Tiberias, 7, 9, 11, 73, 75, 101, 191, 195, 205, 282
Tivon, 123
Trumpeldor, Yosef, 99, 104, 322
Tuberculoses, 104
Tul Karem, 79
Turkey, 9, 55-6, 59
Turkish (Ottoman), 7, 9-10, 14-5, 18, 53, 55-7, 67, 69, 75
Tzachor, Zeev, 20, 23, 68, 96, 121, 162-3

U

Uganda Plan, 19, 326
Uganda, 19, 21
Unger, Gerta, 203
United States (U.S.), 47, 54, 56, 72-4, 142, 191, 193, 196, 198
Ussiskin, Menachem, 19, 181, 323

V

Velensky, 138
Venik, Levi, 99
Vensiani, Emanuel, 14
Vienna, 86, 159

W

War of Independence, 201
Washington, 181
Wauchope, Sir, Arthur, 244
Weinschel, Y., 272
Weizmann, Chaim, 70-1, 138, 141, 163, 239, 269
Western Europe, 47
Worker's Health Fund (Judean, Galilee, Samaria), 35, 39-40, 57-67, 66, 68, 82, 84, 178, 250

Y

Yaakobi, Shoshana, 188, 199
Yafe, Eliezer, 65, 68-9
Yafe, Hillel, 14, 16, 19, 24, 66-8, 74, 323
Yardenai, Yitzhak, 68
Yaski, Chaim, 153, 200-1, 212, 216, 323
Yavniel, farm, 267
Yavnieli, Shmuel, 66, 68, 96
Yishuv, 7, 11, 16, 18-9, 31, 53, 55-6, 60, 67-8, 70-2, 75-6, 78, 81-2, 90-1, 98, 116, 124-5, 131, 134-5, 139, 141, 144, 152, 155-160, 162-3, 165-6, 178-9, 181-2, 185-6, 188, 190, 194-9, 201, 216, 221-2, 224, 226-7, 230, 232, 234,

238-9, 243, 255, 259, 262, 266, 268, 271-2, 275-7, 284, 289, 291, 294, 298-9, 326
Yishuv Health Committee, 128-9, 131, 136-8, 142, 156, 159, 190-1, 194, 197, 209-210, 214, 216-7, 267, 273
Yishuv medical community, 34

Z

Zakai, David, 106, 111, 118
Zartal, Idit, 98-9, 217
Zichron Yaakov, 15-6, 24, 67-8, 261
Zion community group in Afula, 206
Zionism, Modern, 20, 326, 315n12, 317n1
Zionist Congress, 19, 77, 98, 138-142, 188-9, 194, 209, 211, 244, 257, 269, 273, 326
Zionist Executive Committee, 88-9, 100, 104, 114, 116-7, 125-9, 131-2, 139, 156, 159, 193-4, 198-9, 204-7, 210-4, 215-6, 222, 237-8, 245-6, 256-7, 259, 264, 273, 297-9
Zionist Federation, 19, 38, 70-2, 88, 91-2, 103, 138, 142, 177, 181-2, 185, 197
Zionist Movement, 13, 19, 21, 28, 71, 90, 100, 103, 114, 131, 137-8, 163, 180, 182, 200, 205, 239, 269, 283, 293
Zionist Settlements, 13, 293
Zionist, World Organization, 12, 156, 326
Zmora, Moshe, 232, 235, 241